Lecture Notes in Computer Science 9456

Commenced Publication in 1973
Founding and Former Series Editors:
Gerhard Goos, Juris Hartmanis, and Jan van Leeuwen

More information about this series at http://www.springer.com/series/7409

José Bravo · Ramón Hervás
Vladimir Villarreal (Eds.)

Ambient Intelligence
for Health

First International Conference, AmIHEALTH 2015
Puerto Varas, Chile, December 1–4, 2015
Proceedings

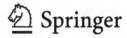 Springer

Editors
José Bravo
Castilla-La Mancha University
Ciudad Real
Spain

Ramón Hervás
Castilla-La Mancha University
Ciudad Real
Spain

Vladimir Villarreal
Technological University of Panamá
Panama
Panama

ISSN 0302-9743   ISSN 1611-3349 (electronic)
Lecture Notes in Computer Science
ISBN 978-3-319-26507-0   ISBN 978-3-319-26508-7   (eBook)
DOI 10.1007/978-3-319-26508-7

Library of Congress Control Number: 2015954353

LNCS Sublibrary: SL3 – Information Systems and Applications, incl. Internet/Web, and HCI

Springer International Publishing AG Switzerland is part of Springer Science+Business Media
(www.springer.com)

Preface

The international conference on Ambient Intelligence for Health (AmIHEALTH) has become established as the premier academic and research conference in ubiquitous computing, ubiquitous communication, and natural interfaces applied to the health knowledge field. Since ambient intelligence (AmI) promotes environments surrounded by intelligent interfaces embedded into everyday objects to support human activities and achieve a better quality of life, it is crucial to still maintain a holistic view: AmI focuses on users, beyond the technology. In these terms, health issues are one of the main challenges to improving the quality of life and the AmiHEALTH conference covers specifically this core topic.

This year we celebrated the first edition of AmIHEALTH as a joint event with the 9th International Conference on Ubiquitous Computing and Ambient Intelligence (UCAmI 2015) and the 7th International Work-Conference on Ambient Assisted Living (IWAAL 2015) held in Puerto Varas, Chile. In order to increase the visibility of the contributions to AmiHEALTH, selected papers were invited to be published as extended versions in the journals: *Biomedical Informatics, Sensors, Journal of Medical Systems,* and *Health Informatics.* As such we would like to thank the distinguished editors of these journals for providing us with this opportunity.

The program of this event covered a variety of topics, including infrastructures and technologies to implement health environments, applied algorithms in e-Health systems, metrics for health systems, interactions with health environments, and applied case studies. This year's event included keynotes from internationally recognized researchers in their fields: Dr. Julita Vassileva from the University of Saskatchewan (Canada) gave a talk entitled "Towards the Personalized Persuasive Technologies for Behavior Change" and Dr. Chris Nugent from Ulster University (Northern Ireland, UK) spoke on "Design, Development, and Evaluation of Mobile Reminding Technologies." We would like to thank our distinguish keynote speakers for their participation and contribution to this joint event.

In this first edition of AmIHEALTH, we received a notable response from researchers who submitted their contributions for consideration to AmIHEALTH. We received 33 submissions involving 139 authors from 14 different countries. Following the review process we had an acceptance rate for long papers of 61 %. A total of 87 reviews were undertaken by 39 reviewers from 18 countries. We would like to thank all the authors who submitted their work for consideration and also the reviewers for providing their detailed and constructive reviews.

Finally, we would like to express our deepest thanks to our colleagues for assisting in organizing this event, particularly Professor Sergio Ochoa from the University of Chile. We would also like to thank all the Program Committee members for their time and contributions.

December 2015

José Bravo
Ramón Hervás
Vladimir Villarreal

Organization

General Chair

José Bravo   University of Castilla-La Mancha, Spain

Local Organizing Chair

Sergio F. Ochoa   University of Chile, Chile

AmIHEALTH Program Committee Chairs

Ramón Hervás   University of Castilla-La Mancha, Spain
Vladimir Villarreal   Technological University of Panamá, Panama

Publicity Chair

Jesús Fontecha   University of Castilla-La Mancha, Spain
  Diezma

Webmaster

Iván González Díaz   University of Castilla-La Mancha, Spain

Steering Committee

Xavier Alaman, Spain
José Bravo, Spain
Jesus Favela, Mexico
Juan Manuel García Chamizo, Spain
Luis Guerrero, Costa Rica
Ramón Hervás, Spain
Rui Jose, Portugal
Diego López-De-Ipiña, Spain
Chris Nugent, UK
Sergio F. Ochoa, Chile
Gabriel Urzáiz, Mexico
Vladimir Villarreal, Panama

Organizing Committee

Nelson Baloian, Chile
Javier Bustos, Chile
Francisco Gutiérrez, Chile
Valeria Herskovic, Chile
José Pino, Chile
Gustavo Zurita, Chile
Tania Mondéjar, Spain
Iván González, Spain
Justyna Kidacka, Spain

Program Committee

Mariano Alcañiz	UPV - LabHuman, Spain
Rosa Arriaga	Georgia Institute of Technology, USA
Frank Biocca	MIND Lab, USA
Stephane Bouchard	Département de psychoéducation et de psychologie, Canada
Fatima Boujarwah	Kuwait University, USA
José Bravo	Castilla La Mancha University, MAmI Research Lab, Spain
Giorgio Carpino	University Campus Bio-Medico of Rome, Italy
Luis Carriço	University of Lisbon, Portugal
Filippo Cavallo	The BioRobotics Institute, Italy
Diane Cook	School of Electrical Engineering and Computer Science, USA
Hariton Costing	University of Medicine and Pharmacy, Iasi, Romania
Michael Craven	University of Nottingham, UK
Fabio De Felice	Università degli Studi di Cassino, Italy
Giuseppe de Pietro	ICAR - CNR (Italian National Council of Research), Italy
Jesus Favela	CICESE, Mexico
Giuseppe Fico	Universidad Politécnica de Madrid, Spain
Andrea Gaggioli	Catholic University of Milan, Italy
Maria Haritou	Institute of Communication and Computer Systems - National Technical University of Athens, Greece
Jan Havlík	Department of Circuit Theory, Faculty of Electrical Engineering, Czech Technical University in Prague, Czech Republic
Ramón Hervás	Castilla La Mancha University, MAmI Research Group, Spain
Alina Huldtgren	Eindhoven University of Technology, Denmark
Lenka Lhotska	Czech Technical University in Prague, Department of Cybernetics, Czech Republic
Vincenzo Loia	Università degli Studi di Salerno, Italy
Ratko Magjarevic	Faculty of Electrical Engineering and Computing, Croatia
Stephen Makonin	Simon Fraser University, Canada
Oscar Mayora	CREATE-NET, Italy
Paolo Melillo	University of Bologna, Italy

Nicolas Palliakarakis	University of Patras, Greece
Leandro Pecchia	University of Warwick, UK
Antonella Petrillo	University of Cassino and Southern Lazio, Italy
Octavian Postolache	Instituto Universitario of Lisbon, Portugal
Giusepe Riva	Università Cattolica del Sacro Cuore, Italy
Marcela Rodríguez	UABC, Mexico
Cristian Rotariu	Faculty of Medical Bioengieering, Romania
Javier Sanchez Galan	Technological University of Panamá, Panama
Monica Tentori	CICESE, Mexico
Gabriel Urzáiz	Universidad Anahuac Mayab, Mexico
Vladimir Villarreal	Technological University of Panamá, Panama
Rainer Wieching	University Siegen, Denmark

Additional Reviewers

Konstantin Aal (Germany)
Jesús Fontecha (Spain)
Iván González (Spain)
Irvin Hussein Lopez-Nava (Mexico)
Daryoush Daniel Vaziri (Germany)

Contents

Metrics for Health Environments

Technologies for Implementing AmIHealth Environments

Real-Time Recognition of Arm Motion Using Artificial Neural Network Multi-perceptron with Arduino One MicroController and EKG/EMG Shield Sensor

Luis A. Caro[✉], Camilo Silva, Billy Peralta, Oriel A. Herrera, and Sergio Barrientos

Computer Science Department, Universidad Católica de Temuco, Rudecindo Ortega, 02950 Temuco, Chile
{lcaro, csilva, bperalta, oherrera, sbarrientos}@uct.cl

Abstract. Currently, human-computer interfaces have a number of useful applications for people. The use of electromyographic signals (EMG) has shown to be effective for human-computer interfaces. The classification of patterns based on EMG signals has been successfully applied in various tasks such as motion detection to control of video games. An alternative to increasing access to these applications is the use of low-cost hardware to sample the EMG signals considering a real-time response. This paper presents a methodology for recognizing patterns of EMG signals given by arm movements in real time. Our proposal is based on an artificial Neural Network, Multilayer Perceptron, where the EMG signals are processed by a set of signal processing techniques. The hardware used for obtaining the signal is based on Ag/AgCl connected to the EKG/EMG-Shield plate mounted on a Arduino One R3 card which is used to control a video game. The implemented application achieves an accuracy above 90 % using less than 0.2 s for recognition of actions in time of testing. Our methodology is shown to predict different movements of the human arm reliably, at a low cost and in real time.

Keywords: Neural networks · Action recognition · Arduino · Microcontrollers

1 Introduction

During the last decades, a breakthrough in research and development of applications related to human-computer interfaces has been experienced [1]. In particular, if we focus on EMG signals (electromyography), we can see interesting work related to the detection of nervous system and neuromuscular diseases [2], control of orthopedic prosthesis [3], video games [4] and robotics [5].

In terms of classification of myoelectric signals, many techniques exist that address this subject [6]. However, the methodology presented in this work is based on techniques that blend computational resources in a balanced matter so as to minimize the delay of muscular activation as well as pattern classification.

© Springer International Publishing Switzerland 2015
J. Bravo et al. (Eds.): AmIHEALTH 2015, LNCS 9456, pp. 3–14, 2015.
DOI: 10.1007/978-3-319-26508-7_1

In this context, our proposal deals with distinct stages that comprise the detection and classification of four basic muscular movements of the forearm: pronation, supination, extension and flexion, which simulate the events produced by the keys: left, right, up and down. The obtained model was tested to control the simple and popular video game called Snake in real time via a person's forearm.

The development of the paper will address an introduction, a model, methodology proposal, the tests and results and the conclusions.

2 State of the Art

Biosignal measurement devices are of great importance in the medical field, generally in the detection of physiological muscular diseases. However, some bioinstrumental applications can currently be found outside of the health sector.

In this context and thanks to the great processing capacity and the low-cost that some current smart devices offer such as: PC Tablets, RasBerry Pi, SmartPhones, Microcontrollers and Biometric Sensors, the application portability facilitates monitoring of the human body's bioelectric activity anywhere and anytime [7]. Likewise, device size is no longer a problem, since bioinstruments as small as the size of a postal stamp have been developed [8]. Nevertheless, for processing purposes, neither the methodology utilized nor the objective of the application matters. This is because the techniques used for biopotential processing are practically the same and have been studied by various authors relating techniques to the digital processing of signals [9–11] and implementing innovative devices with myoelectric signal acquisition [12, 13].

Moreover, works such as [14, 15] have focused attention on the comparison of analysis methods and the classification of EMG signals in order to evidence the effectiveness and approximation of diverse techniques commonly used in this field. It is concluded that Artificial Neural Networks (ANNs) are the best classifiers for this purpose, affirming their superiority over other machine learning classifiers such as: Support Vector Machines (SVMs), Decision Trees (DTs), Radial Basis Functions (RBFs), Linear Discriminant Analysis (LDA), among others.

3 Model

The construction of an EMG pattern recognition system is based on a series of components that involve hardware as much as software. Figure 1 shows the bioinstrumentation model proposed for the project development, which is formed by three fundamental components: (1) Acquisition and Analog Signal Pre-processing, (2) Digital Signal Processing and (3) Classification and Control.

The Acquisition and Analog Signal Pre-processing box models the obtaining of EMG signals through electrodes, amplification, filtering and analog to digital conversion (A/D) done through an EKG/EMG Shield digital card and the Arduino One microcontroller, responsible for processing the data and implementing the communication protocol for the data dispatch to a computer.

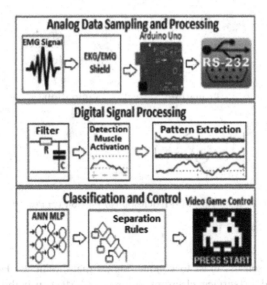

Fig. 1. Bioinstrumentation system model

The second box models the Digital Signal Processing stage, which is comprised of the utilization of smoothing and filtering techniques, which permit the detection of the muscle activation states in order to extract characteristic patterns free of noise and interference.

Finally, the Classification and Control box utilizes an ANN (Artificial Neural Network), Multilayer Perceptron (MLP), for pattern recognition. These outputs are associated with a series of keyboard events that simulate the pressing of the keys: left, right, up and down, to control the classic video game, Snake.

3.1 EMG Signals

The contractile unit of the human skeleton's muscle mass is muscle fiber; cells that upon being stimulated contract, building up force and emitting myoelectric activity in the active muscle [16]. This signal can be sensed through an electromyographic system that is responsible for measuring and registering these biopotentials generated by the activation of a muscle through electrodes, whether they be invasive (needle electrodes) or non-invasive (superficial).

In this work, four forearm movements have been selected which generate biopotential signals. In Fig. 2, one can see the selected movements: pronation, supination, flexion and extension.

The choice of these movements is due to the similarity that they share with their associated action, meaning that, extension, flexion, pronation and supination simulate the actions of up, down, left and right respectively. Additionally, the physiological reason that supports this selection is based on the fact that such movements share similar muscles upon activating [17]. This simplifies the location of the electrodes: above the superficial flexor muscle and above the superficial extensor [18].

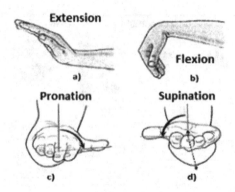

Fig. 2. Movements to distinguish: (a) Extension (b) Flexion (c) Pronation (d) Supination

3.2   Electrodes

A great variety of sensors exist to conduct signal measurements. However, *surface electrodes* are used in surface electromyography (SEMG), usually fabricated from *Ag/AgCl*. It is precisely this type of electrode utilized in this work.

The main function that this sensor carries out is as a transducer since it is responsible for transforming an ion current, generated by living tissue, into an electric current measured in millivolt *(mV)* [19]. In Fig. 3, this sensor is shown.

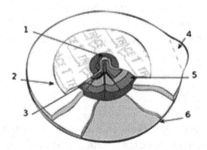

Fig. 3. Structure location of the electrodes. (1) Metallic cone, (2) Foam backing, (3) Ag/AgCl sensor, (4) Flap, (5) Electrolyte gel, (6) Glue

3.3   Hardware

The electronic card used in this project is the EKG/EMG-Shield. It has six data acquisition analog channels by means of three electrodes: positive, negative and one of reference, a digital analog converter, an amplifier circuit and analog filters. This plate is mounted on an Arduino One R3 card, which samples the signals at a frequency of 256 Hz, sending packets of data through serial communication at 57,600 bps-8N1 to a RaspBerry Pi.

In Fig. 4, the three components of the hardware utilized in the project can be observed. The three electrodes, positive and negative above the superficial flexor and extensor muscles respectively and the reference electrode, are shown. The Arduino One R3 unit can also be seen, which sends the sampled data to the RaspBerry Pi through serial communication.

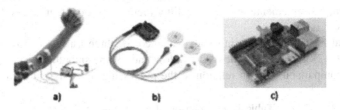

a)   b)   c)

Fig. 4. Hardware utilized. (a) Positioning of the electrodes (b) Arduino plate with EKG/EMG Shield and (c) RaspBerry Pi

4   Methodology

As mentioned previously, the attempted objective in this work is the classification of EMG signals in real time, generated by the forearm muscles to control a video game. To reach this goal, the solution to this problem has been addressed through the following steps.

4.1   Protocol Decoding

The initial phase contains the decoding of the packets sent by the Arduino One R3 microcontroller in conjunction with the EKG/EMG (electrocardiogram) card. This protocol is composed of four bytes under the bytes storage system little-endian, which can be seen in Fig. 5, where bytes 2 and 3 correspond to synchronization and bytes 0 and 1 correspond to the value read between 0 and 1023.

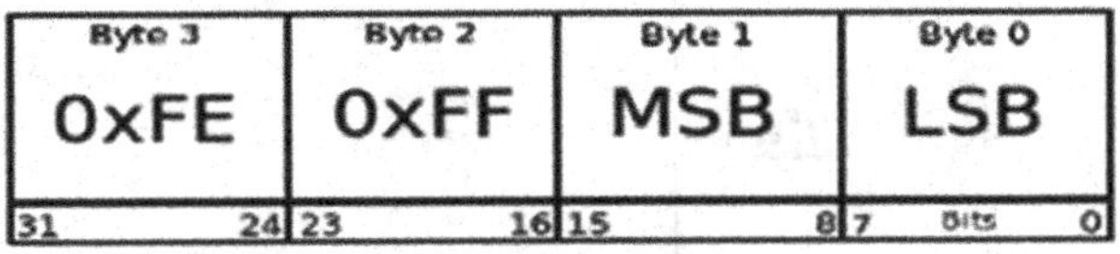

Byte 3	Byte 2	Byte 1	Byte 0
0xFE	0xFF	MSB	LSB
31 24	23 16	15 8	7 bits 0

Fig. 5. Communication protocol structure.

4.2   Filtering

After the decoding stage, the signals are obtained without being filtered, which should be smoothed to remove the crossing with other bioelectric signals and electromagnetic interferences coming from the environment in which the bioinstrument is being used. Various techniques exist for this, like centralization, which consists of deducing the middle point of the value range in which the signal moves. However, the EKG/EMG-Shield plate already incorporates centralization and delivers the signal in the middle point of the resolution which is measured (center = 1024/2).

Diverse algorithms exist for smoothing and filtering, such as: moving average, RMS, sliding windows based on Hanning, Hamming, Bartlett, Flat, Blackman, Kalman filter, Notch, Complementary, the last filter being the one that yielded the best performance.

The final result of the filtering was evaluated for three aspects: (1) required processing time, (2) the length of the data window and (3) the smoothing quality. Table 1 shows the comparison done in relation to the processing times measured in seconds.

Table 1. Comparison of processing time.

Filter	Processing time	Window size	End time
Flat	0.00038	11	0.04339
Hamming	0.00044	11	0.04345
Blackman	0.00046	11	0.04344
Kalman	4.32645	1	4.36946
Complementary	0.00379	1	0.00771

Another very important subject is the data filtering quality. Figure 6 shows a comparison between a real signal (raw) and the application of the filtering algorithms before signals.

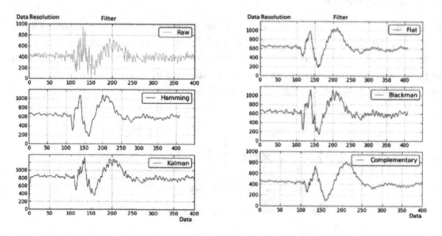

Fig. 6. Comparison of the filtering algorithms.

It can be observed that the Flat, Hamming and Complementary filters present a better smoothing than the rest. Nonetheless, upon analyzing the signal at rest, the Complementary filter minimized the noise the best. Therefore, the best alternative for this project is to use this filter.

4.3   Full-Wave Rectification

Full-wave rectification [20] is a simple technique that reflects the negative values below 512 and the positive values above 512. Figure 7 shows the full-wave rectification with and without a filter.

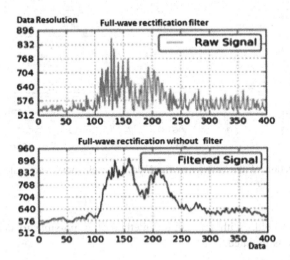

Fig. 7. Comparison between the rectification of a raw signal and a filtered one.

The utility that this technique offers is centered on two essential objectives: (1) bring all the values to one plane and (2) simplify the following stage that corresponds to determining a *triggering threshold*.

4.4   Calibration Mode to Determine the Triggering Threshold

The triggering threshold corresponds to the maximum limit that the signal reaches upon being at rest, for which exceeding this threshold indicates that one is in the presence of a movement.

To graphically visualize this procedure, in Fig. 8 the signals generated by each movement (blue line) and the triggering threshold (red line) are shown. One can observe that the threshold is the same for all of the movements since all the lines initially show a growing tendency due to the full-wave rectification done previously.

4.5   Detection of the Start of Activation

Having determined the triggering threshold, the detection of the beginning of muscular activity is relatively simple since any register above this threshold corresponds to a strong movement. Figure 8 shows this idea clearly with the green vertical line, which marks the intersection between the threshold and the moment in which the signal

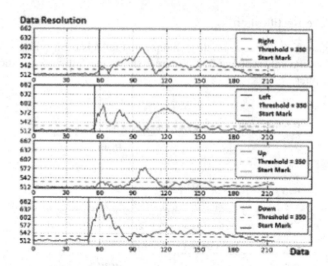

Fig. 8. Representation of the activation threshold for each movement pattern (Color figure online).

exceeds said threshold. With this simple method it is possible to detect when the muscular activity is initiated.

4.6   Generation of the Datasets with Training Patterns

Having the starting point for the movement, all that remains is storing the amount of necessary data that represent each movement. In works such as [21, 22] it is mentioned that the first milliseconds (interval of [3, 5]) are sufficient to distinguish one movement from another. Nonetheless, the sampling frequency in our project is 256 Hz, which implies that new data is being obtained every 3.906 ms.

In Fig. 8 it can be seen that after the reading of 120 data, starting at the *activation point*, the muscles finish their activity. Based on the previous information, the length of all of the patterns was 120 data and the quantity of the samples for each movement was 20 data.

4.7   Creation of the ANN

The pattern recognition was achieved through a MLP neural network utilizing the back-propagation learning algorithm. The initial structure of the network has *120* entries corresponding to the length of the training patterns, one hidden layer with 20 neurons, an output layer with 4 nodes (one for each movement) and a bias in the intermediate layer. The model representation of this network is shown in Fig. 9 and described mathematically in Eq. 1.

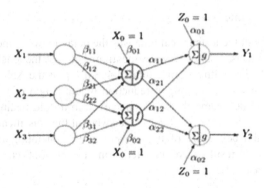

Fig. 9. ANN MLP structure.

$$\mu_k(X) = g_k\left(\alpha_{0k} + \sum_{j=1}^{t} \alpha_{jk} f_i\left(\beta_{0j} + \sum_{m=1}^{r} \beta_{mj} X_i\right)\right) \tag{1}$$

with activation function g and f, connection matrix α between the entrance layer and hidden layer, β the connection matrix between the hidden and output layer, X the entrance vector, Y the outputs and X_0 and Z_0 bias in the intermediate layer and output layer respectively.

5 Test and Results

5.1 Network Training and the Matrix Creation for the Synaptic Weights

The parameter adjustment was done mainly by trial and error. The training data set was 75 % for training and 25 % for validation. Of all of the tests done, the selected parameters to form the matrix of the synaptic weights are shown in Table 2, with which an error was reached in the test groups equal to *0.032639*.

Table 2. Final parameter adjustment for the ANN MLP.

ANN MLP parameters	Values
Input neurons	60
Hidden neurons	18
Output neurons	4
Sample movements	60
Reading rate	0.01
Momentus	0.003
Bias	2
Max iterations	2000
Activation function	tanh()

5.2   Tests in Real Time

The main problem with the tests in real time was the delay between the detection of the movements and their classification. As was mentioned earlier, the length of the samples were made up of 120 data with a storage time of 468 ms, plus the ANN calculation time with a time of 300 ms. However, upon reduction of the length of the patterns to 60, interaction with the video game Snake was achieved in a fluid manner.

Table 3 shows the percentages of correct answers in the classification and the time that it takes from the beginning of the movement to generating the action or the classified output. These results were gathered from a total of 50 consecutive tests for each movement in real time.

Table 3. Percentages of correct classifications and required time to compute the output.

Movement	Success rate	Calculation time
Up	86 %	234 ms + 4.5 ms
Down	98 %	234 ms + 4.6 ms
Right	94 %	234 ms + 4.2 ms
Left	86 %	234 ms + 4.7 ms
Total	91 %	238.5 ms

In Table 3, it is possible to observe that the Up and Left movements possess the lowest performance, while the down and right movements are more robust.

Finally, Fig. 10 exhibits the control of the video game Snake in real time through the project carried out.

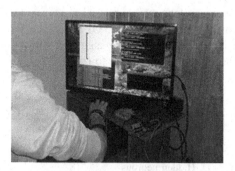

Fig. 10. Controlling the game Snake in real time with the project

Due to the fact that the results in the classification process are not exact, some erroneous movements are sporadically presented. Nevertheless, the delay between movement-action is imperceptible to the naked eye and the video game control is rather robust.

6 Conclusion

The application of the methodology proposed in our work showed its validity by yielding robust results in the detection and classification of biometric signals in spite of utilizing low-cost devices. This without a doubt emphasizes the power that software offers for signal processing.

In this context, the proposed methodology, in spite of its simplicity with regard to calculations and signal transformation, generated sufficient results in the classification of EMG patterns. The main objective was to reduce, if possible, the total time that the system takes to classify without losing quality in the success rate, an objective that reached 91 % achievement.

In relation to the inconveniences presented, the environment where the hardware is located provokes interference, which conditioned that the tests were done in places free of the presence of electronic devices. This situation could be improved in future works through a wireless data transmission system between the processing unit and the sample collection hardware.

The ANN MLPs have a high standard of prestige in reference to EMG pattern classification. However, they are still valid to test other types of recognition models to evidence a comparison of results in the context of suggested development. Likewise, the application of other transformation types to a signal like Wavelet or Fourier Transform with the purpose of extracting characteristics with a higher level of detail is an interesting project. Nevertheless, these are excluded with the purpose of decreasing the calculation time.

Finally, it is valid to emphasize that the Arduino One R3 microcontroller together with the EKG/EMG-Shield card are excellent elements of development to produce prototypes and projects in the area of devices controlled by EMG signals.

References

1. Seungchan, L., Younghak, S., Soogil, W., Kiseon, K., Heung-No, L.: Review of wireless brain-computer interface systems. In: Intech, pp. 215–238 (2013)
2. Donofrio, P.: Abnormal Nerve Conduction Patterns. In: 3nd Biennial Contemporary Clinical neurophysiological Symposium. Vanderbilt University Medical Center (2013)
3. Mateo, A., Giuseppina, G., Michele, F.: Clasification of EMG signals throudg wavelet analysis and neural networks for controlling an active hand prothesis. Department of Electronics and Information, Politecnico di Milano, Italy (2007)
4. Lennart, E., Michael, K., Calvin, L., Regan, L.: Biofeedback game design: using direct and indirect physiological control to enhance game interaction. In: Vancouver, pp. 103–112 (2011)
5. Panagiotis, K., Kostas, J.: An EMG-based robot control scheme robust to time-varying EMG signal features. IEEE Trans. Inf. Technol. Biomed. **14**(3), 581–688 (2010)
6. Chen, X., Zhang, D., Zhu, X.: Application of a self-enhancing classification method to electromyography pattern recognition for multifunctional prosthesis control. JNE 1–13 (2013)

7. Hornos, T.: Wireless ECG/EEG with the MSP430 Microcontroller. Department of Electronics and Electrical Engineering, University of Glasgow (2009)
8. Lessard, C.: Signal Processing of Random Physiological Signals (First). Morgan & Claypool (2006)
9. Reyes, Y.: Procesamiento Digital De Señales Mioeléctricas. Universidad De Las Américas, Puebla. Capítulo, vol. 3, pp. 42–57
10. Alva, C., Castillo, J., Gómez M., Samamé, A.: Procesamiento de Señales Mioeléctricas Aplicado a un Robot de Cinco Grados de Libertad. In: IEEE UNI, pp. 1–6 (2011)
11. Vijay, R.: EMG signal noise removal using neural networks, advances in applied electromyography. In: InTech, pp. 77–99 (2011)
12. López, M., Toranzos, V., Lombardero, O.: Sistema de adquisición y visualización de señales mioeléctricas (2011)
13. González, I., Cifuentes, A.: Diseño y Construcción de un Sistema para la Detección de Señales Electromiográficas. In: UADY (2010)
14. Hong-Bo, X., Tianruo, G., Siwei, B., Socrates, D.: Hybrid soft computing systems for electromyographic signals analysis: a review. In: Biomed Central, pp. 1–19 (2014)
15. Chowdury, R.H.: Surface electromyography signal processing and classification techniques. In: MDPI, pp. 12432–12466 (2013)
16. Palastanga, N., Field, D., Soames, R.: Anatomy and Human Movement: Structure and Function, pp. 91–94 (Paidotribo, Editorial). Butterworth-Heinemann, Oxford (2007)
17. Joseph, S.: Distal Radioulnar Joint Biomechanics and Forearm Muscle Activity. University of Kentucky Doctoral Dissetations. Paper 825 (2011)
18. Stegeman, D., Hermens, H.: Standards for surface electromyography: the European project Surface EMG for non-invasive assessment of muscles (SENIAM), Institute of Neurology, Department of Clinical Neurophysiology, University Medical Centre Nijmegen, Graduate Institute for Fundamental and Clinical Human Movement Sciences (2014)
19. Muhammad, Z.: Signal acquisition using surface EMG and circuit design considerations for robotic prosthesis. In: InTech, pp. 428–448 (2012)
20. Petter, K.: The ABC of EMG. Noraxon Inc., USA (2006)
21. Angkoon, P., Chusak, L., Pornchai, P.: A novel feature extraction for robust pattern recognition. J. Comput. 1, 71–80 (2009)
22. Guanglin, L.: Electromyography pattern-recognition-based control of powerd multifuctional upper-limb prostheses. In: InTech, pp. 100–116 (2011)

Fully-Wireless Sensor Insole as Non-invasive Tool for Collecting Gait Data and Analyzing Fall Risk

Guillermo Talavera[1], Joan Garcia[1], John Rösevall[2], Cristina Rusu[2],
Carlos Carenas[3], Fanny Breuil[3], Elisenda Reixach[3], Holger Arndt[4],
Stefan Burkard[4], Richie Harte[5], Liam Glynn[5],
and Jordi Carrabina[1(✉)]

[1] Universitat Autònoma de Barcelona, CEPHIS, Barcelona, Spain
jordi.carrabina@uab.cat
[2] Department of Sensor Systems, Acreo Swedish ICT AB, Gothenburg, Sweden
[3] CETEMMSA, Av. d'Ernest Lluch 36, 08302 Mataró, Spain
[4] Spring Techno GmbH & Co. KG, Hermann-Köhl-Str. 7,
28199 Bremen, Germany
[5] National University of Ireland, University Road, Galway, Ireland

Abstract. This paper presents the final results and future projection of the European project WIISEL (Wireless Insole for Independent and Safe Elderly Living), that reached to build the first full-wireless insole (that include both wireless communication and wireless charging). These insoles provide a new set of non-invasive tools that can be used either at the clinical installations or at home. That solution improves the usability and user experience compared with traditional tools (smart carpets, wired insoles, etc.) that are oriented to clinical installations. And hence, provide a powerful tool for Ambient Intelligent for Health, especially for elderly people, increasing their autonomy and providing means for long term monitoring.

Health parameters analysed are fall risk and gait analysis. Both are assessed on the establishment of clinical parameters such as fall risk index, and gait pattern and fall detection and algorithms. All those can be obtained thanks to our fully-wireless flexible insole that contains the sensors, embedded processing and wireless communications and charging. Pressure and inertial sensors are embedded into the insoles and a smartphone collects data utilizing Bluetooth Low Energy that is later sent to a main server analysis for its management, analysis and storage. This provides the selected information to the corresponding platform users being either end-users/patients, their relatives or caregivers and the related clinicians.

Keywords: Fall risk · Gait analysis · Wireless insole · Sensors · Bluetooth low energy · Qi wireless charging · Software tools for gait analysis · Fall risk index (FRI)

1 Introduction

Falls are a major health problem for elderly causing both immediate effects as well as long term loss of independence [1]. Non-invasive continuous monitoring allows early detection of risk of falling for individuals under analysis. This is important for the

© Springer International Publishing Switzerland 2015
J. Bravo et al. (Eds.): AmIHEALTH 2015, LNCS 9456, pp. 15–25, 2015.
DOI: 10.1007/978-3-319-26508-7_2

health providers and for the global health systems since therapy avoids accidents and therefore improves person's quality of life.

The main goal of WIISEL [2] was to develop a flexible research tool to collect and analyze gait data from real users, being either elderly or patients recovering from previous fractures or diseases that affect its mobility. The developed tool consists of a combination of a wearable insole device collecting data related with gait together with flexible software platform. Risk of falls is assessed based on multiple gait parameters and gait pattern recognition. WIISEL allows quantifying activity, assessing the quality of gait under real life conditions and enable researchers to evaluate and monitor fall risk in elderly patients, in the home and community environment, mostly reflecting everyday life behaviour.

The potential utility and impact of using the WIISEL system on the research and clinical community is the following: (i) allowing for remote and quantitative assessment of a user's fall risk, (2) measuring activity and mobility in daily living conditions, (3) as a clinical assessment tool, allowing its use as part of any research and assessment of gait parameters, (4) enabling the early identification of functional mobility decline in performance (i.e. assessment of motor fluctuations and disease progression), (5) enabling fall detection in the home setting.

2   Solutions for Motion Detection and Gait Analysis

During the last few years, an increasing number of research works aimed at developing wearable gait analysis systems have been developed and published, demonstrating the large interest to find technological solutions for ubiquitous gait analysis. Our classification of those systems (that include both indoor and outdoor systems) is related to their inner usage model that leads to different products such as: (1) HomeSafe and GoSafe from Philips (pendant) [3], (2) MoveTest and The MoveMonitor from McRoberts (belt) [4], (3) Fall Detector (Wrist Worn) From Chubb [5]. Many other products are following these 3 different strategies [6–8] to wear the fall detectors and gait analysis tools. We considered that integrating higher number of sensors, for both feet offer much more information that those alternatives.

Therefore, we started looking at plantar sensory systems, and specifically to smart insoles, according to their properties such as: embedded sensors for gait measurements, software for monitoring gait, communications technology, power consumption and related autonomy and also cost. The result obtained from the surveillance on the above fields has been structured as follows: Table 1 shows the current list of commercial systems available and its comparison with our current system. This table is indicative and is extracted from the corresponding publically accessible product web pages.

We have to mention that one has to take into account that those prices should be reviewed in detail according to each specific cost models for the insoles and the complete data management system.

Table 1. Current smart insole systems

Device name and company	Application	Sensors	P [kPa] Range	RA[1] [KPa]	IE[2]	Acq[3] [Hz]	D[4]	BA[5] [h]	Price
WIISEL	Continuous gait monitoring, analysis and fall risk assessment	piezoresistive (14) Inertial	350	0.34	Yes	33.3	BLE	16	Pending
Pedar By Novel	Footwear design and injury prevention	pressure (99)	600	2.5	No	100	BT	1	15,450€
F-Scan (insole) By Tekscan	gait analysis & biomechanics, diabetic offloading, sports medicine	pressure (960)	862		No	165	USB Wifi	0.2	16,000$
BioFoot By IBV	Sports Gait analysis Footwear design	pressure (64)	1200	0.1	No	500	Wire WiFi	1	12,995 €
paroLogg/paro Tec by paromed	Foot pressure analysis	Pressure (32) Inertial	625		No	300	Wifi	1.5	
FootPressure MS By Medilogic	Gait, Sports, Health Prevention, Prosthesis and Orthotics, Diabetics rehabilitation process	SSR sensors (240)	640		No	300	Wirel ess		
SmartStep™					No		Card		6,000$
SmartInsoles™ By 24eight, LLC	medical, sports and gaming	Pressure (4) Inertial	241		Yes		wirel ess	~100	
OpenGo science By Moticon	Medical and sports science Rehabilitation and training analysis	Pressure (13) Inertial, Temp	400	2.5	Yes	100	Wire-less		2,000€
Footswitches Insole from B&L Engineering	Gait analysis	4 pressure sensors			No		Wire-less		299$ + 9,000$ SW

[1] Resolution & Accuracy; [2] Integrated Electronics; [3] Max Data acquisition rate; [4] Data Transfer Type; [5] Battery Autonomy

3 System Description

Our platform is composed of the following elements (depicted in Fig. 1):

- A **wearable and unobtrusive sensing insole** that continuously captures spatial–temporal data related to human gait and balance: stride time, single support time, swing time, double support time, cadence, n° steps per day, stride length, gait speed, heel acceleration slope, maximum pressure values on heel and toe.
- **Large data-base** with real-life and long-term human gait data useful for the scientific community.
- A **fall detection algorithm** to feed gait pattern recognition.
- **Intelligent algorithms**, which utilizes data analysis including pattern recognition to quantify fall risk and provide useful information on fall risk assessment. A self-learning analysis framework has been implemented as a basis for further research in optimizing fall risk prediction and identifying fall risk factors.
- A **Fall Risk Index** based on multiple gait parameter pattern to assess and quantify the risk of fall of elderly population. It is based on single support, double support, acceleration amplitude ML, heel strike force slope.
- From a components and related architecture point of view, the system consists of:
- A **pair of** electronic electrically isolated **insoles**. Electrical isolation is reached through wireless charging using the Qi standard and a Bluetooth low energy transmission to a Bluetooth 4.0 (or above) device.
- A **smartphone** that stores data locally and sends it to the main server for its management according the desired policy.
- A **server** that contains the Gait Analysis Tool and the corresponding administrative web application.
- The **user access devices**.

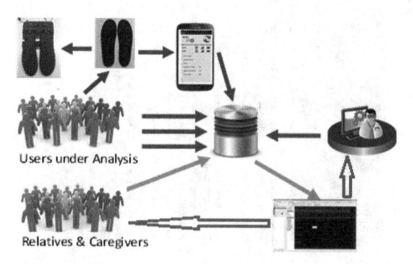

Fig. 1. Gate analysis system architecture

The data from the sensors are sent wirelessly to a Smartphone using Bluetooth Low Energy protocol where the data is stored over the day, before it is sent to a server, which distributes it to instances of the Gait Analysis Tool for further analysis. Researchers and clinicians will be able to analyse data via the Gait Analysis Tool with the help of embedded algorithms, which calculate compute gait behaviour and calculate the current risk of fall. An administration tool on the server allows configuring users, access rights, relationships between insole users and researchers/clinicians. The complete WIISEL system is shown in Gate Analysis System Architecture.

4   Wireless Insoles

The insoles were designed for all day, every day use. At the same time, the insoles are complex multi-layered structures that contain the different electrical and mechanical elements.

The electronics of the WIISEL system is basically composed of three main blocks: (1) the signal acquisition and conditioning system, charged of getting the data from the sensors, (2) the global control of the system including local storage and communication (with antenna), (3) the energy management related with the battery and the wireless Qi protocol.

The pressure sensor layer is made by 14 commercial sensors from Tekscan. These sensors are integrated in a Kapton printed circuit. This layer is interconnected to the electronics layers. An encapsulation material is integrating these layers into comfortable but robust materials (Fig. 2).

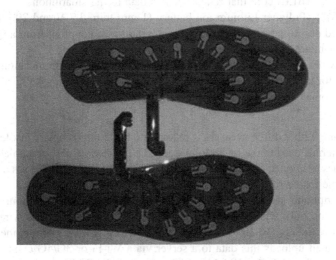

Fig. 2. Pressure sensor layer of the insoles

The electronic layer is built using industrial rigi-flex technology what allows the required degree of flexibility of the insole (Fig. 3). The components selected for the electronics layer are:

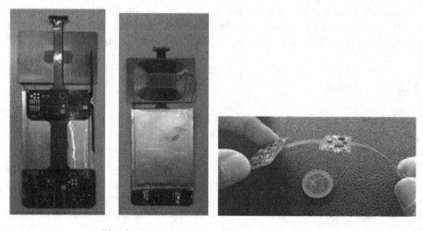

Fig. 3. Electronic layer of the wireless insoles

- Inertial sensors (Gyroscope and Accelerometer) for measuring spatial and temporal parameters (e.g. step length, step frequency).
- A MCU to control the acquisition and ADC for the pressure sensors.
- The main SoC (System-on-Chip) that includes a microprocessor and the Bluetooth Low Energy (BLE) core that relays sensors data to the smartphone.
- Semi-flexible Polymer Lithium-ion battery (1 mm thin, 3.7 V and 200 mAh).
- Embedded coil to power the battery through inductive coupling from a Qi charger.
- The Qi standard commercial Energizer external charger.
- 30 mm wire antenna 2.4 GHz Bluetooth for short range communication.
- Memory for local data storage (for the case of off-line functioning of insole when no wireless connection is available to the smartphone).

A structure with 7 different layers is required to build the complete insole including different materials used in the integration step. The finished insole is completely closed without cables or connectors. In this way, the Qi base charger (Fig. 4) uses a magnet to disconnect the insole from the smartphone system in its stand-by mode.

The smartphone serves two primary functions. First, the smartphone acts as a communications hub, whereby data from the insole sensors are sent wirelessly via Bluetooth Low Energy (BLE) to the Smartphone, which will be worn by the user. The Smartphone then uploads this data to a server via a Wi-Fi or 3G/4G connections.

Second, the Smartphone acts as a system interface for the user wearing the insole. A WIISEL application on the phone provides a number of features such as: battery power status and signal strength status, error messages if problems occur with the

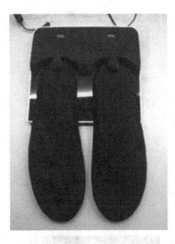

Fig. 4. Example of a final insole in the charging station

insole or communications system, summary of the user's gait and activity, such as steps per day counts, distance measurements and the current fall risk (customisable), and a fall detection system interface.

The Smartphone is used to collect data wirelessly from the insoles using the Bluetooth Low Energy standard. Most of the current smartphones are compatible with Bluetooth 4.0 or above and therefore have built-in Bluetooth low-energy communication. Incoming data is processed locally at reception in order to detect falls. Alarm messages via SMS and email can be configured individually, via the administration tool on the server. In the current implementation, the Smartphone is not used to compute gait parameters. Instead, all data collected from the insoles will be stored locally on the Smartphone memory and transferred via wireless internet to a backend server once per day. Current smartphone app is shown in Fig. 5.

The maximum data transfer rate per insole is 2 kbps. Collecting data at this rate from two insoles for 24 h would require in total 330 Mbytes to be stored. This represents the extreme (unrealistic) condition. Since common smartphone have around 8 Gbytes of flash memories, we do not expect that internal memory space will limit the amount of collected data.

5   Gait Analysis Tools

WIISEL gait analysis tool consists in all-in-one software which covers the whole process of gait analysis. It offers the following functionalities: (1) raw data input in different data formats; (2) raw data filtering with flexible filter settings; (3) gait parameter definition via an editor (oriented to clinicians); (4) automatic pattern extraction; (5) customizable evaluation matrix for the computation of the Fall risk index which helps classify an individual's fall risk and (6) individual subject fact sheets.

A core building block of the system is an intelligent pattern recognition algorithm. The algorithm compares a data population of known fallers with one of known

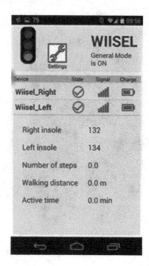

Fig. 5. Screenshot of the current user app at the Smartphone

non-fallers. Relevant classifiers are then extracted, using self-learning algorithms, which are based on a modified Pearson Correlation method. The modification adds a non-linear component that weights elements of the recent past in a stronger way. A Fall Risk Index which aggregates multiple gait parameters (e.g., stride time, gait speed, step length, double support time, variability, non-linear metrics) and gait pattern recognition has been defined. The fall risk index provides quantitative information on possible gait trends and risk of fall.

Figure 6 shows the raw data filtering section in which the subject's data can be previewed. This section facilitates an up to milliseconds study of data values, data filtering and gait parameter extraction shows the fall-risk index definition section, in which weighted clusters of selected patterns (classifiers) can be built and be applied to the data. The result is a classification of each data set in a Fall-risk-index that ranges from zero (meaning no fall risk) to 100 (meaning high risk of falls) (Fig. 7).

Figure 8 shows an example of individual Fact Sheet. Furthermore, the system also provides an import function which allows researchers to insert and analyse their own data or third party data.

6   Validation and Results

Our system has been tested during the validation studies with elderly volunteers at three different clinician sites: TASMC in Israel, INRCA in Italy and NUI-Galway in Ireland. The objective of the validation studies was mainly to assess the feasibility, usability and functionality of the system and the ability of the potential target user to use the system and receive valuable information from it to help them address their risk of falls. Important improvements in usability and user acceptance were achieved after the system was adjusted according to the feedback from experts and users.

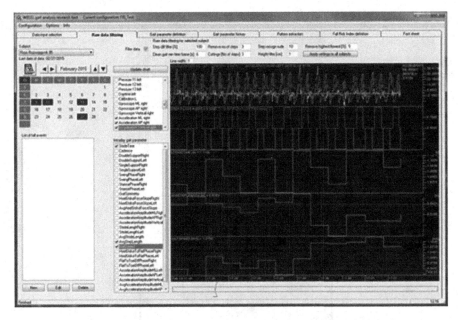

Fig. 6. Screenshot for data filtering of the gait analysis and monitoring tool.

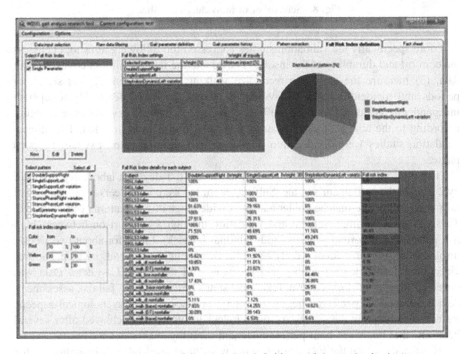

Fig. 7. Screenshot of the fall-risk index definition tool (set and selection).

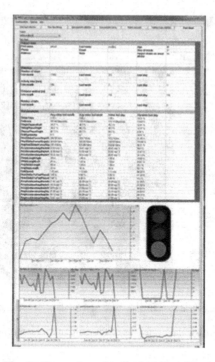

Fig. 8. Screenshot of individual Fact Sheet.

More specifically the validation studies addressed the following aims to: (1) assess the comfort and durability of the insole, (2) evaluate the functionality in collecting gait data, (3) measure the ability to recognize walking patterns, activity and sedentary periods and to identify risky behaviors, (4) assess the users' feasibility to operate independently at home (donning, doffing, charging, ...) and (5) evaluate the usability according to the ability of users to understand the information provided. The clinical validation studies were divided into pilot (assisted) and validation (weaker support) phases.

The pilot phase consisted of 3 days of assessment: 1 day in a laboratory followed by 2 days in the participant's home. Subjects recruited were volunteers with a history of falls and healthy age-matched older adults. A wide range of gait patterns was collected. These allowed the improvement and validation through a comparison between 'high risk patterns' and normal patterns (with minimal fall risk). Later, for about two weeks, insoles were used in patient's daily living environment. At the end, participants provided their feedback on usability and acceptance of the WIISEL system. Data was collected for gait, postural control, functional status of the subjects, fall risk assessment, device acceptance, perceived degree of safety, and social and psychological aspects. Results clearly show the success of the wireless insole system achieved after several iterations that improved both performance and usability.

Results show that the FRI predicts quite well the clinical fall risk identified by the cluster in a statistically significant way. These initial findings suggest that the fall risk level assignment based on the new FRI is valid, as it performs similarly to conventional fall risk tests.

7   Conclusion

The present results support the idea that the WIISEL system can, potentially, be useful as a tool for studying fall risk and as a clinical tool for long-term monitoring of fall risk in the home and community setting, advancing research in this area and leading to relevant savings in terms of time and money.

The wireless insoles are much easier to use than conventional wired insoles that can be almost exclusively used in the laboratory. User's acceptance of this new technology is encouraging. Many aspects of the insole and the smartphone interface were already deemed to be acceptable by most users. The implemented SW platform is flexible and can be adjusted and tailored to the group of users. The new Fall Risk Index proposed apparently captures fall risk to a degree that is achieved using conventional, widely used performance-based tests of fall risk like the Tinetti gait and balance test and the Dynamic Gait Index.

Acknowledgements. Authors would like to thank the clinician partners of the WIISEL project for the fruitful collaboration, especially in the clinician and usability validation of the technology developed. Among then to those that had major interaction in the final part of the project J. Hausdorff and A. Mirelman (TASMC), R. Harte, M. Casey, L. Glynn, (NUI Galway), M. Di Rosa, L. Rossi and V Stara (from INRCA) and J. Chamague (from Geisa). Authors would like to acknowledge the financial support from EU-FP7 grant WIISEL Wireless Insole for Independent and Safe Elderly Living (FP7-ICT 288878). The UAB team would like to acknowledge the support of the Spanish government funded project ASPEC-TDK (TEC2011-29800).

References

1. World Health Organization. WHO global report on falls prevention in older age. WHO, Geneva (2007)
2. Wiisel site. http://www.wiisel.eu/
3. http://www.lifelinesys.com/content/
4. https://www.mcroberts.nl/products
5. http://www.chubbcommunitycare.co.uk/products/info/fall-detector-wrist-worn/
6. Aminian, K., et al.: Spatio-temporal parameters of gait measured by an ambulatory system using miniature gyroscopes. J. Biomech. **35**, 689–699 (2002)
7. Czerwosz, L., et al.: Recognition of gait disturbances in patients with normal pressure hydrocephalus using a computer dynography system. J. Physiol. Pharmacol. **59**(Suppl 6), 201–207 (2008)
8. Rösevall, J., et al.: A wireless sensor insole for collecting gait data. Stud. Health Technol. Inform. **200**, 176–178 (2014)

A Mobile Cloud Shared Workspace to Support Homecare for Respiratory Diseases in Chile

Andrés Neyem[1], Nicolas A. Risso[1(✉)], Marie J. Carrillo[2],
Angélica Farías[2], and Macarena J. Gajardo[2]

[1] Department of Computer Science,
Pontificia Universidad Católica de Chile, Santiago, Chile
{aneyem, narisso}@uc.cl
[2] Nursing School, Pontificia Universidad Católica de Chile, Santiago, Chile
{mcarrilb, amfariac, mjgajardo}@uc.cl

Abstract. Respiratory diseases are a group of chronic diseases affecting the airways and other structures of the lungs, which cause thousands of breathing problems in Chile. Respiratory Therapy services comprise a variety of interventions that are related to airway management and maintenance of lung health. In Chile, RTs are predominantly carried out in hospitals, especially in high-intensity areas such as intensive care units. However, RTs also work in outpatient settings, for instance, patients can receive treatment at home in pulmonary rehabilitation programs. RTs at home involve an active role of the caregivers in charge of the patient's health. In the case of informal caregivers, this situation results in a deterioration of the quality of life. At the same time, innovations in mobile and electronic healthcare open up new ways of supporting patients and caregivers. This brings up the question: how can we contribute to the quality of life of a patient's support network and enhance RTs through the use of information technology and communication services? This paper presents a mobile cloud shared workspace to support and improve homecare for respiratory diseases. The platform is the result of research and development work performed during the last two years.

Keywords: Homecare · Respiratory diseases · Mobile shared workspaces · Cloud workspaces · Design guidelines

1 Introduction

A global population with an increased life expectancy, combined with the rise of chronic diseases and economic factors, is driving the increased provision and prevalence of healthcare at home. Chronic diseases and conditions, such as heart diseases, strokes, cancer, diabetes, obesity, and arthritis, are among the most common, costly, and preventable kinds of health problems in the world population [18].

In Chile, the most common health problems are respiratory diseases. These diseases are a group of chronic diseases affecting the airways and other structures of the lungs. Common chronic respiratory diseases are asthma, bronchiectasis, chronic sinusitis, lung fibrosis, and lung cancer, among others. Respiratory Therapy (RT) services comprise a

J. Bravo et al. (Eds.): AmIHEALTH 2015, LNCS 9456, pp. 26–36, 2015.
DOI: 10.1007/978-3-319-26508-7_3

variety of interventions that are related to airway management and maintenance of lung health. These include oxygen therapy, ventilation, tracheostomy care, medication management, and teaching of and support with inhaler-use techniques. Eligible patients can be funded fully or partially to receive RT home visits for home oxygen, which is usually indicated during some stage of the disease. Table 1 describes the most common respiratory diseases and breathing disorders in Chile and if they are eligible for national RT programs at home [2, 3].

Table 1. Chronic respiratory diseases and other breathing disorders in Chile

Disease	International classification of diseases (ICD-10)	Home respiratory therapy (AVNI, AVNIA)
Asthma	J45	
Bronchiectasis	J47	
Muscular dystrophy (Duchenne, Becker, etc.)	G71.0	✓
Thoracic deforming dorsopathies	M40	✓
Chronic obstructive lung disease, including chronic obstructive pulmonary disease, bronchitis, and emphysema.	J40-J44	✓ (Type 2 respiratory failures)
Sleep apnea syndrome	G47.3	✓
Congenital malformations of trachea and bronchus	Q32	✓
Chronic sinusitis	J32	
Lung fibrosis	J84.1	
Pneumonia	J12 – J18	

This type of homecare service began to emerge in Chile in 2000, with respiratory therapies and special programs focused on children and adolescents, such as the SAVED [24] and AVNI [3] programs. Based on the good results of these programs, in 2015 the Ministry of Health of Chile created the AVNIA program for noninvasive ventilation of adult patients [3]. One of the main issues of RTs at home is that it involves an active role of the caregivers (formal or informal) in charge of the patient's health. Several studies show that caregivers experience significant stress and depression [11, 13, 28]. In the case of informal caregivers, this situation imposes a deteriorating quality of life not only for the caregiver, but also for the patient's support network [32].

Nevertheless, innovations in mobile healthcare (mHealth) and electronic healthcare (eHealth) are revolutionizing the interaction among patients, caregivers, and the medical team in the modern healthcare system [5, 12, 21, 22]. On one hand, they create new opportunities for individuals to actively monitor themselves and improve their health. Indeed, a number of studies have underlined that a well-informed patient is more likely to participate in healthy behaviors and to better manage his or her condition [10, 16]. As a result, patients can enjoy a better quality of life and seek less medical attention from the medical team. This creates new opportunities for caregivers to remotely monitor patients' health and to manage many, especially chronic, diseases. Therefore, mHealth and eHealth, such as tele-monitoring platforms and mobile health applications [14], can be integrated into routine care of acute and chronic diseases and provide essential information for their management among patients, caregivers, and medical providers.

This paper proposes the development of a Mobile Cloud Shared Workspace (MCSW) to provide a healthcare solution at home using mobile, embedded healthcare devices and cloud computing. The research is focused on improving the Family Quality of Life (Family QoL) for informal caregivers within RTS. To measure this, the Impact on Family Scale (IFS) is used to quantify the platform's impact.

This project is trying to take the first step in Chile towards understanding how we are able to improve quality of life not only for patients, but also for the family caregiver support network. The next section describes the status of information technology in healthcare. Section 3 presents the proposed system and Sect. 4 presents conclusions and future work.

2 Mobilizing Healthcare Services

Mobile, embedded, and cloud computing technologies are converging in the new, rapidly growing field of mobile ecosystems. These technological advances are changing how healthcare services are provided. For instance, there has been a trend linked to the Quantified Self movement [5], which is characterized by the use of wearable sensors in wireless technologies to monitor, analyze, and improve health outcomes. It exposes the effect of motivation on changes in health behavior through quantitative measurement and analysis of personal health parameters [5].

Wearable sensors nowadays have been successfully tested in wellness and fitness. These devices provide an opportunity for patients to meet their needs by administering information online to their mobile computing device or other wearable devices. Besides providing health parameters, these wearable sensors also have the potential to influence a patients' behavior (feedback motivates better self-management) [10]. They are easily managed and are becoming increasingly more accurate and reliable for patient care [5, 31]. Indeed, these devices could be utilized in the modern healthcare system as a diagnostic tool to aid in identifying and managing several diseases [16, 29]. Therefore, vital signs monitoring systems could have an important impact on public health and healthcare costs through the implementation of specific disease prevention programs and through improved disease management programs [7].

In summary, advances in information and communication technology services (ICT) have changed how healthcare services can be provided. This will lead to the healthcare industry becoming more patient- rather than doctor-centric. Hence, it is important for healthcare providers to provide services in line with the customers' requirements without jeopardizing their safety and lives.

3 The Proposed Mobile Cloud Shared Workspace

The previous sections have shown that the implementation and management of ICT solutions in the healthcare sector could enhance public health and healthcare at home. We propose the design of a MCSW as the best approach to addressing the challenge of implementing a homecare service for chronic respiratory diseases. Shared workspaces are virtual spaces focused on supporting cooperative tasks in a group [30]. A number of studies and projects have shown that workspaces are also valuable for distributed collaboration [19, 30]. Typically, these groupware applications consider distributed users communicated by networks.

Developing software for mobile work contexts is different from other areas of software development. Thus, developing shared workspaces for mobile environments has always been a challenging task for software developers as they are typically unaware of several requirements and limitations of the frontend and backend of the shared workspace system [15, 19]. Taking into account these limitations, we propose the design of a MCSW as the best approach to address these challenges for designers.

We consider a novel computing model called Mobile Cloud Computing (MCC) in order to approach this. MCC is an infrastructure where both the data storage and data processing may be performed outside of the mobile device if necessary [9]. This way, it is possible to leverage cloud computing technologies and principles to increase, enhance, and optimize computing capabilities of mobile devices by executing resource-intensive mobile application components in resource-rich cloud-based resources, augmenting mobile hardware capabilities and overcoming its limitations. This process is known as Cloud Mobile Augmentation (CMA) [4]. Another reason for incorporating cloud computing into the design is that cloud-connected applications generate compelling crowdsourced output that could not otherwise be easily obtained [6].

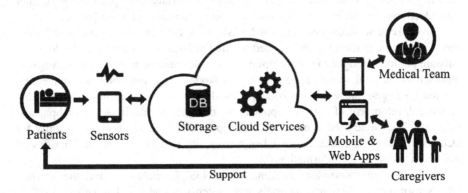

Fig. 1. General architecture of the mobile cloud shared workspace

The proposed platform aims to provide help to the patient's primary caregiver and support network. Figure 1 shows the general architecture of the MCSW, separating its functionality into three basic concerns: (a) Cloud-based backend services for computation and data storage, (b) Mobile and Web applications to enhance collaboration and analysis among patients, caregivers, and medical providers, and (c) Embedded and mobile applications to support the vital signs monitoring and improve the communication channel in the family caregiver support network.

3.1   Cloud-Based Backend Services

Cloud-based backend services are designed to be universally interoperable with different devices and applications. Using the cloud as a service platform has the following advantages:

- *High availability.* The cloud provides a set of features that permit a highly available application. Disaster recovery techniques and self-managed Content Delivery Networks (CDN) are among such features.
- *Storage.* Benefits of storage in a cloud platform include data loss recovery, geo-replication, and flexible capacity.
- *Flexibility.* Adding and removing servers and databases is almost instantaneous.
- *Processing power.* The cloud reduces the running cost for computing-intensive processes that take a long time when performed on limited resource devices.
- *Ease of integration.* Multiple services from different service providers can be integrated.
- *Security and privacy.* Cloud computing users prove their identities with passwords and digital certificates.

The cloud-based backend service that powers the platform gathers the data from multiple sensors and together with an authentication model builds a Personal Health Record (PHR) for each patient. A PHR is a health record where the health data is maintained by the patient, who manages access to that information. Most articles regarding PHRs have been published since 2000 and discuss their practicality together with Electronic Health Records (EHRs) and the barriers for adoption [26].

The backend services powering our MCSW were built on top of several technologies. The service platform itself is coded within the Node.js environment. Node.js is a software platform designed for developing fast and scalable networking and server-side applications. Several studies have shown that Node.js is a well-rounded architecture solution for large-scale sensor networks [8]. Node.js provides an event-driven API that suits the development of network applications designed to maximize throughput and efficiency. The Node.js backend service layer provides authentication and security for each sensor data entry, fires alarms when a risky situation is detected, and notifies all users with access to the information.

For storage, our cloud-based backend uses a NoSQL database to store the patient's data. Sensor data collection is naturally write-intensive, and it is known that NoSQL solutions can outperform traditional relational database systems in these situations [27]. The backend uses an open-source MongoDB distribution, chosen from all the available NoSQL storage options.

The Node.js services and MongoDB instances are hosted on Microsoft's Azure cloud platform. Both components use Azure's Platform as a Service (PaaS) solution, which allows us to manage applications without the complexity of building and maintaining the infrastructure. Azure provides a way to scale the backend painlessly through many instances.

The backend service needs to distribute data to several users (medical experts and caregivers) and through several platforms (mobile and web). To achieve this, several technologies need to be adopted. Push services for web applications commonly use the web socket protocol, while a mobile application can use an array of push notification services (Google Cloud Messaging, Apple Push Notifications). For the cloud-based backend we opted to use the *PubNub* push service that combines these technologies into a single service. *PubNub* provides an API to deliver a high amount of real-time messages without regards to scaling or the infrastructure used. *PubNub* has been used effectively in various research applications [17].

3.2 Mobile and Web Monitoring Applications

The monitoring solutions provide a virtual space where patients, caregivers, and medical providers share information and visualize data in different ways. The workspace presents two specialized interfaces to deliver the patient's vital signs information, a web application and a mobile application.

Our web application is targeted towards medical teams and experts for continuous monitoring. This component focuses on displaying three key pieces of information: the most recent oxygen saturation value (the percentage of oxygen-saturated hemoglobin relative to total hemoglobin in the blood), the most recent heart rate (measured in beats per minute), and the patient's connection to the sensor (connected or disconnected).

The web application is built using common web technologies (Javascript, HTML, and CSS) and is presented as a single page application. The framework of choice is Google's AngularJS platform. This JavaScript library works by reading custom tag attributes embedded into the HTML page. AngularJS interprets these attributes as directives to bind input or output parts of the page to a model that is represented by standard JavaScript variables. AngularJS implements the MVC pattern to separate presentation, data, and logic components.

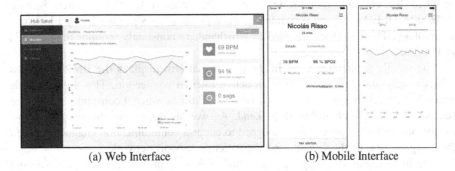

    (a) Web Interface   (b) Mobile Interface

Fig. 2. Vital signs monitoring

Figure 2a shows a screenshot of the monitoring interface. The values of the latest heart rate and oxygen saturation can be seen on the right side, while in the middle the application displays the data captured within the last hour and can be scrolled to access past values.

The workspace's mobile application aims to enable other members of the patient's support network to monitor vital signs and receive risk alerts. The interface focuses on displaying the same three key pieces of information as before but is meant for spot checks rather than constant monitoring.

The mobile application is available on iOS and Android and was built using the open-source Ionic hybrid mobile SDK. Ionic is built on top of the Cordova and AngularJS platforms and enables developers to target multiple platforms within a single JavaScript code base.

Figure 2b shows a screenshot of the mobile application displaying the sensor's data. The screen on the left displays the main interface and is designed to immediately display the most relevant information for spot checks. The screen on the right displays the last hour's sensor data and can be accessed through a side menu.

3.3   Sensor Platform and Embedded Applications

The embedded application is designed to enhance the process of collecting data from wearable vital signs devices. The sensor platform is composed of two components: the sensor device itself and a mobile application focused on vital signs monitoring and communication with the cloud platform.

For the respiratory therapies that are eligible for homecare, the most important vital sign is oxygen saturation, referring to the percentage of oxygen-saturated hemoglobin relative to total hemoglobin in the blood. Peripheral capillary oxygen saturation (SpO_2) is an estimation of the oxygen saturation level, usually measured with a pulse oximetry device. For RTs, the SpO_2 level of a patient needs to be constantly monitored. Any drop for its normal value needs an intervention ranging from an adjustment in the mechanical respirator to an emergency transfer.

The sensor platform is built to support multiple models of pulse oximetry devices; they must measure the SpO_2 levels and heart rate and use Bluetooth for communication. Preferably, these devices should use Bluetooth Low Energy (BLE) and be designed for constant monitoring. The devices chosen for the research include BM2000A OLED wrist pulse oximeters, manufactured by Shanghai Berry Electronic Technology. These devices are used as wristbands to constantly monitor the patient's vital signs.

The mobile application used in the sensor platform displays the BM2000A data values locally and does not require an active Internet connection. This application is meant to be used on a tablet and be powered at all times, since it constantly pushes the sensor's data to the cloud-based backend. As well as displaying the sensor's information, the mobile application is designed to act as a communication channel between the caregiver, the medical team, and the patient's support network.

The local monitoring application is built natively on the Android platform and requires a device running Android 4.0 or newer for the use of BLE. We chose to natively build this application to manage in detail the sensor's data and guarantee that the values are being sent to the backend, even if the patient closes it.

Figure 3 shows a screenshot of the local monitoring application and a photo of a BM2000A device. The interface is designed to display the information the sensor is capturing in a simple fashion. It begins by constantly scanning the nearby area for a compatible sensor. When a device is found, the application starts reading the vital signs data.

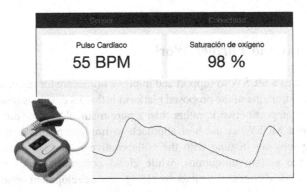

Fig. 3. Local vital signs monitoring application and BM2000A sensor device

3.4   Preliminary Results

This research takes the definition of Family Quality of Life to be "Conditions where the family's needs are met, and family members enjoy their life together as a family and have the chance to do things which are important to them" [20]. The Impact on Family Scale is a generic instrument that assesses the impact of chronic diseases on a family. It describes four factors: financial burden (4 items), family/social impact (9 items), personal strain (6 items), and coping (5 items). Scores are set on a 4-point scale in which 1 represents major impact and four represents minor impact. The score is set by the algebraic sum of the answer given by the family caregivers globally and per item [23].

This project conducted a descriptive analysis of 10 families included in the program of home care and ventilator support TEVEUK. Ltd before the intervention. The inclusion criteria corresponded to those described for AVNI and AVNIA programs. The average age for this program is 11.3 ± 4.7 years and patient diagnoses, according to ICD-10, are: M40; 6 patients (60 %), J43; 3 patients (30 %), and Q32; 1 patient (10 %). The families have been included in the ventilator support program an average of 7.1 ± 1.7 years. The IFS applied to the families resulted in 53.8 ± 2 global points. Analysis by factor showed a high relative impact of the financial burden (8.6 ± 2 points) and social burden (14.5 ± 1.7).

Even though families included in the study have spent over 7 years in their situation, there are still high-impact factors in the Family QoL, namely, financial and social burden factors. Under this condition ICTs have proved useful for promoting social and economic development. In order to estimate the impact of the proposed MCSW in the quality of life in the informal caregiver, we gave each family access to the platform and performed a semi-structured question. The interview was recorded, transcribed textually, and analyzed with the Colaizzi strategy [25]. All patients within our study had access to a Wi-Fi Internet connection and smartphones. The preliminary results show promise of positive adoption of the technology. For instance, when the caregivers answered the question "Do you think having immediate information about the health of your child on a mobile device can improve your quality of life? Why?" this common feedback revealed the following meanings: *Having freedom and autonomy* and *Peace and security*.

4   Conclusions and Further Work

This paper proposes a MCSW to support and improve homecare for respiratory diseases. One of the major strengths of the proposed platform is that its design is based around the patient and their support network, rather than a pure medical tool for diagnosis.

We propose a MCSW as the best approach to implement this homecare system because workspaces are in tune with the collaborative nature of homecare. Mobile devices make the system ubiquitous, while cloud computing helps overcome the limitations of mobile devices, as well as providing new development opportunities. For example, future work for this research includes incorporating machine learning to automatically determine the most probable cause of a drop in oxygen saturation levels given the patient's PHR and offer a set of advices.

The initial research conducted on patients and caregivers shows promise for a smooth adoption of the MCSW and evidences the impact of RTs in the Family QoL. The next step within this track involves performing a quasi-experiment with patients in RTs and a comprehensive study after the intervention.

Finally, this proposal targets specifically patients with respiratory problems and could be used for other chronic diseases at home. Furthermore, the MCSW could potentially have an important impact on public health and healthcare costs through the implementation of specific disease prevention programs and through improved disease management programs. Taking this into account, we are working with the public policy center of *Pontificia Universidad Catolica de Chile* and the health ministry of Chile to bring the ICTs to the Chilean public healthcare system.

For instance, in April 2015, Chile's Calbuco volcano erupted, sending vast clouds of ash into the sky that caused serious respiratory illnesses among other problems [1]. A MCSW could play an important role in this extreme event in order to treat patients with chronic diseases remotely. The workspace encourages collaboration and self-care among patients and their support network, and can stay operational even in a disaster. Patients with no means of mobilization could keep their treatments unaltered and new users could be included.

Acknowledgements. This work was partially supported by VRI-PUC Interdisciplinary Grant No. 03/2013 and UC Center for Public Policies Grant 2015. Finally, we'd like to give special thanks to Claudio Jerez, CEO of TEVEUK Ltd, for providing the connection with homecare patients.

References

1. Minsal prepara planes para tratar efectos postraumáticos en vecinos del volcán calbuco, el mercurio online (2015). http://goo.gl/YgTA8B. Accessed May 2015
2. National department for health statistics, DEIS (2015). http://www.deis.cl/. Accessed May 2015
3. National respiratory therapy programs, Ministry of Health, Chile (2015). http://respiratorio.minsal.cl/. Accessed May 2015
4. Abolfazli, S., Sanaei, Z., Ahmed, E., Gani, A., Buyya, R.: Cloud-based augmentation for mobile devices: motivation, taxonomies, and open challenges. Commun. Surv. Tutorials IEEE **16**(1), 337–368 (2014)
5. Appelboom, G., Yang, A.H., Christophe, B.R., Bruce, E.M., Slomian, J., Bruyère, O., Bruce, S.S., Zacharia, B.E., Reginster, J.Y., Connolly, E.S.: The promise of wearable activity sensors to define patient recovery. J. Clin. Neurosci. **21**(7), 1089–1093 (2014)
6. Bahl, P., Han, R.Y., Li, L.E., Satyanarayanan, M.: Advancing the state of mobile cloud computing. In: Proceedings of the Third ACM Workshop on Mobile Cloud Computing and Services, pp. 21–28. ACM (2012)
7. Berkelman, R.L., Sullivan, P., Buehler, J.W., Detels, R., Beaglehole, R., Lansing, M., Gulliford, M., et al.: Public health surveillance. In: Oxford Textbook of Public Health: The Methods of Public Health, vol. 2, 5 edn., pp. 699–715 (2009)
8. Casini, E., Depree, J., Suri, N., Bradshaw, J.M., Nieten, T.: Enhancing decision-making by leveraging human intervention in large-scale sensor networks. Presentation at the Military Communications Conference (MILCOM 2014), AFCEA International (2014)
9. Dinh, H.T., Lee, C., Niyato, D., Wang, P.: A survey of mobile cloud computing: architecture, applications, and approaches. Wirel. Commun. Mob. Comput. **13**(18), 1587–1611 (2013)
10. Dobkin, B.H., Dorsch, A.: The promise of mhealth daily activity monitoring and outcome assessments by wearable sensors. Neurorehabilitation Neural Repair **25**(9), 788–798 (2011)
11. Escarrabill, J.: Calidad de vida de los pacientes respiratorios: aportación de los sistemas domiciliarios e importancia de la formación de cuidadores. Informe INESME Terapias respiratorias domiciliarias: ¿gasto o inversión en salud? (2008)
12. Eysenbach, G.: What is e-health? J. Med. Internet Res. **3**(2), e20 (2001)
13. Fernández-Alvarez, R., Rubinos-Cuadrado, G., Cabrera-Lacalzada, C., Galindo-Morales, R., Gullón-Blanco, J.A., González-Martín, I.: Ventilación mecánica domiciliaria: dependencia y carga de cuidados en el domicilio. Archivos de Bronconeumología **45**(8), 383–386 (2009)
14. Hayakawa, M., Uchimura, Y., Omae, K., Waki, K., Fujita, H., Ohe, K., et al.: A smartphone-based medication self-management system with realtime medication monitoring. Appl. Clin. Inform. **4**(1), 37–52 (2013)
15. Herskovic, V., Ochoa, S.F., Pino, J.A., Neyem, H.A.: The iceberg effect: behind the user interface of mobile collaborative systems. J. UCS **17**(2), 183–201 (2011)
16. Hibbard, J.H., Greene, J.: What the evidence shows about patient activation: better health outcomes and care experiences; fewer data on costs. Health Aff. **32**(2), 207–214 (2013)
17. Lin, C.Y., Chu, E.T.H., Ku, L.W., Liu, J.W.: Active disaster response system for a smart building. Sensors **14**(9), 17451–17470 (2014)
18. Lorig, K.R., Sobel, D.S., Ritter, P.L., Laurent, D., Hobbs, M.: Effect of a self-management program on patients with chronic disease. Effective Clin. Pract. ECP **4**(6), 256–262 (2000)
19. Neyem, A., Ochoa, S.F., Pino, J.A., Franco, R.D.: A reusable structural design for mobile collaborative applications. J. Syst. Softw. **85**(3), 511–524 (2012)

20. Park, J., Hoffman, L., Marquis, J., Turnbull, A., Poston, D., Mannan, H., Wang, M., Nelson, L.: Toward assessing family outcomes of service delivery: validation of a family quality of life survey. J. Intellect. Disabil. Res. **47**(4–5), 367–384 (2003)

21. Phillips, G., Felix, L., Galli, L., Patel, V., Edwards, P.: The effectiveness of m-health technologies for improving health and health services: a systematic review protocol. BMC Res. Notes **3**(1), 250 (2010)

22. Ricciardi, L., Mostashari, F., Murphy, J., Daniel, J.G., Siminerio, E.P.: A national action plan to support consumer engagement via e-health. Health Aff. **32**(2), 376–384 (2013)

23. Salinas, P., Farias, A., González, X., Rodríguez, C.: Calidad de vida rela-cionada en salud: Concepto y evaluación en pacientes con ventilación mecánica no invasiva. Neumol. Pediatr. **3**(Suppl 1), 34–39 (2008)

24. Sánchez, D., Valenzuela, S., Bertrand, N., Alvarez, G., Holmgren, P., Linus, N., Vilches, J., Jerez, T., Ronco, M., et al.: Apoyo ventilatorio domiciliario en niños con insuficiencia respiratoria crónica: Experiencia clínica. Revista chilena de pediatría **73**(1), 51–55 (2002)

25. Speziale, H.S., Streubert, H.J., Carpenter, D.R.: Qualitative Research in Nursing: Advancing the Humanistic Imperative. Lippincott Williams &Wilkins, Philadelphia (2011)

26. Tang, P.C., Ash, J.S., Bates, D.W., Overhage, J.M., Sands, D.Z.: Personal health records: definitions, benefits, and strategies for overcoming barriers to adoption. J. Am. Med. Inform. Assoc. **13**(2), 121–126 (2006)

27. van der Veen, J.S., van der Waaij, B., Meijer, R.J.: Sensor data storage performance: Sql or nosql, physical or virtual. In: 2012 IEEE 5th International Conference on Cloud Computing (CLOUD), pp. 431–438. IEEE (2012)

28. Vidal, A., Duffau, G., Ubilla, C.: Calidad de vida en el niño asmático y su cuidador. Revista chilena de enfermedades respiratorias **23**(3), 160–166 (2007)

29. Villarreal, V., Fontecha, J., Hervas, R., Bravo, J.: Mobile and ubiquitous architecture for the medical control of chronic diseases through the use of intelligent devices: using the architecture for patients with diabetes. Future Gener. Comput. Syst. **34**, 161–175 (2014)

30. Whittaker, S., Geelhoed, E., Robinson, E.: Shared workspaces: how do they work and when are they useful? Int. J. Man-Mach. Stud. **39**(5), 813–842 (1993)

31. Yang, C.C., Hsu, Y.L.: A review of accelerometry-based wearable motion detectors for physical activity monitoring. Sensors **10**(8), 7772–7788 (2010)

32. Zarit, S.H., Whetzel, C.A., Kim, K., Femia, E.E., Almeida, D.M., Rovine, M.J., Klein, L.C.: Daily stressors and adult day service use by family caregivers: effects on depressive symptoms, positive mood, and dehydroepiandrosterone-sulfate. Am. J. Geriatr. Psychiatry **22**(12), 1592–1602 (2014)

Extracting Information from Electronic Medical Records to Identify Obesity Status of a Patient Based on Comorbidities and Bodyweight Measures

Rosa L. Figueroa and Christopher A. Flores$^{(\boxtimes)}$

Departamento de Ingeniería Eléctrica, Facultad de Ingeniería,
Universidad de Concepción, Concepción, Chile
{rosa.figueroa, chrisflores}@udec.cl

Abstract. Obesity is a chronic disease with an increasing impact on the world's population. In this work, we present a method to identify obesity using text mining techniques and information related to body weight measures and obesity comorbidities. We used a dataset of 2412 de-identified medical records that contains labels for two classification problems. The first classification problem recognizes between obesity, overweight, normal weight, and underweight. The second problem of classification corresponds to the obesity types under the obesity category to recognize between super obesity, morbid obesity, severe obesity and moderate obesity. We used a Bag of Words approach to represent the records together with unigram and bigram representation of the features. We used Support Vector Machine and Naïve Bayes together with ten-fold cross validation to evaluate and compare performances. In general, our results show that Support Vector Machine obtains better performances than Naïve Bayes for both classification problems. We also observed that bigram representation improves performance compared with unigram representation.

Keywords: Machine learning · Natural language processing · Obesity · Comorbidities

1 Introduction

Obesity is a chronic disease with an increasing impact on the world's population. According to the World Health Organization, by 2014 1.9 billion adults were overweight and from this 600 million were obese [1]. In Chile, according to the National Health Survey, 25.1 % of the adult population is affected by this condition [2]. Obesity not only affects the quality of life, but is also accompanied by some health risks, called comorbidities, such as diabetes, hypertension, cardiovascular disease, and even depression [3].

Health information technology introduction has changed the way health information is documented and stored. Electronic Health Records (EHR) are an example of such technologies. EHR allows the centralized storage of the patient's medical history in a digital version. The use of EHR has enabled researchers to develop information

© Springer International Publishing Switzerland 2015
J. Bravo et al. (Eds.): AmIHEALTH 2015, LNCS 9456, pp. 37–46, 2015.
DOI: 10.1007/978-3-319-26508-7_4

extraction systems to obtain information about different health risks and conditions that may affect patients [4].

Since obesity has become a major global challenge, there is a growing interest in studying this disease and its related comorbidities. In [5] Üzuner describes a challenge in creating information extraction systems for automatically identify and extract information on obesity and its comorbidities organized by the Informatics for Integrating Biology and the Bedside (i2b2) in 2008. They released a set of de-identified medical discharge records from Partners HealthCare Research Patient Data Repository. The records were annotated by two obesity experts who identified and assigned labels to obesity and each of its fifteen more frequent comorbidities. These labels classify each disease as Present, Absent, Questionable, or Unmentioned based on the textual documented information or intuitive judgment. Yang et al. [6] and Solt et al. [7] obtained the best results in this challenge both in textual extraction and intuitive judgment. Yang et al. [6] used a set of lexical and semantic resources to identify a disease, such as concepts, sub-concepts, synonyms, treatments and related symptoms, most of them from the Unified Medical Language System (UMLS). The resultant features were exploited by dictionary look-up, rule-based and machine learning methods. They applied their methods to 507 unseen discharge summaries and evaluated using a manually prepared gold standard. In the textual task, they obtained a macro-averaged F-measure of 81 % and a macro-averaged F-measure of 63 % for the intuitive task. On the other hand, Solt et al. [7] used a context-aware rule-based semantic classifier. To perform a semantic analysis of the records, they include a set of clue terms for each disease such as synonyms, frequent typos, abbreviations among others. First, they eliminated some irrelevant and misleading content, then partitioned the records according to its classes, and finally, applied a set of binary classifiers. In the textual task they obtained a macro-averaged F-measure of 80 % and a macro-averaged F-measure of 67 % for the intuitive tasks. The work of Murtaugh et al. in [8] describe a more recent approach to extract information related to obesity. They developed a Regular Expression Discovery Extractor (REDEx) to extract body weight-related measures, such as weight, height, abdominal circumference and BMI from clinical notes. The aim was to complement the data that is obtained from structured fields for research purposes. The algorithm was trained on a set of 268 outpatient primary care records and tested on separate records. They obtained an accuracy of 98.3 %, and an F- measure of 98.5 %.

In this work, we present a method to identify obesity automatically, using text mining techniques and information related to body weight measures and obesity comorbidities. As our dataset, we used structured and narrative fields present in outpatient reports obtained from Guillermo Grant Benavente Hospital (HGGB). Our work will face two main challenges: to identify obesity based on its comorbidities and other associated information and to process medical records in Spanish.

2   Materials and Methods

2.1   Dataset

As our dataset, we used a set of 65780 outpatient records obtained from the HGGB EMR system. These notes include records from 43 medical specialties that were registered between 2011 and 2012. Each medical record has structured fields to report risks factors, habits, and vital signs and also has narratives or non-structured fields to report physical examination, medical history, observations, and indications. Some of the structured fields also included a small space for the doctor to write comments and observations. For the purpose of this work, we considered structured and narrative fields.

2.2 Preprocessing

First, we normalized each report by changing words to lower cases, non-alphanumeric characters and stop words (e.g. a, the, on, etc.) were removed. Second, we replaced all the BMI values present in the text to its minimum value, according to its category [9]. For example, underweight values were replaced with 0, normal weight values were replaced with 18.5, overweight values replaced with 25, moderate obesity values with 30 and so on (see Table 1). The two steps mentioned were done to facilitate the feature extraction process. Third, in this stage we created a list of comorbidities associated with obesity. To create this list, we used the fifteen diseases provided in [5], however, after the annotation process we added two more diseases: Cushing disease and hypothyroidism.

Table 1. BMI and nutritional status

Nutritional status	BMI	Minimum value
Underweight	<18.5	0
Normal weight	18.5–24.9	18.5
Overweight	25–29.9	25
Moderate obesity	30–34.9	30
Severe obesity	35–39.9	35
Morbid obesity	40–49.9	40
Super obesity	≥50	50

Finally, we filtered out records that were not relevant to this study. To do that, we used a custom-made dictionary together with regular expressions that could filter out records that do not contain information related to obesity or body weight measures. Our dictionary included a set of key terms, such as underweight, normal weight, overweight, obesity and BMI, synonyms of the key terms, and frequent typos. After the filtering process, we recovered a total of 2462 records (out of 65780) containing relevant information to the study.

2.3 Annotation

For this work, we defined two classification problems. Classes for the first problem were: obesity (O), overweight (OW), normal weight (NW), and underweight (UW). The second classification problem corresponds to the obesity types under the Obesity category. The classes for this problem were: super obesity (S), morbid obesity (M), severe obesity (SO), and moderate obesity (MO).

To generate a gold standard for classification, we asked two students with biomedical background to revise and annotated a total of 2462 records using an annotation tool designed in QT-designer[1] and programmed in Python. This tool allows the annotator to assign a specific label to a record and suggest possible features for classification. For each record, they first assigned a label within the first classification problem. In the case that Obesity label was assigned to a record, the reviewer was asked to annotate the record with a label of the second classification problem. We also asked the evaluators to provide information about keywords related to obesity, body weight or obesity comorbidities that were not considered in the list of keywords but were present in the records.

When all the documents were annotated, we filtered out records that reviewers deemed as possible false positives. These are records that mentioned keywords related to obesity but were not relevant to the study (e.g. records mentioning "low molecular weight"). Finally, we asked a third evaluator to solve any disagreement and to validate the assigned classes.

At the end of the annotation process, we obtained a total of 2412 annotated records for the first classification problem and 920 annotated records for the second problem. We evaluated inter-annotator agreement using Cohen's kappa coefficient [10]. Cohen's kappa is a statistical index to measure agreement between two raters. When an inter-annotator agreement is poor, values closer to zero are expected, on the other hand, when the agreement is almost perfect, values between 0.81–1 are expected. Table 2 describes the datasets distribution after the annotation process ended.

Table 2. Class distribution

	Class I	Class II	Class III	Class IV	Total
Nutritional status	264 (UW)	37 (NW)	247 (OW)	1864 (O)	2412
Obesity types	166 (MO)	133 (SO)	589 (M)	32 (S)	920

2.4 Feature Extraction and Selection for Classification

To extract features for classification, first we filtered out records that do not contain information related to obesity comorbidities. The filtering process used a dictionary of obesity comorbidities that contains 17 diseases and regular expressions. The dictionary contains fifteen diseases taken from the list provided in [5], and two diseases suggested by the annotators. After this process, we obtained a total of 2082 records. Second, we tokenized the resultant records using unigrams (N1) and bigrams (N2). We defined unigrams as single word tokens and bigrams as sequences of two word tokens. We obtained a total of 3274 unigram tokens and 8927 bigram tokens. Before using this tokens as features for classification, we applied feature selection using the

---

[1] QT-designer is a Qt tool to design and build graphical user using widgets. http://doc.qt.io/qt-5/qtdesigner-manual.html.

InfoGainAttributeEval filter together with Ranker available from Weka[2]. The InfoGainAttributeEval filter selects features by measuring the information gain with respect to the class. The Ranker method sorts the features by their individual evaluations scores obtained in the InfoGainAttributeEval. Using both methods we reduced our feature set to 500 for the first classification problem for both unigram and bigram tokens. For the second classification problem, we have 532 unigrams and 548 bigrams. These features contain the selected 500 features plus some tokens related to obesity types, such as "BMI 20", "obesity degree", and "severe obesity", that we manually added to the set.

2.5 Feature Representation

For each classification problem, we used Bag of Words (BoW) representation. We used term frequency-inverse document frequency (TF-IDF) weighting schema to represent the occurrences of the selected features in each record [11]. Equations (1) and (2) describe the TF-IDF schema where TF is the term frequency, IDF is the inverse document frequency, N is the number of documents, and N_i the number of documents that contain the token t_i.

$$TF - IDF = TF_{t,d} \times IDF_{t,D} \qquad (1)$$

$$IDF_{t_i} = \log_{10}\left(\frac{N}{n_i + 1}\right). \qquad (2)$$

2.6 Classification and Evaluation

To classify the records, we built models using the implementations of Naïve Bayes (NB) and Support Vector Machines (SVM) classifiers. NB classifiers are a family of probabilistic classifiers that use the Bayes' theorem. This classifier assumes that features in the dataset are mutually independent [12]. SVM are supervised learning models that build a set of hyperplanes in a high dimensional space that can separate the classes and find the one that maximize the margin between the members of the classes [12]. Both classifiers were implemented using the scikit tool for machine learning in Python [13]. In the case of NB, we use a multinomial approach together with TF-IDF matrix representation. In the case of SVM, we used a linear kernel together with the one by one multiclass classification setting, the rest of the parameters were kept at their default values.

To evaluate the classification models, we implemented ten-fold cross validation and repeated each experiment 10 times. Performance measures used to evaluate the classifiers' predictive capacity were Accuracy (ACC), F-measure, False Positive Rate (FPR) and False Negative Rate (FNR). We averaged all the performance measures over

---

[2] Weka is an open source software for data mining tasks. http://www.cs.waikato.ac.nz/ml/weka/.

the ten runs. Equations (3)–(6) show how each performance measures were calculated, where TP: true positives, TN: true negatives, FP: false positives, and FN: false negatives. In order to compare performances, we calculated the weighted average of each performance measure using as weights the amount of examples per class and used a paired t-test (significance level of 0.05).

$$\text{Accuracy} = \frac{TP + TN}{TP + FP + TN + FN} \tag{3}$$

$$\text{F} - \text{measure} = \frac{2 \cdot TP}{2TP + FN + FP} \tag{4}$$

$$\text{FPR} = \frac{FP}{FP + TN} \tag{5}$$

$$\text{FNR} = \frac{FN}{FN + TP}. \tag{6}$$

3 Results

Once all the documents were annotated we used Cohen's kappa coefficient to evaluate the inter-rater agreement. For the first classification problem, where evaluators have to decide between O, OW, NW, and UW, we obtained a Cohen's kappa coefficient of 0.97. For the second classification problem, where evaluators have to decide between the obesity types S, M, SO, and MO, we obtained a Cohen's kappa coefficient of 0.96. Both classification problems presented Cohen's kappa coefficients representing an almost perfect agreement between the annotators. Thus, our gold standard can be considered reliable and useful to build models and evaluate classification results.

From the annotated records, we found that most of them were written by physicians of endocrinology and general surgery (adult) specialties. In terms of gender, 78.49 % of the annotated records belong to women that present some degree of obesity.

Tables 3 and 4 show the classification results for both classification problems. We can observe from Table 3 that both unigram and bigram representations together with SVM, perform better than NB in terms of ACC, except for the O class in bigram representation. In terms of F-measure, unigram representation together with SVM, performs better than NB, except for the OW class. We also observe that the O class obtains the highest values of FPR for both unigram and bigram representations. On the other hand, the class OW and NW have the highest values of FNR. In terms of weighted average, ACC and F-measure of unigram representation together with SVM, are better than NB. Finally, we observe that bigram representation together with NB performs slightly better than SVM.

Table 3. Classifiers' performance measures for the first classification problem

	Class	Accuracy	F-measure	FPR	FNR
N1					
NB	UW	97,63	89,12	1,28	11,25
	NW	97,69	51,41	2,03	**20,27**
	OW	89,73	**51,64**	6,15	**46,44**
	O	88,42	92,39	**20,27**	9,02
	Weighted average	89,70	87,23	**16,47**	13,27
SVM	UW	**99,32**	**96,93**	**0,43**	**2,65**
	NW	**98,83**	**63,71**	**0,68**	32,70
	OW	**90,93**	46,07	**3,01**	62,19
	O	**89,95**	**93,64**	29,60	**4,30**
	Weighted average	**91,21**	**88,67**	23,24	**10,48**
N2					
NB	UW	98,82	94,49	0,42	**7,39**
	NW	98,74	67,24	1,02	**16,22**
	OW	92,90	**61,07**	2,70	**45,63**
	O	**92,48**	95,19	20,78	3,62
	Weighted average	**93,31**	**91,19**[a]	16,40	8,53
SVM	UW	**99,65**	**98,38**	**0,14**	2,08
	NW	**99,33**	**78,74**	**0,38**	19,19
	OW	**92,95**[a]	54,75	**1,20**	58,34
	O	92,19	95,10	28,01	**1,87**
	Weighted average	93,19	91,08	21,79	**7,94**

[a]Not statistically better

From Table 4 we can observe that both unigram and bigram representations together with SVM, perform better than NB in terms of single and weighted ACC and F-measure. We also observe that the M class obtains the highest values of FPR for both unigram and bigram representations. On the other hand, the class S has the highest values of FNR.

In general, from Tables 3 and 4 we observe that bigram representation obtains better values of performance when compared with unigram representation.

4 Discussion and Conclusion

This work shows a method to extract obesity from clinical records in Spanish by studying the disease, its comorbidities, body weight measures and BMI.

To classify obesity, the records don't have any explicit negation for the condition. Thus, we had to add counterexamples based on the nutritional information of the patient. However, we only recover a 3.67 % out of the total number of records that contain relevant information to the study. From the 3.67 %, only a 38.14 % contains information about obesity types.

Table 4. Classifiers' performance measures for the second classification problem

	Class	Accuracy	F-measure	FPR	FNR
N1					
NB	MO	82,02	55,17	13,42	38,67
	SO	83,70	37,40	7,85	66,32
	M	83,88	87,38	21,99	12,82
	S	95,84	31,64	1,71	72,19
	Weighted average	83,93	72,40	17,69	27,28
SVM	MO	82,26[a]	55,76[a]	13,28[a]	38,01[a]
	SO	85,91	50,02	7,81[a]	51,20
	M	87,57	90,13	14,50	11,27
	S	96,87	44,57	0,95	63,75
	Weighted average	86,70	76,55	12,84	23,69
N2					
NB	MO	97,07	91,83	1,68	8,61
	SO	94,96	83,25	3,65	13,31
	M	91,97	93,77	12,33	5,62
	S	97,18	44,74	0,50	67,19
	Weighted average	93,50	90,19	8,74	9,41
SVM	MO	98,85	96,76	0,38	4,64
	SO	98,37	94,30	0,76	6,77
	M	95,61	96,64	9,73	1,39
	S	97,85	58,53	0,20	56,25
	weighted average	96,67	95,00	6,41	4,66

[a]Not statistically better

According to the annotated records, women have the highest prevalence of obesity with a 78.49 % of the total of the reported cases. These results are comparable to the information reported by the National Health Survey in 2010, where 30.7 % of women have obesity [2]. We think the highest prevalence of obesity in women might be because women tend to visit health centers more frequent than men.

In general, the highest percentages of ACC can be explained by the high amount of TN obtained by both classification problems. We believe this result is due to the class imbalance observed for both classification problems (see Table 2). For this reason, we calculated a weighted average for Accuracy and F-measure. The weighted average showed, in general, lower ACC values when compared with single ACC values.

As we mentioned in Sect. 3, in most of the cases SVM outperforms NB for both classification problems. In general, N2 representation shows better performance values than N1 representation. We believe that using N2 representation helps to capture more informative features (e.g.: blood pressure, Gastroesophageal reflux disease, Type I, BMI 40, etc.). However, the computational cost of programming N2 is highest than programming N1 to extract features.

It is worth mentioning that the comorbidities are not exclusive of Obesity which could have generated ambiguities in the classifiers' learning. In the first classification problem, the system tends to classify more often examples in the class O, which generates a high percentage of FPR. We believed this affected the detection of examples of the NW and OW classes that present a high FNR. We can observe something similar for the M class, which has the highest percentages of FPR while the S class shows a high FNR. For the second classification problem, we observe that for both classifiers, N2 shows lowest FNR, except for the S class, when compared with N1. We have observed ambiguities in the use of the class S in the medical records. Sometimes the physician identifies a patient as having morbid obesity when it should be a super-obese patient. We believe that if we merge S class with the M class, our classification results may improve.

Classifiers' performance highly depends on the selected features. Thus, we applied feature selection as explained in Sect. 2.4. Applying feature selection improved the performance of the classifiers when compared with classifiers built without feature selection. For this reason, we decided to report in this work the results obtained with feature selection.

To extend and maybe improve our research, we plan - as a future work- to do a more extensive feature selection for classification. We also plan to perform classifier tuning once we obtain a bigger database of medical records.

Acknowledgment. The authors want to thank the informatics division of the HGGB, Universidad de Concepcion, and FONDECYT (Grant N°11121463) for their support of this research.

References

1. Curtis, M.: The obesity epidemic in the pacific islands. J. Dev. Soc. Transform. **1**, 37–42 (2004)
2. Atalah, E.: Epidemiología de la obesidad en Chile. Rev. Med. Clin. Condes. **23**(2), 117–123 (2012)
3. Markowitzs, S., Friendman, M., Arent, S.: Understanding the relation between obesity and depression: causal mechanism and implications for treatment. Clin. Psychol. Sci. Pract. **15** (1), 1–20 (2008)
4. Crawford, A., Cote, C., Cuoto, J., et al.: Prevalence of obesity, type II diabetes mellitus, hyperlipidemia, and hypertension in the United States: findings from the GE centricity electronic medical record database. Popul. Health. Manag. **13**(13), 151–161 (2010)
5. Üzuner, O.: Recognizing obesity and comorbidities in sparse data. J. Am. Med. Inform. Assoc. **16**(4), 561–570 (2009)
6. Yang, H., Spasic, I., Keane, J.A., Nenadic, G.: A text mining approach to the prediction of disease status from clinical discharge summaries. J. Am. Med. Inform. Assoc. **16**(4), 596–600 (2009)
7. Solt, I., Tikk, D., Gál, V., Kardkovács, Z.: Semantic classification of diseases in discharge summaries using a context-aware rule-based classifier. J. Am. Med. Inform. Assoc. **16**(4), 580–584 (2009)
8. Murtaugh, M., Smith, B., Redd, D., Zeng-Treitler, Q.: Regular expression-based learning to extract body weight values from clinical notes. J. Biomed. Inform. **54**, 186–190 (2015)
9. Moreno, G.: Definición y clasificación de la obesidad. Rev. Med. Clí. Condes. **23**(2), 124–128 (2012)

10. Viera, A., Garret, J.: Understanding interobserver agreement: the kappa statistic. Fam. Med. **37**(5), 360–363 (2005)
11. Gebrekidan, B., Zampieri, M., Wittenburg, P., Heskes, T.: Improving native language with TF-IDF weighting. In: 8th NAACL Workshop on Innovative Use of NLP for Building Educational Applications (BEA8), Atlanta, USA, pp. 216–233 (2013)
12. Rennie, J., Rifkin, R.: Improving multiclass text classification with the support vector machine. Technical report, AIM, pp. 2001–2016 (2001)
13. Buitinck, L., Louppe, G., Blondel, M., et al.: API design for machine learning software: experiences from the scikit-learn project. In: ECML PKDD Workshop on Languages for Machine Learning (2013)

Daily Activity Monitoring for Prevention of Pressure Ulcers in Long-Term Wheelchair Users

Diego E. Arias[1], Esteban J. Pino[1(✉)], Pablo Aqueveque[1], and Dorothy W. Curtis[2]

[1] Universidad de Concepción, Concepción, Chile
{diegoarias, pablo.aqueveque}@udec.cl, epino@ieee.org
[2] Massachusetts Institute of Technology, Cambridge, MA, USA
dcurtis@csail.mit.edu

Abstract. This paper presents an assistive device for assessment and prevention of pressure ulcers in long-term wheelchair patients. The system consists of several sensors deployed on the wheelchair non-invasively for monitoring pressure changes and tilt usage during daily activities. A pilot study was conducted to evaluate the potential capabilities of the system and the feasibility of implementing alarms based on clinical recommendations. During two weeks, six full-time wheelchair users with severe disability were monitored. Their wheelchairs were electric-powered and equipped with tilt-in-space systems and pressure relief cushions as methods for relieving pressure. Results show that the system is able to capture tilt usage and pressure changes during daily life. Also, it provides relevant information regarding to wheelchair occupancy and activity level. The study shows that most of the subjects spent long hours on the wheelchair without performing pressure relief as often as recommended, confirming the usefulness of a personalized alarm system.

Keywords: Activity monitoring · Assistive device · Caregiver · Disability · Electric-powered wheelchair · Mobile health care · Monitoring system · Pressure relief · Pressure ulcer · Tilt-in-space

1 Introduction

According to the World Health Organization, around the world there are more than 785 million people with a disabling condition [1]. Currently, people are spending more years of their life with some kind of disability produced to a great extent by the population aging and the increase in chronic diseases [2]. This global scenario challenges researchers to develop new technological solutions to improve quality of life for people living with a disability.

People who are unable to walk and need a wheelchair to move independently are estimated at about 10 % of disabled people worldwide [3]. Wheelchair users spend long hours sitting, which can increase the probability of pressure ulcers (PU). PU are injuries on the skin produced by excessive pressure during long periods of time. Excessive pressure, usually over bony prominences, reduces the blood flow producing tissue

© Springer International Publishing Switzerland 2015
J. Bravo et al. (Eds.): AmIHEALTH 2015, LNCS 9456, pp. 47–58, 2015.
DOI: 10.1007/978-3-319-26508-7_5

ischemia and death, resulting in an ulcer. Parts of the body in contact with the wheelchair such as the ischial tuberosities, coccyx and pelvis bones are more likely to develop PU. The proper way to avoid PU is to change position regularly. This way, the excessive pressure is relieved and blood can flow through the tissues. Clinicians recommend patients to perform push-ups, side-to-side leans or lean forward over the knees as methods to relieve pressure. However, people who suffer severe mobility impairment cannot relieve pressure by themselves. Usually, they need help from other people, either family members or specialized caregivers, to change positions regularly. In those cases powered wheelchairs equipped with seat functions such as a tilt-in-space system, are often prescribed. The tilt-in-space system allows the seat angle orientation to be changed in relation to the ground while maintaining the seat to back angle [4]. This mechanism redistributes the seat pressure, transferring it from the seat to the back.

The use of a tilt-in-space system depends on patients as well as caregivers. Patients need to understand why it is important to relieve pressure and to be reminded how often they should tilt the wheelchair. Caregivers should be aware of reminding patients when to tilt the wheelchair and assist them. However, for example, patients with Spinal Cord Injury (SCI) and Multiple Sclerosis (MS) can suffer loss of awareness, sensory impairment and cognitive loss which can result in patients forgetting to tilt their wheelchairs [5, 6]. Also, the high workload in nursing homes can lead caregivers to forget to tilt the patient's wheelchair or to remind them to tilt by themselves. The same can happen when a family member is responsible for the patient's care. In those cases, it would be valuable to be able to alert the patient and/or the caregiver when such action is necessary.

Clinicians and nursing staff have used simple techniques as reminders for PU prevention. For example, audible broadcast reminders have being implemented playing music every 2 h through the paging system to remind caregivers [7, 8]. An issue in this approach is that the reminders are not well received by the staff. Also beepers and clock watches alarms have been used by caregivers to remind help patients. On the other hand, several research groups have designed assistive devices with the goal of averting PU in people who use wheelchairs. Some authors have used commercial pressure mapping systems to monitor pressure changes during daily activities. In [9, 10], alarm devices based on commercial pressure mapping systems, have been proposed to warn patients and/or caregivers when a change in position is necessary. Both systems generate an audible alarm if any of the sensors exceed an established threshold for 15 or 30 min. The advantage of using this kind of system is that it allows capturing a reliable pressure distribution due to the high number of sensors. This is why they are extensively used in clinical and laboratory research. However, pressure mapping systems are deployed on top of the pressure relief cushion, interfering with its performance. Patients have expressed their concern that the cushion would lose its effectivity, increasing the probability to develop PU [11]. This technology is unsuitable for unobtrusive long-term monitoring. In [12], the authors propose a custom pressure mapping system embedded into the cushion. However, the matrix of 8 × 8 sensors is made with rigid copper electrodes which can produce discomfort to the patient. Other projects have designed systems where the sensors are deployed under the pressure relief cushion, to avoid interfering with its function and making them imperceptible to patients. For instance, in [13] the authors use 8 piezoresistive sensors which are the same used by FSA Seating Assessment system, a commercial pressure mapping device. In this case, the sensors are put under the cushion and distributed around the ischial tuberosities to capture pressure relief over this region. A similar project is presented in [14]. In this case, 6 force sensitive resistor (FSR) sensors deployed around the ischial tuberosities and the thigh are used to study pressure relieving patterns in SCI patients using manual wheelchairs. In [15], the authors propose an alarm system based on capturing pressure relief movements using FSR sensors. When the system detects that the patient has not moved during 15 min, a band put on the patient's arm vibrates, warning that it is necessary to move. The systems presented in [11, 12], reduce the number of sensors in comparison with commercial pressure mapping devices, affecting the capacity to capture a reliable pressure distribution. However, they are able to detect when patients relieve pressure on the buttocks which is the key to avoid PU. In addition, reducing the number of sensors, less memory capacity and processing power is required which is ideal for continuous and real-time monitoring.

Another approach to detect pressure relief is used when the patients use powered wheelchairs equipped with a tilt-in-space system. Some projects focus on monitoring the tilt-in-space usage as way for relieving pressure during daily activities. In [16, 17] the authors describe a device composed of a data logger with three tilt sensors to monitor seat tilt and backrest recline. Also, the system uses a linear transducer to capture seat elevation and three FSR sensors to monitor wheelchair occupancy. A similar system is used in [18, 19]. It consists of an accelerometer to detect tilt and a ribbon switch under the cushion to detect wheelchair occupancy all stored in a data logger. In [20], authors also use an accelerometer but the processing stage is performed on a Raspberry Pi®.

For patients who are unable to relieve pressure by themselves and users of powered wheelchairs with a tilt-in-space system, a more reliable system to detect pressure relieving patterns must combine both approaches: monitoring pressure changes as well as the tilt-in-space usage during daily activities. This way, it is possible verify that a tilt is actually producing a pressure relief. The system provides sufficient data to generate personalized alarms/recommendations regarding how often the patients should tilt their wheelchair. It also collects valuable clinical information for a proper pressure management, as well as general activity monitoring. The objective of this study is to present a non-invasive assistive device able to reliably capture pressure changes and tilt-in-space usage for powered wheelchair users during daily activities. This project focuses on patients affected by severe mobility impairment who are more prone to develop PU.

2 Methods

2.1 Instrumentation

The designed system consists of several pressure sensors and an accelerometer to capture pressure relieving tilt (PRT) during daily activities. To this end, nine FSR (model FSR 406 manufactured by Interlink Inc.) are deployed on the wheelchair distributed as follow: 4 sensors are put on seat (FSR_S), under the pressure relief cushion, and 5 on the backrest (FSR$_B$), inside a piece of foam. This way it is possible to detect weight shifting produced by tilt-in-space system with a good spatial resolution. Also, this setup allows us to capture the information in a non-invasive way without discomfort to the user, because the sensors do not touch the patient directly. To detect the wheelchair tilt and to capture information related to subject activity, an accelerometer (ADXL335 chip) is fixed to the wheelchair. The ADXL335 has analog output and a resolution of ±3 g. All information acquired by the sensors is send to a microcontroller which samples the data at 100 Hz with 11 bits of resolution. Then, the data are transmitted through the serial port to a small laptop mounted on the wheelchair. Finally, the data are stored in a PostgreSQL [19] database for further analysis. All the system is powered from the wheelchair batteries. The power consumed by the hardware is minimal and does not affect the wheelchair performance. Figure 1 shows the implemented system mounted on the wheelchair.

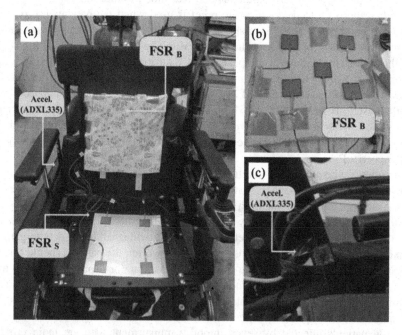

Fig. 1. Pictures of the implemented system. FSR$_S$ are deployed under the pressure relief cushion (a) and FSR$_B$ are deployed inside a foam (b) to detect pressure changes. An accelerometer fixed to the wheelchair detects the tilt-in-space usage (c).

2.2   PRT Detection Algorithm

A PRT detection algorithm is designed to find when the wheelchair user relieves pressure by tilting. PRT is defined as a wheelchair tilt due to the operation of the tilt-in-space system which produces relief of pressure over the buttocks area. According to the study presented in [20], a pressure relief is achieved if the skin is unloaded for at least 3 min and 30 s, this way the tissues are oxygenated. For increased safety, in our project, a threshold of 5 min is used.

The detection algorithm uses the accelerometer data and the pressure sensors deployed on the seat. Accelerometer data is filtered using a low pass filter to extract the static component of acceleration and this way transforms it into a tilt angle. The angle is averaged using a 10 s sliding window to detect angle changes. When the tilt angle is reduced by at least 5 degrees, which means that the wheelchair is tilted back, and the pressure sensors reduce their level sharply, the tilt is marked as possible PRT. To consider the tilt as a PRT, the subject should maintain this position or increase the tilt angle for at least 5 min. Otherwise, the algorithm is restarted. When the subject returns to the initial position, the tilt is finished. Figure 2 shows an example of PRT detection. This full day record shows 4 PRT detections. Vertical lines marked with an 'X' indicate the start of a tilt. Lines marked with an 'O' indicate the end of a tilt. It is possible to observe how pressure over the buttocks area is transferred to the back during a PRT. Also, the pressure sensors allow detecting when the subject is using the wheelchair which is useful for calculating the wheelchair occupancy duration. In the Fig. 2 example, the volunteer is on the wheelchair for 6:41 h.

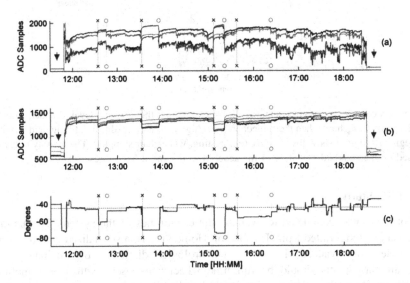

Fig. 2. PRT detection algorithm. FSR_B (a), FSR_S (b) and tilt angle obtained with the accelerometer (c) allows capturing pressure relieving patterns during the day. Vertical lines marked with 'x' and 'o' indicate the PRT detected. Arrows on the FSR sensors mark the beginning and end of the wheelchair occupancy.

2.3 Activity Level Estimation

An activity index (AI) was designed to quantify the activity level of each subject during the time spent on the wheelchair. The AI is defined as the percentage of the wheelchair occupancy duration where the subject shows high activity. The AI is estimated based on the dynamic component of the accelerometer data which reflects the subject's movement and the wheelchair vibration during driving. To extract this component, the standard deviation of the accelerometer data is calculated using a sliding window. High standard deviation values reflect periods of time where the subject shows a high level of activity. Using a fixed threshold, it is possible to distinguish between high and low levels of activity. Figure 3 shows an example of the activity level estimation.

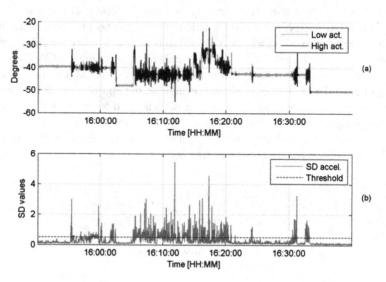

Fig. 3. Processing the accel. data (a) allow estimating the activity level of each subject. Segments in black show when the subject presents high activity (e.g. driving, tilting, and moving) and segments in grey show low activity (e.g. resting, wheelchair stopped). The activity detection is based on the standard deviation of the accel. data (b) and a fixed threshold.

2.4   Pilot Study

A pilot study was conducted to evaluate the capabilities of the system. To this end, volunteers were recruited from The Boston Home (TBH), a specialized care residence for people with advanced MS and other neurological diseases. To participate in this study all participants should be full time wheelchairs users with severe mobility impairment. Also, their wheelchairs should be electric-powered and equipped with at least a tilt-in-space system and a pressure relief cushion as methods to relieve pressure.

The protocol consists of deploying the prototypes on the wheelchairs at the beginning of the study. Every day, before the volunteers start to use their wheelchairs, the prototypes are checked to avoid technical issues. Then, prototypes collect data continuously, thus they are able to capture tilting habits during daily activities. Neither the caregivers nor the research personnel interfered in the tilting habits of the participants. This study was approved by The MIT Committee on the Use of Humans as Experimental Subjects.

3   Results

The study was conducted during two weeks. Six eligible TBH residents consented to participate in this study: 4 women and 2 men (hereafter called S1 to S6) with a mean age of 56 ± 12 years. All of them were diagnosed with a progressive form of MS. The mean time after diagnosis was 24 ± 6 years. The Expanded Disability Status Scale [24], which is used to quantify the level of disability in MS, varies between 7.5 and 8.5 indicating a high level of disability. All participants use an inflatable pressure relief cushion manufactured by ROHO®.

Figure 4 shows the AI and the wheelchair occupancy distribution from all subjects during 39 days of data collection. On average, the participants presented a level of activity of 18.6 ± 11.3 % with a maximum of 61.1 % and minimum of 5 %. Most cases (29 days), the subjects showed an AI between 10 % and 30 %. Only in 2 days (2.2 % of time), they presented an AI greater than 30 %.

Regarding to the wheelchair occupancy, the participants spent 6.38 ± 1.72 h per day in their wheelchair. The maximum wheelchair occupancy registered was 10.58 h and the minimum was 2.17 h. Most days (17 days) the subjects spent between 4 and 6 h (44 %) on their wheelchairs. Only in 3 days (7.7 %) the wheelchair occupancy was less than 4 h. The rest of the days, the occupancy time was distributed as follow: 6–8 h in 12 days (31 %), 8–10 h in 6 days (15.4 %) and over 10 h in 1 day (2.6 %).

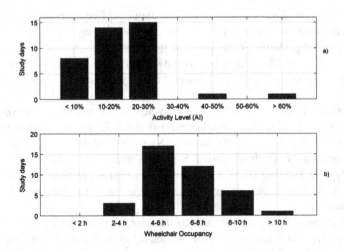

Fig. 4. AI level (a) and wheelchair occupancy (b) for all subjects representing 39 days of data collection.

Figure 5 shows an example of the AI level and the wheelchair occupancy registered for S1 during 9 days. S1 occupied the wheelchair on average 7.47 ± 0.92 h per day and the AI level was between 20 % and 30 % during 8 of 9 study days, except for day 3 where AI level reached 48 %. The increase in the AI is coincidental when S1 left the nursing home to go to a shopping mall.

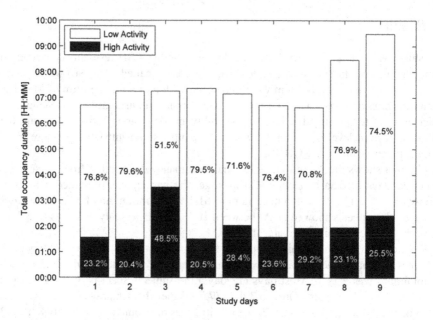

Fig. 5. Wheelchair occupancy and AI level registered by S1 during 9 days of study.

There are several clinical recommendations about the frequency to relieve pressure. Some guidelines for prevention of PU recommend performing a pressure relief every 15 min [25], other guidelines recommend longer intervals such as every 1 h or every 2 h [26]. Only 2.1 % of PRT performed by the subjects meet the recommendation if the interval is every 15 min, 25.8 % if the interval is every 1 h and 57.7 % if the interval is every 2 h.

Figures 6 and 7 show two different cases where it is possible to observe a subject who performs several PRT and another who doesn't. Figure 6 shows a full record obtained from S1 during day 9. In that day, S1 performed 10 PRT during 9.47 h of wheelchair occupancy. Each tilt lasted 5 min on average. Figure 7 shows S4 performing only 1 PRT during 10.58 h spent on the wheelchair. In this case, the tilt lasted 1.25 h. In Fig. 7, we can also observe that the subject only touches the sensor on the backrest when tilting.

Figure 8 shows a histogram that reflects the time intervals spent by the subjects on the wheelchair without performing a PRT. S1 and S2 spend the shorter intervals. 18.9 % of the time intervals for S1 and 5.1 % for S2 were under 1 h. For S1, most of the intervals (41.7 %) were between 1 and 2 h. On the other hand, more than 50 % of the intervals spent by the rest of the subjects (S2 to S6) were longer than 3 h exceeding all the recommendations to avoid PU. The maximum was registered by S6 reaching 93.9 %. There were days when S2 to S6 did not perform PRT at all. For instance, S3 spent 3.57 h in the wheelchair during day 6 without performing a PRT. If this situation is frequent the subject is prone to develop PU. However, the situation is more risky when the wheelchair occupancy duration is high. For instance, S6 spent 9.18 h on the wheelchair without performing a PRT during day 1, four hours more than S3. The average duration

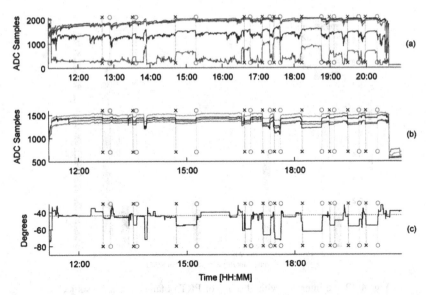

Fig. 6. Full record obtained from S1. (a) FSR$_B$, (b) FSR$_S$, and (c) angle data are labeled with the PRT detections. In this case, the subject presents 10 PRT in 9:28 h and 21 min on average tilted.

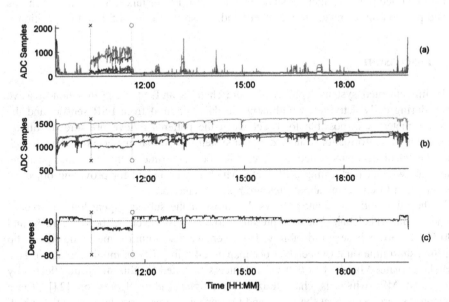

Fig. 7. Full record obtained from S4. (a) FSR$_B$, (b) FSR$_S$, and (c) angle data are labeled with the PRT detections. In this case, the subject presents only one PRT in 10:35 h and 1:34 h tilted.

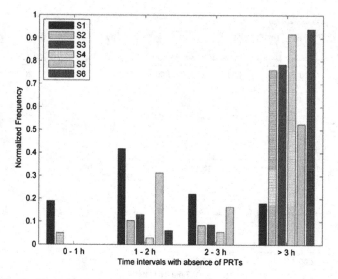

Fig. 8. Time intervals with absence of PRT obtained from all subjects.

in a PRT position is 1.57 h. However, those who perform frequent PRT spent a shorter time in a tilted position than the subjects who don't. For instance, S1 spent 21 min in a tilted position on average. On the other hand, S6 spent around 4.5 h in this position.

4   Discussion

The implemented system captures pressure changes and tilt usage in a non-invasive way during daily activities. Combining the data acquired from FSR sensors and the accelerometer, it is possible to detect when the patients relieve pressure by tilting. Analyzing the information collected by our system, useful parameters are obtained such as wheelchair occupancy, activity level, PRT per day, time spent in a tilted position, intervals without performing a PRT etc. which can be useful for providing objective information to clinicians about pressure relieve behavior.

The pilot study conducted shows that most of the subjects spent long periods of time on the wheelchair, but they present a low activity level (AI between 10 % and 30 %) due to their severe disability. However, we also found some participants who spent a short time on it (wheelchair occupancy < 4 h in 7.7 % of monitored days). This can be explained by the fact that the volunteers recruited for this study are affected by advanced MS, which is characterized by fatigue and/or depression [24]. These symptoms seriously affect the mood and the capacity to perform daily activities which can lead to spending more time in bed. In this case, the usage of this assistive device could be complemented with nursing cares and/or assistive devices focused on the time spent in bed.

The results also show that the subjects did not relieve pressure in a proper way using the tilt-in-space system. This result is similar to those presented in [14, 16]. In most cases, the subjects did not comply with the recommendations related to the frequency of pressure relief. They spent long periods (intervals without PRT > 3 h) without performing a PRT. In addition, during the study, there were entire days when the subjects did not perform PRT. If these situations recur frequently and the subjects spend long hours on the wheelchair without relieving pressure, the probability of developing PU increases.

No pressure changes and tilt absence during long period of time should cause a warning to be sent to caregivers/family member or patient to avoid pressure ulcers. The designed system will allow implementing an alarm system which helps remind the subjects when they should tilt their wheelchair. The collected data shows the feasibility of implementing personalized alarms or reminders for PRT with a much better expected outcome than general broadcast reminders or 'once in a while' nursing reminders. In this study, the system was deployed for wheelchair users living in a nursing home, however it can also provide valuable assistance in a home-care environment.

Acknowledgment. E.P. would like to acknowledge project Fondecyt Iniciación 11130340 for the financial support.

References

1. World Health Organization: World Report on Disability, p. 325. WHO, Geneva (2011)
2. Vos, T., Flaxman, A.D., Naghavi, M., Lozano, R., Michaud, C., Ezzati, M., et al.: Years lived with disability (YLDs) for 1160 sequelae of 289 diseases and injuries 1990–2010: a systematic analysis for the global burden of disease study 2010. Lancet **383**, 2163–2196 (2012)
3. World Health Organization: Guidelines on the Provision of Manual Wheelchairs in Less Resourced Settings, p. 129. World Health Organization, Geneva (2008)
4. Dicianno, B.E., Arva, J., Lieberman, J.M., Schmeler, M.R., Souza, A., Phillips, K., et al.: RESNA position on the application of tilt, recline, and elevating legrests for wheelchairs. Assist. Technol. Off. J. RESNA. **21**, 13–22 (2009)
5. Byrne, D.W., Salzberg, C.A.: Major risk factors for pressure ulcers in the spinal cord disabled: a literature review. Spinal Cord **34**, 255–263 (1996)
6. Hagisawa, S., Ferguson-Pell, M., Herbert, J.: Reactive hyperemia response to pressure-induced localized ischemia in patients with multiple sclerosis. Neurorehabil. Neural Repair **8**, 193–201 (1994)
7. Institute for Healthcare Improvement: How-to Guide: Prevent Pressure Ulcers. Institute for Healthcare Improvement, Cambridge, MA (2011). www.ihi.org
8. Courtney, B., Ruppman, J., Cooper, H.: Save our skin: initiative cuts pressure ulcer incidence in half. Nurs. Manage. **37**, 36–45 (2006)
9. Russo, J.L., Cezeaux, J.L.: Design of a wheelchair pressure monitoring system. In: Proceedings of the 2010 IEEE 36th Annual Northeast Bioengineering Conference, pp. 1–2 (2010)
10. Kozniewski, B.S., Cezeaux, J.L.: Wheelchair pressure monitoring alert system for the reduction of the occurrence of pressure sores. In: 2011 IEEE 37th Annual Northeast Bioengineering Conference (NEBEC), pp. 1–2 (2011)

11. Bain, D., Ferguson-Pell, M.: Remote monitoring of sitting behavior of people with spinal cord injury. J. Rehabil. Res. Dev. **39**, 513–520 (2002)

12. Rocha, J.G., Carvalho, H., Duarte, F.M., Carvalho, M.A.F., Moreira, V.M.: System providing discomfort monitoring for people in wheelchairs. In: 2008 IEEE International Symposium on Industrial Electronics, pp. 961–916. IEEE (2008)

13. Dai, R., Sonenblum, S.E., Sprigle, S.: A robust wheelchair pressure relief monitoring system. In: 2010 Annual International Conference of the IEEE Engineering in Medicine and Biology Society (EMBC), pp. 6107–6110 (2012)

14. Yang, Y.-S., Chang, G.-L., Hsu, M.-J., Chang, J.-J.: Remote monitoring of sitting behaviors for community-dwelling manual wheelchair users with spinal cord injury. Spinal Cord **47**, 67–71 (2009)

15. Rush, R.: Sensation augmentation to relieve pressure sore formation in wheelchair users. In: Proceedings of the 11th International ACM SIGACCESS Conference on Computers and Accessibility, pp. 275–276 (2009)

16. Ding, D., Leister, E.: Usage of tilt-in-space, recline, and elevation seating functions in natural environment of wheelchair users. J. Rehabil. Res. Dev. **45**, 973–983 (2008)

17. Ding, D., Cooper, R.A., Cooper, R., Kelleher, A.: Monitoring seat feature usage among wheelchair users. In: 2010 Annual International Conference of the IEEE Engineering in Medicine and Biology Society (EMBC), Lyon, France, pp. 4364–4367 (2007)

18. Sonenblum, S.E., Sprigle, S., Maurer, C.L.: Use of power tilt systems in everyday life. Disabil. Rehabil. Assist. Technol. **4**, 24–30 (2009)

19. Sonenblum, S.E., Sprigle, S.: Distinct tilting behaviours with power tilt-in-space systems. Disabil. Rehabil. Assist. Technol. **6**, 526–535 (2011)

20. Yang, T., Hutchinson, S., Rice, L.: Development of a scalable monitoring system for wheelchair tilt-in-space usage. Int. J. Phys. Med. **1**, 1–6 (2013)

21. The PostgreSQL Global Development Group: PostgreSQL database. http://www.postgresql.org. Accessed 5 August 2013

22. Coggrave, M.J., Rose, L.S.: A specialist seating assessment clinic: changing pressure relief practice. Spinal Cord **41**, 692–695 (2003)

23. Fehr, L., Langbein, W.E., Skaar, S.B.: Adequacy of power wheelchair control interfaces for persons with severe disabilities: a clinical survey. J. Rehabil. Res. Dev. **37**, 353–360 (2000)

24. Kurtzke, J.F.: Rating neurologic impairment in multiple sclerosis: an expanded disability status scale (EDSS). Neurology **33**, 1444–1452 (1983)

25. Consortium for Spinal Cord Medicine: Pressure Ulcer Prevention and Treatment Following Spinal Cord Injury: A Clinical Practice Guideline for Health-care Professionals, p. 80. Paralyzed Veterans of America (2000)

26. Porter, R.S., Kaplan, J.L., Homeier, B.P.: The Merck Manual Home Health Handbook. Merck, New Jersey (2009)

27. Janardhan, V., Bakshi, R.: Quality of life in patients with multiple sclerosis: the impact of fatigue and depression. J. Neurol. Sci. **205**, 51–58 (2002)

Frameworks Related with AmIHealth Environments

ReApp – A Mobile App for the Rehabilitation of Ankle Sprains

Jonathan Synnott[1](✉), Katy Pedlow[2], Chris Bleakley[3],
Richard Davies[1], Chris Nugent[1], José Antonio Moral-Muñoz[4],
Adele Boyd[1], Joseph Rafferty[1], and Suzanne McDonough[2]

[1] School of Computing and Mathematics, University of Ulster, Belfast, UK
{j.synnott, rj.davies, cd.nugent, a.boyd,
j.rafferty}@ulster.ac.uk
[2] School of Health Sciences, University of Ulster, Belfast, UK
{k.pedlow, s.mcdonough}@ulster.ac.uk
[3] Sport and Exercise Sciences Research Institute,
University of Ulster, Belfast, UK
c.bleakley@ulster.ac.uk
[4] Department of Library Science, University of Granada, 18071 Granada, Spain
jamoral@ugr.es

Abstract. Musculoskeletal injuries are common and costly. Ankle sprains are one of the most common such injuries, carrying significant risk of persistent disabling symptoms. Rehabilitation has been shown to be more effective than standard conservative approaches for musculoskeletal injuries. The use of a mobile app to present rehabilitation guidance may offer a more accessible, engaging and effective solution to ankle sprain rehabilitation. Many existing apps target the prevention and rehabilitation of ankle sprains, however, evaluation details are limited. This paper presents ReApp, a novel app for the rehabilitation of ankle sprain. Full details of the app implementation are provided, in addition to details of the results from a three phase evaluation process involving technical (n = 5), clinical (n = 6) and end-users (n = 7). Results from the evaluation were positive, and feedback was used to improve the app.

Keywords: Rehabilitation · Mobile apps · Ankle sprain

1 Introduction

Musculoskeletal injuries in the UK are common and costly [1]. Ankle sprains which are one of the most common musculoskeletal injuries, have been estimated to incur an annual cost of $2 billion in the United States [2]. They also carry significant risk of persistent disabling symptoms such as: pain, instability and recurrent injury [3, 4] and are also a common pre-disposing factor for post-traumatic arthritis [5]. Musculoskeletal treatment guidelines advocate that rehabilitation should be initiated as quickly as possible post injury and should continue until full functional recovery has been achieved. Our previous research findings show that rehabilitation is more effective than standard conservative approaches for ankle injuries [1]. Nevertheless, current constraints within

© Springer International Publishing Switzerland 2015
J. Bravo et al. (Eds.): AmIHEALTH 2015, LNCS 9456, pp. 61–67, 2015.
DOI: 10.1007/978-3-319-26508-7_6

the National Health Service (NHS) in the UK mean that practitioners are unable to invest large amounts of time treating musculoskeletal injuries. The majority of service users are discharged without further follow-up. As a direct result, service users have requested more comprehensive and directed rehabilitation advice [6, 7].

One way to address this need is through the use of mobile phone applications specifically designed to act as an adjunct to clinician directed management of those recovering from musculoskeletal injury. Many apps currently exist for the management of medical conditions, however, many are limited by app quality, inaccurate information, absence of evidence-based content and lack of user and clinician engagement in their development [8, 9]. A comprehensive review of Apple's App store, the Google Play store and academic publications was conducted to examine the current state of the art for apps in relation to ankle sprains. The results indicated a selection of free and paid apps, which focused on either prevention or rehabilitation. Crucially, many of these existing apps had no scientific support and evaluation details were limited.

The research described in this paper was funded by a Knowledge Transfer Scheme from the Public Health Agency's Health and Social Care Research and Development Division in Northern Ireland. This Knowledge Transfer Scheme was designed to support knowledge transfer that delivers benefits to practice, and was to be used to transfer previously generated knowledge and develop effective engagement with the users of research outputs. With this in mind, the aim of the research described in this paper was to transfer our existing research in the domain of rehabilitation [1] into a mobile platform capable of delivery by clinicians to service users.

The remainder of the paper is structured as follows. Section 2 details the ReApp consortium and the implementation of the app. Section 3 outlines the evaluation methodology and provides details of the results from technical, clinical and end-user evaluations. Section 4 provides concluding remarks.

2 Methods and Implementation

The ReApp research project is supported by a multidisciplinary research team whose backgrounds included biomedical engineering, computer science, connected health, mobile app development, physiotherapy and rehabilitation. The development of the app was managed by a Project Steering Group (PSG) including expert academics, an industrial partner with specialization in commercial mobile app development, medical clinicians and service users.

2.1 ReApp Implementation

Android was chosen as the development platform to maximize the potential user base. The platform commanded a global market share of 78.0 % in Q1 2015, compared to 18.3 % for iOS and 2.7 % for Windows Phone [10]. A minimum target SDK version of 2.2 (Froyo) was chosen in order to support over 99 % of Android devices that are currently on the market. The main menu (Fig. 1a) facilitates access to and information for each level of exercise. For each exercise level, users can select either the information

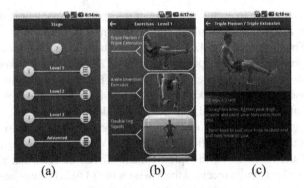

Fig. 1. The main components of the ReApp user interface: (a) the rehabilitation level selection screen. (b) The exercise list for level 1. (c) Exercise video playback and text description.

page or the exercise list. The information page for each exercise level identifies the target user and describes the focus of the level, for example mobilization or proprioception. The exercise list for each level (Fig. 1b) is presented as a scrollable list of exercise names with thumbnail images. In total, the app provides 4 stages of rehabilitation, with a total of 21 exercises. The content of the app and exercise progression was informed by our existing research into staged rehabilitation of ankle sprain.

If the device is held in portrait, selected exercises are displayed as shown in Fig. 1c. An exercise video automatically plays at the top of the screen. These videos were recorded and edited to loop seamlessly where possible to allow a user to watch them continuously while performing the exercise. Underneath the video, additional information includes the recommended maximum number of reps, number of sets and a breakdown of the required steps. If the device is held in landscape orientation, the video expands to fill the entire screen.

3   Evaluation and Results

The evaluation of ReApp was performed in three phases: a technical evaluation, a clinical evaluation, and an end-user evaluation. This Section provides details of the methodology and results obtained for each phase.

3.1   Technical Evaluation

The purpose of the technical evaluation was to assess the usability of the app by a technical user group who had significant and sustained experience with the use of mobile apps. Feedback received from this phase was used to inform app improvements prior to the clinical evaluation. Five participants were recruited, consisting of technical developers from Ulster University's School of Computing and Mathematics. These participants had a minimum of 5 years of experience in ICT or a related discipline. Participants were invited to complete a list of tasks within the app, designed to ensure participants had exposure to each key feature of the app. On completion of the task list, each participant was asked to complete a questionnaire. The questionnaire consisted of two sections. The first section asked participants about their experience with smart phones and the various available operating systems. The next section asked participants for feedback on the app's features and usability. The majority of these questions required responses on a 5-point Likert scale. Additionally, participants were invited to provide details of additional useful functionality or desirable changes.

The results from the technical evaluation were predominantly positive. Nevertheless, some areas that could benefit from improvement were identified. Figure 2 provides an overview of the results from the questionnaire. It can be seen that all areas were scored positively. Text clarity received the lowest score (3.6). This was justified through quantitative feedback which stated that the text was too small. Quantitative feedback indicated participants shared an interest in being able to manually track the rehabilitation process by adding completion checkboxes and counters beside each exercise.

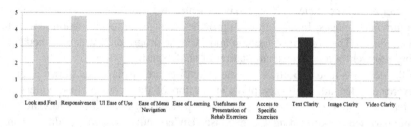

Fig. 2. An overview of the quantitative results from the technical evaluation phase in which 5 = very good and 1 = very bad.

3.2 Clinical Evaluation

The purpose of the clinical evaluation was to assess the usability and clinical content of the app by an expert clinical user group who worked in the NHS or private practice. These users had professional experience in delivering care and management of patients presenting with acute ankle sprains. A sample of doctors (n = 3) and physiotherapists (n = 3) were recruited from professional networks; each had a minimum of 5 years of experience in acute management of ankle sprains. Participants were asked to use all sections and features of the app for a one week period before completing an anonymous questionnaire to assess usability and clinical application.

All participants stated that they had access to a mobile phone and experience of using mobile applications. Overall the results for usability of the app were positive (0 = low rating, 5 = high) as presented in Fig. 3. All participants reported that the app would be useful to use for rehabilitation purposes (n = 6 min 4/5), and rated the usability high in terms of reaching specific exercises (n = 6, min 4/5), clarity of the images and clarity of videos (n = 6, min 4/5). The clinical content results were equally positive. All participants agreed that the app content was evidence based, was suitable for ankle rehabilitation and they would use it in their clinical practice.

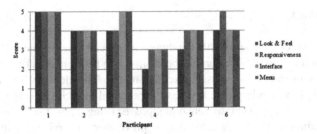

Fig. 3. An overview of the results obtained from each participant in the clinical evaluation.

Qualitative responses to the questionnaire highlighted the need for more guided progression through stages in addition to a voice over function to be included for exercises.

3.3   End-User Evaluation

The purpose of the final phase of evaluation was to assess the usability of the app with a patient population who had a history of ankle sprain. A sample of 7 participants was recruited. Participants were required to be over 18 years old and have more than 12 weeks of history of lateral ankle sprain which required medical assessment and was now completely recovered. Additionally, they were required to have no concomitant injury and no existing medical conditions. Participants who met these criteria were provided with instructions detailing how to use the app to perform exercises on alternative days for a one week period. Participants were asked to anonymously complete a questionnaire to provide feedback on app usability.

Once participants had completed the one week usage period, usage data collected during the evaluation was extracted from each smartphone. Baseline demographics indicated participants had a mixed demographical profile including male (n = 3) and female (n = 4) with different levels of physical activity (sedentary n = 1, moderate n = 3, high n = 3). The app was used on 3 or more days by 4 participants and on 2 days by 3 participants, with the most common usage days being Monday and Tuesday. Across the entire week, the amount of usage time varied from 3 min 49 s to 29 min 5 s; most of this use was in the evening. An analysis of the total time spent on each exercise level by all participants revealed that Level 1 was used the most (2775 min) compared to Levels 2, 3 and Advanced (681, 1187 and 855 min, respectively). Analysis of quantitative questionnaire feedback revealed that the look and feel of the app was rated as very good (3.6/5 mean) and it was reported as easy to learn to use (4.6/5 mean). Qualitative feedback indicated further refinements in the app, including voice over to accompany the video clips and more direct guidance on acute injury management.

4 Conclusion

Ankle sprains are common and costly conditions which carry significant risk of persistent disabling symptoms. Rehabilitation has been shown to be more effective than standard conservative approaches for musculoskeletal injury. The delivery of rehabilitation guidance through a mobile phone app has the potential to facilitate a more accessible, engaging, effective approach to rehabilitation. Existing apps make some progress towards providing solutions to ankle sprain prevention and rehabilitation; however, details of their evaluation are limited. This paper has detailed ReApp, a novel app for the staged rehabilitation of ankle sprain injury. The paper also includes discussion of the results obtained from a three phase trial involving technical users, clinical users and end users. Results from each phase resulted in improvements to the app, and positive feedback was received throughout. A limitation of this work is the small number of participants in each phase. Future work will address this limitation by completing evaluations of future iterations of the app with larger numbers of participants with acute ankle sprain.

Acknowledgements. This work was funded by the Public Health Agency (HSC R&D Division) Knowledge Transfer Scheme (RES/4598/11) and the Ulster University's Research Challenge Fund. Additionally, Invest Northern Ireland is acknowledged for supporting this project under the Competence Centre Program Grant RD0513853 - Connected Health Innovation Centre.

References

1. Bleakley, C.M., O'Connor, S.R., Tully, M.A., Rocke, L.G., Macauley, D.C., Bradbury, I., Keegan, S., McDonough, S.M.: Effect of accelerated rehabilitation on function after ankle sprain: randomised controlled trial. BMJ **340**, c1964 (2010)
2. Waterman, B.R., Owens, B.D., Davey, S., Zacchilli, M.A., Belmont, P.J.: The epidemiology of ankle sprains in the United States. J. Bone Joint Surg. Am. **92**, 2279–2284 (2010)
3. Bleakley, C.: Oxford Handbook of Sport and Exercise Medicine, 2nd edn. Oxford University Press, Oxford (2012)
4. Kobayashi, T., Gamada, K.: Lateral ankle sprain and chronic ankle instability: a critical review. Foot Ankle Spec. **7**, 298–326 (2014)
5. Golditz, T., Steib, S., Pfeifer, K., Uder, M., Gelse, K., Janka, R., Hennig, F.F., Welsch, G. H.: Functional ankle instability as a risk factor for osteoarthritis: using T2-mapping to analyze early cartilage degeneration in the ankle joint of young athletes. Osteoarthritis Cartilage **22**, 1377–1385 (2014)
6. Bridgman, S.A.: Population based epidemiology of ankle sprains attending accident and emergency units in the West Midlands of England, and a survey of UK practice for severe ankle sprains. Emerg. Med. J. **20**, 508–510 (2003)
7. Richardson, B., Shepstone, L., Poland, F., Mugford, M., Finlayson, B., Clemence, N.: Randomised controlled trial and cost consequences study comparing initial physiotherapy assessment and management with routine practice for selected patients in an accident and emergency department of an acute hospital. Emerg. Med. J. **22**, 87–92 (2005)
8. Huckvale, K., Car, M., Morrison, C., Car, J.: Apps for asthma self-management: a systematic assessment of content and tools. BMC Med. **10**, 144 (2012)

9. Reynoldson, C., Stones, C., Allsop, M., Gardner, P., Bennett, M.I., Closs, S.J., Jones, R., Knapp, P.: Assessing the quality and usability of smartphone apps for pain self-management. Pain Med. **15**, 898–909 (2014)

10. International Data Corporation. http://www.idc.com/prodserv/smartphone-os-market-share. jsp

A Sensorized and Health Aspect-Based Framework to Improve the Continuous Monitoring on Diseases Using Smartphones and Smart Devices

Jesús Fontecha[✉], Ramón Hervás, and José Bravo

MAmI Research Lab, University of Castilla-La Mancha, Ciudad Real, Spain
{jesus.fontecha,ramon.hlucas,jose.bravo}@uclm.es

Abstract. Growth of mobile technologies and smart devices in Health-care domains leads to patient self-control of chronic and non-chronic diseases, facilitating the real time communication with the physician. This work describes the basis of a health aspect-based framework to monitor multiple diseases by using the smartphone and the interaction with smart devices. Aspects comprise information about patient and disease, and these are used to study monitoring behaviors and goals depending on the disease.

Keywords: Mobile monitoring · Ubiquitous computing · Health aspect-based framework · Sensors · Chronic disease · mHealth

1 Introduction

Nowadays, technological advances provide new oportunities for disease monitoring. Mobile devices allow users to keep many vital signs under control, however, many other factors should be taken into account in monitoring tasks. Prediction, prevention and treatment of chronic and non-chronic diseases depend on a group of factors which can be analyzed through software systems. Thus, there are many studies focused on frameworks development in healthcare environmens, some of these focused on monitoring tasks. In this sense, Al-Zoube [1] showed the benefits of a cloud-based mobile health monitoring framework for heart rate data analysis. In [2], Memon et al. present a review of frameworks, platforms and standards in Ambient Assisted Living (AAL). Their work identified essential data to be collected, and also several pros and cons of current systems in which technologies are used in a limited and isolated manner because of lack of interoperability between devices.

This paper presents a proposal of modular framework based on health aspects for monitoring multiple diseases. The framework determines the interaction with smart devices and smartphones, facilitating patient self-monitoring and clinical treatment. Two groups of aspects were defined, primary and complementary. The information gathered from aspects is used to determine monitoring behavior and

© Springer International Publishing Switzerland 2015
J. Bravo et al. (Eds.): AmIHEALTH 2015, LNCS 9456, pp. 68–73, 2015.
DOI: 10.1007/978-3-319-26508-7_7

objectives which keep the disease under control. Several study cases have been identified from the general proposal.

2   Clinical Variables and Disease Monitoring

Many diseases require the analysis of certain variables for their prevention and treatment, whose importance depends on the disease. However, most diseases take into account common variables from a clinical viewpoint. Some of these features can be measured by means of clinical devices and others depend on physician criteria. For example, Fontecha et al. [3] studied a set of factors which affect to frailty syndrome in adults. In their work, they also used the smartphone as a complement to collect more accurate data from the functional domain. Also, Villarreal et al. [4] used the smartphone and a bluetooth glucometer in diabetes monitoring tasks. The glucose monitor gathered glucose data and it was combined with information introduced manually about diet and exercise.

Technology helps to monitor some clinical data in a more accurate way, however, other data must be analized by clinicians.

Furthermore, each patient could require different action levels on his illness. The amount of clinical variables to consider determines that action level. The greater number of considered variables, the more monitoring complexity and intensity, and the greater requirement for further clinical supervision.

3   Sensorized and Health Aspect-Based Framework

In this section, the framework proposal is presented taking into account identified aspects, monitoring devices and sensors, and the principles to monitor behavior and objectives of a disease.

3.1   Definition of Health Aspects

An health aspect is defined as a set of variables, not only clinical, related to a disease which can be monitored. We have considered two groups of aspects: primary and complementary. The identified primary aspects are the following:

Vital Signs. It refers to the vital signs to be monitored. The smartphone gathers data directly from sensors and smart devices associated with the person.

Physical Activity. It is another monitoring aspect, and its measures also come from smart devices and sensors.

Clinical. It defines relevant variables from the patient record for disease treatment and assessment.

Diet. Nutrition fundamentals are considered as important aspects in most cases. Commonly, diet works in combination with physical activity aspect.

Education. It represents education and knowledge of the disease as a support to the patient. Smartphone can promote and manage this aspect.

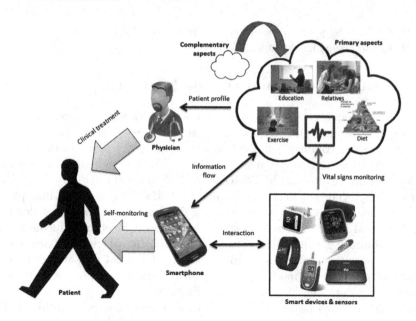

Fig. 1. Disease monitoring cycle. Interactions and information flows between framework parts and patient

Relatives and Caregivers. Communication between patient and relatives is essential in most diseases. This aspect allows monitoring of the patient by relatives helping to keep the patient independence.

Physician. This aspect leads to the patient supervision, decision making, and treatment taking into account the monitored disease at real time.

Each primary aspect can be studied by a simple software module (or mobile application), sharing information generated with other aspects or software pieces. Communication between health aspects helps monitoring tasks.

Complementary aspects form the other group of identified health aspects. The difference between primary and complementary aspects is that primary are common to all monitored diseases. However, secondary aspects could be added to the system to complement and improve the monitoring behavior of a particular disease. Some domains of complementary aspects are the following: social, environmental, psychological, habits & lifestyle, emotions or stress. Sometimes, several aspects (primary and/or complementary) work together or require information from other aspects. Thus, dependence between aspects is considered, and it is defined by the disease. For example, in case of obesity, diet and physical activity are extremely dependent for the patient, however, physical activity and relatives can be considered independent.

3.2   Sensorization and Smart Devices

Advances in mHealth paradigm [5] provide new ways of self-monitoring of chronic and non-chronic diseases. In recent years, smartphones, built-in sensors and

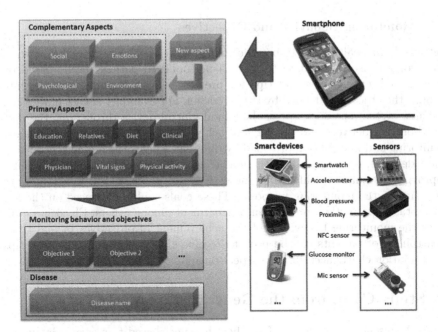

Fig. 2. Aspect-based framework for disease monitoring. A general overview (Color figure online)

smart devices have been integrated in healthcare processes. Sensors and external devices send information to the smartphone. Smartphone gathers information from aspects and some aspects receive data from sensors and smart devices. Due to non-intrusive approach of this work, we use the sensors included in the smartphone and the minimum of smart devices to achieve monitoring goals (see Sect. 3.3).

All aspects, including those from smart devices and sensors generate information flows to physicians and patients. Figure 1 shows the patient monitoring cycle of a disease. The smartphone interacts with smart devices to gather data about vital signs, it is combined with the rest of primary and complementary aspects, to generate an information flow as support for self-monitoring. Besides, the physician uses data from these aspects and the patient profile to improve the patient treatment.

Smartphone groups all procedures and mechanisms to carry out a disease self-control. Results from some aspects require to collect data from external devices. Currently, there are many smart devices such as bracelets or smartwatches among others, depending on the purpose, which send data to the smartphone. These devices are an independent solution, however, a richer approach is provided when they work in combination with others to, for example, assess the disease behaviour or determine specific objectives, making a multidisciplinary framework.

3.3   Monitoring Behavior and Objectives

Outputs from health aspects provide information about the disease behavior. Our proposal uses these data to make a personalized patient profile based on recommendations, alarms and tips for prevention and treatment, taking into account the objectives defined by the physician. For example, in case of diabetic patients, system should keep regular blood glucose levels throughout the day. Collaboration between aspects helps to achive these goals. In this case, glucose monitoring and information provided by different aspects (including sensors and smart devices), making possible the management the glucose trend of a patient, improving his quality of life. Many objectives can be defined in the framework according to the monitoring purposes. These goals could be focused on the following tasks: prediction, prevention or treatment among others. Physician evaluates the monitoring behavior and the achievement of objectives in real time. Smartphone of patients can be used to receive alarms, recommendations, tips and evolution charts according to aspect outputs.

4   Study Cases from the General Framework

Figure 2 presents an overview of the health aspect-based framework, including blocks which represent the identified primary and complementary aspects, and monitoring objectives (defined by the physician). Besides, examples of smart devices and sensors are shown. These devices communicate with the smartphone to gather variables from *vital signs* and *physical activity* aspects (colored in green). Smartphone works with the rest of aspects for goal achievement.

Table 1. Example of framework aspects and elements for three specific diseases.

	Diabetes	Hypertension	Obesity
Sensors & smart devices	Smartwatch, Accelerometer, NFC sensor, Glucose monitor	Smartwatch, Accelerometer, Blood pressure monitor	Smartwatch, Accelerometer, Activity bracelet, NFC sensor, Smart scale
Primary aspects	Education, Relatives, Diet, Patient profile, Endocrine, Glucose level, Physical activity	Education, Relatives, Diet, Patient profile, Physician, Blood pressure level, Physical activity	Education, Relatives, Diet, Patient profile, Endocrine, Weight level, Physical activity
Complementary aspects	Social, Emotions, Environment	Social, Environment, Stress	Psychological, Environment, Social
Monitoring goals	Diabetes behavior, Glucose trend	Blood pressure behavior, Heart stroke risk prediction	Weight decrease behavior, Health living motivation

This framework can be adapted to a particular disease. In each case, the framework uses different sensors and smart devices, and the blocks of aspects correspond to specific aspects. Diabetes, hypertension and obesity may be some of these diseases. Table 1 shows differences between aspects according to the characteristics of each disease. Primary aspects are similar in the three diseases, although each aspect is focused in a specific disease. Vital signs aspect depends on the monitoring purpose and monitoring goals are also different in each case. Sensors and smart devices collect data from common aspects (e.g. physical activity, diet) and specific ones (e.g. glucose monitor).

5   Conclusions and Future Work

We have presented a framework proposal with the fundamentals to design and develop software platforms which facilitate the monitoring of chronic and non-chronic diseases. The health aspect-based approach allows the interaction between these aspects and collecting data from sensors and smart devices regarding the monitored disease. From this information, the framework helps to assess illness behavior and achieve goals, supporting a comprehensive clinical treatment and promoting patient self-control as main motivation of the presented approach.

The future work includes the development of several mobile applications to get information from primary and complementary aspects focusing on diabetes disease. Last advances in smart devices communication and interaction, allows us to develop non-intrusive mobile monitoring solutions combining their results with other software pieces as the framework proposes. Besides, framework could get data from sensors and devices of different manufacturers as long as they provide a open communication API[1] (as it is happening with most current smart devices).

Acknowledgements. This work is conducted in the context of "S4U (Smart For You): sensor, sytems and services for a smart world" project at UCLM, and UBIHEALTH project under International Research Staff Exchange Schema (MC-IRSES 316337).

References

1. Al-Zoube, M.A., Alqudah, Y.A.: Mobile cloud computing framework for patients' health data analysis. Biomed. Eng. - Appl. Basis Commun. **26**(2), Article Number 1450020 (2014)
2. Memon, M., Wagner, S.R., Pedersen, C.F., Aysha Beevi, F.H., Hansen, F.O.: Ambient assisted living healthcare frameworks, platforms, standards, and quality attributes. Sensors **14**(3), 4312–4341 (2014)
3. Fontecha, J., Hervás, R., Bravo, J., Navarro, F.C.: A mobile and ubiquitous approach for supporting frailty assessment in elderly people. J. Med. Internet Res. **15**(9), e197 (2013). doi:10.2196/jmir.2529
4. Villarreal, V., Fontecha, J., Hervás, R., Bravo, J.: Mobile and ubiquitous architecture for the medical control of chronic diseases through the use of intelligent devices: using the architecture for patients with diabetes. Future Gener. Comput. Syst. **34**, 161–175 (2014). doi:10.1016/j.future.2013.12.013
5. Fiordelli, M., Diviani, N., Schulz, P.J.: Mapping mHealth research: a decade of evolution. J. Med. Internet Res. **15**(5), Article Number e95 (2013)

---

[1] Application Programming Interface.

Applied Algorithms in e-Health Systems

Real-Time Decision Support Using Data Mining to Predict Blood Pressure Critical Events in Intensive Medicine Patients

Filipe Portela[1,3]($\boxtimes$), Manuel Filipe Santos[1], José Machado[1],
António Abelha[1], Fernando Rua[2], and Álvaro Silva[2]

[1] Algoritmi Centre, University of Minho, Braga, Portugal
{cfp, mfs}@dsi.uminho.pt, {jmac, abelha}@di.uminho.pt
[2] Serviço Cuidados Intensivos, Centro Hospitalar do Porto,
Hospital Santo António, Porto, Portugal
fernandorua.sci@chporto.min-saude.pt,
moreirasilva@me.com
[3] ESEIG, Porto Polytechnic, Porto, Portugal

Abstract. Patient blood pressure is an important vital signal to the physicians take a decision and to better understand the patient condition. In Intensive Care Units is possible monitoring the blood pressure due the fact of the patient being in continuous monitoring through bedside monitors and the use of sensors. The intensivist only have access to vital signs values when they look to the monitor or consult the values hourly collected. Most important is the sequence of the values collected, i.e., a set of highest or lowest values can signify a critical event and bring future complications to a patient as is Hypotension or Hypertension. This complications can leverage a set of dangerous diseases and side-effects. The main goal of this work is to predict the probability of a patient has a blood pressure critical event in the next hours by combining a set of patient data collected in real-time and using Data Mining classification techniques. As output the models indicate the probability (%) of a patient has a Blood Pressure Critical Event in the next hour. The achieved results showed to be very promising, presenting sensitivity around of 95 %.

Keywords: Data mining · Intcare · Intensive medicine · Blood pressure · Critical events · Decision support · Real-Time

1 Introduction

In critical environments the decision needs to be perform quickly and with a high level of accuracy. To help the decision-makers to take the best decision it is fundamental to develop a solution able to predict events before their occurrence. Intensive Medicine (IM) is a critical area of Medicine. Patients in weak conditions and with multiple diseases as is organ failure are cared every day. One of the most common complications is related to Blood Pressure with a constant values changing due to medical diseases, therapeutics or other procedures. Higher Blood pressure is associated to cardiovascular organ failure/diseases [1]. Nowadays the Intensive Care Units (ICU) are filled out with

© Springer International Publishing Switzerland 2015
J. Bravo et al. (Eds.): AmIHEALTH 2015, LNCS 9456, pp. 77–90, 2015.
DOI: 10.1007/978-3-319-26508-7_8

many technical devices allowing a continuous patient monitoring. However these data are only used in the acquisition moment and they are not used to support the decision process. Having in consideration this aspect arises INTCare. INTCare [2] is a Pervasive Intelligent Decision Support System (PIDSS) able to collect and process data in real-time in order to provide new knowledge [3–7] anywhere and anytime. This knowledge is achieved by means of Data Mining (DM) techniques. This work is framed in INTCare project and it wants to develop DM models able to help the Intensivist to act in order to prevent Blood Pressure Critical Events (BPCE). Critical Events are defined as a continuous data acquisition of values out of the normal range for a determined period of time. BPCE can provoke hypotension and hypertension and leverage a set of other diseases as is heart attack, cardiovascular system failure, kidney failure and others. This work is a classification DM problem with the goal to induce DM models in real-time able to predict the probability of a patient has a BPCE in the next hours. The achieved results are promising. The models are very good to predict BPCE (sensitivity around 95 %) however they are not accurate in predicting both classes (accuracy around 75 %). These results are a natural consequence of preventing actions in IM. The predictions are made in an hourly base approach and due to a quick decision by the intensivist, the BP value can change to a normal range in a few minutes resulting in a set of false positives values. In a clinical point of view, these models are very useful because can help to predict a possible CE in the next hours giving the possibility to the intensivist take a decision based on evidences i.e., according to the new knowledge achieved. Supporting Decision-Making process by providing the probability of a patient has a critical event in the next hours in order to prevent and avoid their occurrence is the main goal of this work. The models developed will be included in INTCare system.

This paper is divided in six sections. After a first introduction of the paper, all the concepts and related work are presented in Sect. 2. Section 3 presents the methodologies, materials and methods used in this work. Section four presents all the work made following CRISP-DM phases. Then the results are discussed and a set of last considerations are made including future work.

2   Background

2.1   Blood Pressure

According to the National Institute of Health [8], Blood Pressure (BP) is the force of blood pushing against the walls of the arteries as the heart pumps blood. If this pressure rises and stays high over time, it can damage the body in many ways. BP is measured as systolic and diastolic pressures. "Systolic" refers to BP when the heart beats while pumping blood. "Diastolic" refers to BP when the heart is at rest between beats. BP has a normal pattern of values. Values out of this pattern can provide Hypotension (low pressure) and Hypertension (Higher pressure). In clinical studies [9] was found a strong relationship between prevalence of hypertension and mortality by stroke. Hypertension can provoke several and dangerous diseases to human life [10] as is for example: Heart attack or stroke, Aneurysm Heart failure and others. Hypotension is dangerous and can be a source of other diseases [11] as is for example Kidney Failure, Congestive Heart Failure, Anaemia, and Pulmonary Embolism.

In the literature review there are several works related to BP [12], however the goals are different. This work predicts the probability of occurring a BPCE in the next hours (e.g. Hour1–10 % … Hour4–15 % … Hour24–30 %) by using streaming data and intelligent agents to perform automatically tasks (e.g. data transformation and induce the models.)

2.2 Intensive Care Units

Intensive Medicine (IM) is a critical area with the highest incidences of medical error and patient injuries [13]. Its practices is in Intensive Care Units (ICUs). To the ICUs only patients in a critical condition are transferred. ICUs are endowed with several medical devices (e.g. vital signs monitor, ventilators and infusion pumps) able to monitoring the patient condition in real-time. Additionally a set of clinical data are hourly recorded. Although there are a high number of data available, the information are not fully used to create new knowledge. This fact happens due to the need of having a quick decision in order to avoid worst conditions and save patient life. In this sense the intensivists do not have time to consult or analyse all the collected data. Thus, becomes fundamental having a decision support system able to help them to take the best decision always in the patient best interest by considering all the collected data.

2.3 INTCare

INTCare is a PIDSS able to monitoring the patient condition in real-time and to predict a set of clinical events/diseases using the collected data and adaptive DM models. Online-learning, real-time data processing [14] and system interoperability are others features. Until now, INTCare allows predicting organ failure and patient outcome [7], SEPSIS [15], barotrauma [16], readmissions [5, 17] and length of stay [6, 18] in real-time and with high sensitivities rates. In the past a first study was performed in order to predict critical events. In this study [4] the probability of a patient having a cardiac arrhythmia was predicted (sensitivity = 95 %). Now it is time to explore other areas and tracking the Blood Pressure in order to early detect possible critical events, i.e., possible situations of hypertension or hypotension.

2.4 Critical Events

Critical Events (CE) represents an abnormal value (out of normal range) continuously monitored in a patient. A CE is defined by Álvaro Silva [19] as "a more serious event and it is classified by a longer event or a more extreme out of range measurement". In the ICU the vital signs are collected and processed in real-time [20] in order to categorize a value as critic or not. Then an intelligent agent is used to analyse if the values collected can represent or not a critical event. To understand if an event is critical, two main criteria were used [21]:

- Occurrence and duration should be registered by physiological changes;
- Related physiological variables should be registered at regular intervals.

An event is considered critical, when a longer event occurs or a more extreme physiological measurement is found [21]. In this work the protocol associated to Blood Pressure (Table 1) was followed. For example, a critical event happens whenever the patient's blood pressure is less than 90 mmHg for more than 1 h or the value drops below 60 mmHg.

Table 1. The protocol for the out of range physiologic measurements (adapted from [21])

	Blood Pressure
Normal range	90–180 mmHg
Critical event (continuously out of the normal range)	≥1 h
Critical event (anytime)	<60 mmHg

3 Methodologies, Materials and Methods

In this work the Design Science Research Methodology (DSR) was followed. DSR is fundamental in developing effective solutions – products, services, and systems able to answer to human needs [22]. According to Lunenfeld [23] research for design is the hardest to characterize, its purpose is to create objects and systems that display the results of the research and prove its worth. DSR is based in the creation and assessment of artefacts. To complement this methodology, Cross Industry Standard Process for Data Mining (CRISP-DM) was used. It is divided in six phases: Business Understanding, Data Understanding, Data Preparation, Modelling, Evaluation and Deployment. By crossing DSR and CRISP-DM it was possible develop and assess an artefact (prediction models) able to support the decision-making in the BP field.

This study used the data collected in real-time from 359 patients admitted in the ICU of Hospital Santo António, Centro Hospitalar do Porto, comprising a period between 2012.02.01 to 2014.02.26 (757 days) in a total of 222381 rows. In this project four data systems were considered: Vital Signs Monitors, Laboratory, Electronic Health Record and Pharmacy. Data mining models were induced exploring four different techniques: Decision Trees, Support Vector Machines, Naïve Byes and Generalized Linear Models.

4 Real-Time Decision Support

As already mentioned all the work was developed recurring to CRISP-DM methodology. The main work developed in each phase is presented in this section.

4.1 Business Understanding

The problem and their importance to the environment (service, professionals and patients) was already presented in the Sect. 2.1. In this work to avoid the occurrence of hypertension and hypotension in patients admitted in ICU is the business goal. Developing models with a high level of sensitivity able to support the decision process by predicting the probability of a patient has a BPCV in the next hours is the DM goal.

4.2 Data Understanding

In this phase the initial dataset was analysed in order to prepare it to be used by the DM engine. With the goal to answer to the main question it was used data provided from four data sources: Vital Signs Monitors – {Blood Pressure and Heart Rate}; Electronic Health Records – {Admission variables and Age}; Therapeutic Plan – {Vasopressores}; Laboratory Results – {Bilirubin, Creatinine, Po2/Fio2 and Platelets}.

In Table 2 is presented a distribution (percentage of cases) of the non-numeric variables, age and target (20 % of the records has critical events associated). These variables were not submitted to a processing phase because the value was only associated to a pre-defined class. It represents a simple matching between the DM classes and the values collected for each variable.

Table 2. Variables distribution

ID	Variable	Min	Max	Class	Cases
Age	Age	18	46	1	17.37 %
		47	65	2	35.46 %
		66	75	3	21.32 %
		76	130	4	25.85 %
Admission type	Urgent	–	–	U	80.29 %
	Programmed	–	–	P	19.71 %
Admission provenance	Chirurgic	–	–	1	47.66 %
	Observation	–	–	2	0.05 %
	Emergency	–	–	3	18.44 %
	Nursing room	–	–	4	15.37 %
	Other ICU	–	–	5	2.44 %
	Other hospital	–	–	6	1.32 %
	Other	–	–	7	14.73 %
Insufficiencies cardiac	Yes	–	–	1	91.76 %
Transplant	Yes	–	–	1	10.24 %
Surgical admission	Yes	–	–	1	55.02 %
Cerebrovascular accident (CVA)	Yes	–	–	1	2.20 %
Critical event	Yes	–	–	1	20.00 %

4.3 Data Preparation

In this phase all the variables were validated. First the existence of null values was verified and then it was verified the occurrence of values out of the acceptable range (noise values). Then all transformations rules were executed. Both tasks were performed by intelligent agents. The tasks performed were:

- To verify and group the admission type and admission from;
- To classify the Blood Pressure values as critical or not;
- To create the critical events variable;
- To determine the patient SOFA value for all the organic systems;
- To create a new variable which identifies if the patient has risk factors;
- To determine the last seven Blood Pressure values (BPLV) collected;
- To calculate the accumulated critical events (ACE) and all associated ratios;
- To create classes to numerical values (e.g. ratios and BPLV).
- To create the DM input dataset in a hourly base;

To induce the DM models, several scenarios were prepared using attributes sets. The first set created was Case Mix (CM). All the CM variables were provided by the patient Electronic Health Record (EHR). From the EHR, the variables: age, admission type, admission from, insufficiencies cardiac and risk patient (combination of a set of patient admission variables) were used. These variables were recorded at patient admission phase, being then transformed in accordance with the DM attributes.

The second group of variables used was the Sequential Organ Failure Assessment (SOFA). SOFA is used in ICU to score the degree of dysfunction/failure of the six organic systems (cardiovascular, respiratory, renal, liver, haematological and neurological) [24]. SOFA score varies from 0 (normal function) and 4 (total dysfunction). In this case the transformation made was simple: in case of normal function it was attributed the value 0 otherwise the value was 1. Thus, the attribute SOFA used in DM only considers two values 0 (SOFA = 0) or 1 (SOFA > 0).

The third group was based in the CE concept by creating the Accumulated Critical Events (ACE) variable. ACE includes three physiological variables: Blood Pressure (BP), Saturation of Oxygen (SPO2) and Heart Rate (HR). ACE values are calculated in real-time by counting the number of critical events verified by hour since patient admission. An attribute (TOTAL) that reflects the sum of ACE by each variable was also added. Then and using ACE a set of ratios were introduced.

These ratios allow to determine a relation between the number of ACE verified in a patient and the maximum number of ACE occurred by hour (R1) and a correspondence between the number of ACE verified in a patient and the maximum number of events verified in the past (from all the patients), until the hour in analysis (R2). Both the values were grouped by category and by patient.

Finally another group composed by the last seven BP values (BPLV) collected in a specific hour was created. This attribute is generated all hours by an agent. It analyse the last values collected in the last hour and put them in the same row (hour).

After performing all the transforming tasks, a set of new variables were introduced. These variables and their distribution are presented in the Table 3. For example, the SOFA_HEPATIC attribute is 1 when the bilirubin value collected is higher than the minimum considered (1.2). In the case of Risk Patient, the attribute is 1 when at least one of the symptoms or conditions presented in the Table 3 is verified. These conditions were verified in 21.32 % of the cases.

Table 3. Transformed variables distribution

Attribute	Variable	Min	Max	Value	% cases
SOFA_CARDIO	BP (mean)	0	70	1	72.63 %
	Dopamine or dobutamine	0.0	–	1	
	Epi/Norepi	0.0	–	1	
SOFA_RENAL	Creatinine	1.2	–	1	21.41 %
SOFA_RESPIRAT	Po2/Fio2	0	400	1	67.76 %
SOFA_HEPATIC	Bilirubin	1.2	–	1	21.37 %
SOFA_HEMAT	Platelets	0	150	1	47.76 %
RISK PATIENT	CVA	–	–	1	21.32 %
	Alcoholism or addicted	–	–	1	
	Pacemaker	–	–	1	
	Corticoids	–	–	1	
	Transplanted	–	–	1	
	Vasoactive drug	–	–	1	

In the last step a discretization technique has been considered. Having in consideration all numeric values used by the models, the attributes were transformed and categorized according to an interval (*Min* and *Max*). Using this technique the groups were defined according to the respective average (R1) or higher value (R2) of the data collected. These ranges are flexible and they are updated automatically according to the values collected. The groups were defined using a 7-point-scale adapted by Clinical Global Impression – Severity scale (CGI-S) [25]. The goal of CGI-S is to allow the clinician to rate the severity of illness [26]. The ranges defined [7] has clinical significance and represents the patient condition. A higher value represents a worst patient condition. The standard used to define the percentages concentrate the most part of patient values within a scale between 0 and 5. More severe cases are assigned to the levels 6 and 7. Table 4 presents the rules defined to discretize each continuous value (*values* ϵ *[|R_{0+}])*. The groups are identified at the top of the table and the left column identifies the variable. In the centre of the table are the ranges for each group. These values were obtained after apply the ranges (%) defined.

The attributes of *R1* are determined by the rows (*R1 BP Min* to *R1 TOT Max*). R2 is categorized according to the percentage of the values collected, i.e., level 1 corresponds to 10 % of the cases (values collected between 0 % and 10 % of the Maximum). All attributes of *R2* have the same limits. ACE attributes were grouped in agreement to their importance and the number of occurrences. These values were defined by ICU experts but can be modified in the future.

In case of ACE, if a BP value equal to 2 is verified, this variables is categorized in the second level (value = 1). The same happens to patients who present values of R2 between 0.01 and 0.10 or R1 HR between 0.004 and 0.008. The CGI-S was not used to calculate BPLV. The clinical guidelines and the values defined as normal were considered. Level 2 and 3 corresponds to the acceptable (normal) range.

Table 4. Discretization sets of data mining input

SET		0	1	2	3	4	5	6	7
R1	Min	−0.1	0.000	0.010	0.021	0.041	0.062	0.082	0.123
BP	Max	0.000	0.010	0.021	0.041	0.062	0.082	0.123	2.000
R1	Min	−0.1	0.000	0.018	0.036	0.072	0.108	0.144	0.216
O2	Max	0.000	0.018	0.036	0.072	0.108	0.144	0.216	2.000
R1	Min	−0.1	0.000	0.004	0.008	0.015	0.023	0.030	0.045
HR	Max	0.000	0.004	0.008	0.015	0.023	0.030	0.045	2.000
R1	Min	−0.1	0.000	0.020	0.041	0.081	0.122	0.162	0.243
TOT	Max	0.000	0.020	0.041	0.081	0.122	0.162	0.243	2.000
R2	Min	−0.1	0.000	0.100	0.250	0.500	0.750	0.900	1.000
	Max	0	0.100	0.250	0.500	0.750	0.900	1.000	2.000
ACE	Min	−0.1	0	3	5	8	10	12	15
	Max	0	3	5	8	10	12	15	50
BPLV	Min	−1	60	110	150	170	200	–	–
	Max	60	110	150	170	200	400	–	–

After being accomplished the transformation tasks, the DM input table (DMIT) was created. Finally, in order to prepare the DM scenarios, the values were organized by hour considering the following variables:

- **Hour:** The hour associated to the values collected, all models use this variable;
- **Case Mix (CM)** – Age, admission type, admission provenance, Risk Patient, Insufficiencies Cardiac, CVA, Transplant, Surgical Admission;
- **SOFA** – Cardiovascular, Respiratory, Renal, Hepatic, Hematologic;
- **Accumulated Critical Events (ACE)** – ACE of Blood Pressure (BP), ACE of Oxygen Saturation (SPO2), ACE of Heart Rate (HR) and Total ACE;
- **Ratios 1 (R1)** – ACE of BP/ max number of ACE of BP, ACE of SPO2/ max number of ACE of SPO2, ACE of HR/ max number of ACE of HR;
- **Ratios 2 (R2)** – ACE of BP/ elapsed time of stay, ACE of SPO2/ elapsed time of stay, ACE of HR/ elapsed time of stay, Total of ACE/ elapsed time of stay;
- **Ratios (R)** – Union of the two sets of ratios (R1 and R2).
- **Blood Pressure Last Values** (BPLV): The last seven values collected in an hour, being one value for each column.

4.4   Modelling

In this phase, the data mining models were induced using the data processed and transformed in the preceding phases. A set of Data Mining models (DMM) were induced using four DM techniques (DMT): GLM, SVM, DT and NB and two sampling methods: Holdout sampling (70 % of the data for training and 30 % for testing) and Cross Validation. Additionally the numeric attributes were used in two representation methods (Natural and Categorized). Scenarios 1 to 9 were manually configured.

Scenario 10 (S10) was automatically configured by using variables selected by the DM engine (based in heuristic rules). A total of 160 models were induced.

DMM = {*10 Scenarios, 4 Techniques, 2 Sampling Methods, 2 Representation Methods, 1 Target*}

Where the scenarios are :
S1 : {CM, SOFA, ACE, R, RISK, BPLV}
S2 : {CM, SOFA, RISK, BPLV}
S3 : {CM, ACE, R, RISK, BPLV}
S4 : {CM, RISK, BPLV}
S5 : {CM, R, RISK, BPLV}

S6 : {CM, SOFA, ACE, R, RISK}
S7 : {CM, RISK, BPLV}
S8 : {CM, SOFA, ACE, R, BPLV}
S9 : {CM, ACE, R, RISK, BPLV}
S10 : {Automatic}

Sampling Methods :
SM1 : Holdout Sampling (HS)
SM2 : Cross Validation (CV)

Representation Methods :
RM1 : Natural values (NAT)
RM2 : Categorized values (CATEG)

Techniques :
T1 : Generalized Linear Models (GLM)
T2 : Support Vector Machine (SVM)

T3 : Decision Trees (DT)
T4 : Naive Byes (NB)

Target : TT1 : Blood Pressure Critical Event

All the models were automatically induced in real-time, using streamed data and online-learning. A DM Model (DMM) can be represented by the following tuple.

DMM = <Δ, α, DMT, DMSM, DMRM, DMTG, Hour, Age, AdmissionFrom, AdmissionType, Risk, ace_bp, ace_bp_time, ace_bp_max, ace_hr, ace_hr_time, ace_hr_max, ace_spo2, ace_spo2_time, ace_spo2_max, total_ace, total_ace_time, total_ace_max, SOFA_Respiratory, SOFA_Cardiovascular, SOFA_Hepatic, SOFA_Renal, SOFA_Hematologic, BPLV1, BPLV2, BPLV3, BPLV4, BPLV5, BPLV6, BPV7>
Where,

Δ is the DM rules and α is the DM model configuration,
DMSM is the sampling method and *DMRM* is the representation method,
DMT is the DM technique and *DMTG* is the target,
Hour ... BPLV7 are the variables used by each model

For example if the Model 6 is composed by S6 using SVM, cross validation and categorized values, the tuple can be represented as:

DMM6 = <Δ, α, SVM, SM2, RM2, TT1, Hour, Age, AdmissionFrom, AdmissionType, Risk, ace_bp, ace_bp_time, ace_bp_max, ace_hr, ace_hr_time, ace_hr_max, ace_spo2, ace_spo2_time, ace_spo2_max, total_ace, total_ace_time, total_ace_max,, SOFA_Respiratory, SOFA_Cardiovascular, SOFA_Hepatic, SOFA_Renal, SOFA_Hematologic>
The configurations presented in Table 5 were used to induce Data Mining models.

Table 5. Algorithms configurations

Algorithm name	Configuration	Value
Generalized linear Model	Automatic preparation	On
	Confidence level	0.95
	Enable ridge regression	Enable
	Missing values treatment	Mean for numeric mode for categorical
	Ridge parameter	10.0000
	Variance inflation factor	Disable
Support vector Machine Decision Tree	Active learning	Enable
	Automatic preparation	On
	Complexity factor	0.165605
	Kernel function	Linear
	Tolerance	0.001
	Automatic preparation	On
	Criteria for splits	20
	Criteria for splits (%)	0.1
	Maximum tree depth	7
	Minimum child record count	10
	Minimum records per node	0.05
	Tree impurity metric	Gini
Naive Bayes	Automatic preparation	On
	Pairwise, singleton threshold	0

4.5 Evaluation

After inducing all the models, the results achieved by each one of the 160 models were assessed. To assess the models the confusion matrix (CMX) was used. CMX allows determining the number of True Positives (TP) (predicted 1 and real 1), False Positives (FP) (1, 0), True Negatives (TN) (0, 0) and False Negatives (FN) (0, 1). Using the CMX is possible calculate some measures: Sensitivity = TP/(TP + FN); Specificity: TN/(TN + FP); Accuracy: TP/(TP + FP + TN + FN) and Precision: TP/(TP + FP).

Table 6 presents the best results achieved by each technique and measure. For example, in the case of GLM the best accuracy (72.23 %) and the best sensitivity was achieved by the same scenario (S3) but using different representation methods. The best sensitivity (95.90 %) was achieved by the scenario 7 using SVM. The type of Sampling Methods used are not mentioned because the results are similar for both cases.

To choose the best model, a threshold was introduced. The threshold combine three metrics in order to find the most suitable model to predict the probability of having a critical event (sensitivity) with an acceptable accuracy and precision in order to avoid a high number of false positives. The threshold defined was: Sensitivity ≥ 90 % and Accuracy and Precision ≥ 70 %.

Table 6. Best model for each technique and measure

Technique	Sensitivity		Specificity		Accuracy	
GLM	S3RM2	0.9127	S2RM2	0.3866	S3RM1	0.7223
SVM	S7RM2	0.9590	S6RM2	0.2942	S5RM2	0.5586
DT	S6RM2	0.9316	S6RM2	0.3851	S6 S7 RM2	0.7152
NB	S3RM2	0.9100	S2RM2	0.3829	S7RM2	0.7099

Table 7 presents the best three models which achieved the threshold defined. The ranking was defined according to the sensitivity result.

Table 7. Best models achieving the threshold

Model	Accuracy	Sensitivity	Specificity	Precision
S3T1RM2	0.7120	**0.9127**	0.3792	0.7310
S2T1RM2	0.7038	0.9125	0.3781	0.7346
S5T1RM2	0.7028	0.9120	0.3793	0.7359

5 Discussion

After analysing the models induced it was possible observe that the achieved results were not influenced by the sampling method used. Both approaches presented similar results. However the same consideration cannot be done concerning to the representation method. The achieved results by the models using categorized variables were significantly better. The models using natural values did not achieved the threshold. The model with a best sensitivity (95.90 %) presented an accuracy of 49.26 % using SVM and categorized variables. This model was rejected because did not achieved the threshold defined. In general, the models using categorized values increased the sensitivity in 10–15 % and the accuracy in 1–3 %.

Due the fact of the Intensivist preferring models sensitive to 1 (by predicting the worst scenario it is possible to avoid their occurrence. It is better predicting 1 and verify 0 than the opposite), the precision is a complementary measure to give an idea the number of correct predictions. It is important to note that to the intensivist is presented the probability (confidence rate) of a patient has a critical event in the next hours and not if he will have or not a critical event. It is not presenting a correct result (Yes or No) but the percentage of a critical event appear in the next hours (e.g. the probability of a patient has a BPCE in the next 10 h is 80 %). This reality decreases the significance of false positives (FP), because the main goal is to avoid the occurrence of BPCE. Consequently the number of FP is higher.

In Fig. 1 is possible observing the receiver operating characteristic (ROC) curve for the model which achieved the threshold and presented the best sensitivity (S3T1RM2). The curve is created by plotting the true positive rate (sensitivity) against the false positive rate (specificity) at various threshold settings.

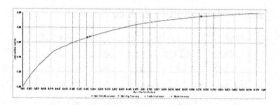

Fig. 1. ROC for the most sensitivity model

6   Conclusions and Future Work

At the end of this work it was possible to assess the viability of using these variables to predict Blood Pressure Critical Events. The goal is not to predict effectively if the patient will have a BPCE or not but the probability of occurring a BPCE in the next hours. It was possible observe that the models using categorization methods presented best results. Only some of these models achieved the threshold defined. To the Intensivist the attained results (sensitivities between 90 % and 95 %) can help the decision and represents an important step in order to help to prevent possible cases of Hypertension or Hypotension. For them the number of False Positives (around 25 %) are quite acceptable, once the goal is to prevent the occurrence of Critical Events. If the system is predicting a high probability of occurring a CE and the Intensivist can prevent it, the occurrence of a False Positive is an inevitable enjoyable. The models developed will be included in the INTCare ensemble engine. Scientifically the models produced can be used by other researchers in order to improve their works. The next step is focused in evaluating the predictions made by the system. In this process the intensivists will assess the clinical results. In addition this concept will be explored to other type of critical events.

Acknowledgments. This work has been supported by FCT - Fundação para a Ciência e Tecnologia within the Project Scope UID/CEC/00319/2013 and the contract PTDC/EEI-SII/1302/2012 (INTCare II).

References

1. Kannel, W.B.: Risk stratification in hypertension: new insights from the Framingham Study. Am. J. Hypertens. **13**, 3S–10S (2000)
2. Portela, F., Santos, M.F., Machado, J., Abelha, A., Silva, Á., Rua, F.: Pervasive and intelligent decision support in intensive medicine – the complete picture. In: Bursa, M., Khuri, S., Renda, M.E. (eds.) ITBAM 2014. LNCS, vol. 8649, pp. 87–102. Springer, Heidelberg (2014)
3. Oliveira, S., Portela, F., Santos, M.F., Machado, J., Abelha, A., Silva, Á., Rua, F.: Predicting plateau pressure in intensive medicine for ventilated patients. In: Rocha, A., Correia, A.M., Costanzo, S., Reis, L.P. (eds.) New Contributions in Information Systems and Technologies, Advances in Intelligent Systems and Computing 354. AISC, vol. 354, pp. 179–188. Springer, Heidelberg (2015)

4. Portela, F., Santos, M.F., Machado, J., Abelha, A., Silva, Á., Rua, F.: Preventing patient cardiac arrhythmias by using data mining techniques. In: 2014 IEEE Conference on Biomedical Engineering and Sciences (2014)
5. Braga, P., Portela, F., Santos, M.F.: Data mining models to predict patient's readmission in intensive care units. In: ICAART - International Conference on Agents and Artificial Intelligence (2015)
6. Veloso, R., Portela, F., Santos, M., Machado, J.M.F., Abelha, A., Silva, Á., Rua, F.: Real-time data mining models for predicting length of stay in intensive care units. In: KMIS 2014-International Conference on Knowledge Management and Information Sharing (2014)
7. Portela, F., Santos, M.F., Machado, J., Abelha, A., Silva, Á.: Pervasive and intelligent decision support in critical health care using ensembles. In: Bursa, M., Khuri, S., Renda, M. E. (eds.) ITBAM 2013. LNCS, vol. 8060, pp. 1–16. Springer, Heidelberg (2013)
8. NIH. http://www.nhlbi.nih.gov/health/health-topics/topics/hbp. Accessed May 2015
9. Wolf-Maier, K., Cooper, R.S., Banegas, J.R., Giampaoli, S., Hense, H.-W., Joffres, M., Kastarinen, M., Poulter, N., Primatesta, P., Rodríguez-Artalejo, F.: Hypertension prevalence and blood pressure levels in 6 European countries, Canada, and the United States. JAMA **289**, 2363–2369 (2003)
10. Mancia, G., Fagard, R., Narkiewicz, K., Redon, J., Zanchetti, A., Böhm, M., Christiaens, T., Cifkova, R., De Backer, G., Dominiczak, A., Zannad, F.: 2013 ESH/ESC guidelines for the management of arterial hypertension: the task force for the management of arterial hypertension of the European society of hypertension (ESH) and of the European Society of Cardiology (ESC). Blood Press. **22**(4), 193–278 (2013)
11. Mahfoud, F., Ukena, C., Kandolf, R., Kindermann, M., Böhm, M., Kindermann, I.: Blood pressure and heart rate predict outcome in patients acutely admitted with suspected myocarditis without previous heart failure. J. Hypertens. **30**, 1217–1224 (2012)
12. Mitsa, T.: Temporal Data Mining. CRC Press, Boca Raton (2010)
13. Bucknall, T.K.: Medical error and decision making: learning from the past and present in intensive care. Aust. Crit. Care **23**, 150–156 (2010)
14. Portela, F., Santos, M.F., Silva, Á., Machado, J., Abelha, A.: Enabling a pervasive approach for intelligent decision support in critical health care. Presented at HCist 2011 – International Workshop on Health and Social Care Information Systems and Technologies, Algarve, Portugal, p. 10 (2011)
15. Gonçalves, J.M.C., Portela, F., Santos, M.F., Silva, Á., Machado, J., Abelha, A.: Predict sepsis level in intensive medicine — data mining approach. In: Rocha, Á., Correia, A.M., Wilson, T., Stroetmann, K.A. (eds.) Advances in Information Systems and Technologies. AISC, vol. 206, pp. 201–211. Springer, Heidelberg (2013)
16. Oliveira, S., Portela, F., Santos, M.F., Machado, J., Abelha, A., Silva, Á., Rua, F.: Intelligent decision support to predict patient barotrauma risk in intensive care units. In: Procedia Computer Science - HCIST 2015 - Healthy and Secure People. Elsevier (2015)
17. Veloso, R., Portela, F., Santos, M.F., Silva, Á., Rua, F., Abelha, A., Machado, J.: A clustering approach for predicting readmissions in intensive medicine. Procedia Technol. **16**, 1307–1316 (2014)
18. Portela, F., Veloso, R., Oliveira, S., Santos, M.F., Abelha, A., Machado, J., Silva, Á, Rua, F.: Predict hourly patient discharge probability in intensive care units using data mining. In: International Conference on Computer Science and Computational Mathematics (ICCSCM 2014). Science Society, Langkawi, Malaysia (2014). ISSN: 1513-1874
19. Silva, A., Cortez, P., Santos, M.F., Gornesc, L., Neves, J.: Mortality assessment in intensive care units via adverse events using artificial neural networks. Artif. Intell. Med. **36**, 223–234 (2006)

20. Portela, F., Gago, P., Santos, M.F., Machado, J., Abelha, A., Silva, Á., Rua, F.: Implementing a pervasive real-time intelligent system for tracking critical events with intensive care patients. IJHISI – Int. J. Healthc. Inf. Syst. Inf. **8**(4), 1–16 (2013). (IGI Global)
21. Silva, Á., Cortez, P., Santos, M.F., Gomes, L., Neves, J.: Rating organ failure via adverse events using data mining in the intensive care unit. Artif. Intell. Med. **43**, 179–193 (2008)
22. Lee, P.: Design research: what is it and why do it? In: The Reboot, vol. 2013. Reboot (2012). http://thereboot.org
23. Lunenfeld, P., Laurel, B.: Design Research: Methods and Perspectives. MIT Press, Cambridge (2003)
24. Vincent, J.L., Moreno, R., Takala, J., Willatts, S., De Mendonca, A., Bruining, H., Reinhart, C.K., Suter, P.M., Thijs, L.G.: The SOFA (sepsis-related organ failure assessment) score to describe organ dysfunction/failure. Intensive Care Med. **22**, 707–710 (1996)
25. Guy, W.: ECDEU Assessment Manual for Psychopharmacology. US Department of Health, Education, and Welfare, Public Health Service, Alcohol, Drug Abuse, and Mental Health Administration, National Institute of Mental Health, Psychopharmacology Research Branch, Division of Extramural Research Program, Rockville (1976)
26. Guy, W.: Clinical global impressions (CGI) scale. In: Psychiatric Measures. APA, Washington, D.C. (2000)

A Real-Time Intelligent System
for Tracking Patient Condition

Filipe Portela[1,2(✉)], Sérgio Oliveira[1], Manuel Santos[1],
José Machado[1], and António Abelha[1]

[1] Algoritmi Research Centre, University of Minho, Braga, Portugal
{cfp,mfs}@dsi.uminho.pt,
sergiomdcoliveira@gmail.com,
{jmac,abelha}@di.uminho.pt
[2] ESEIG, Porto Polytechnic, Porto, Portugal

Abstract. Hospitals have multiple data sources, such as embedded systems, monitors and sensors. The number of data available is increasing and the information are used not only to care the patient but also to assist the decision processes. The introduction of intelligent environments in health care institutions has been adopted due their ability to provide useful information for health professionals, either in helping to identify prognosis or also to understand patient condition. Behind of this concept arises this Intelligent System to track patient condition (e.g. critic events) in health care. This system has the great advantage of being adaptable to the environment and user needs. The system is focused in identifying critic events from data streaming (e.g. vital signs and ventilation) which is particularly valuable for understanding the patient's condition. This work aims to demonstrate the process of creating an intelligent system capable of operating in a real environment using streaming data provided by ventilators and vital signs monitors. Its development is important to the physician because becomes possible crossing multiple variables in real-time by analyzing if a value is critic or not and if their variation has or not clinical importance.

Keywords: Ambient intelligence · Healthcare · Data streaming · Critic events · Intelligent systems · Real-time · Tracking system · Intcare · Intensive care

1 Introduction

The ability to extract useful knowledge from the data collected can provides better working practices tools [1]. Hospitals see in the database an important asset to the decision-making process [2]. The health sector is in constant development and evolution in order to provide better patient care and improving their services delivery. The technologies related to Ambient Intelligence has a great importance in providing health care, not only in the medical care field but also in the administrative and organizational field [3]. The use of appropriate tools by health professionals, can help them to identify causes and more effective treatments focused on patient disease [4].

This work aims to show the importance of developing a system capable of interacting with an intelligent environment system by combining the information needed by the clinician and the patient condition. This system is able to identify critic events for

© Springer International Publishing Switzerland 2015
J. Bravo et al. (Eds.): AmIHEALTH 2015, LNCS 9456, pp. 91–97, 2015.
DOI: 10.1007/978-3-319-26508-7_9

all monitored variables in two ways: detecting critic values by using a table containing the normal values range by attribute (minimum and maximum) and detecting variations in an attribute by analyzing the curve of values. The system was tested in a real environment - Intensive Care Unit (ICU) of Centro Hospitalar do Porto (CHP) and using the data provided by patient sensors: vital signs and ventilation. The achieved results by this new tool were very satisfactory. The intensivists see a big utility in using this tool. Their features help to quickly understand the patient condition more effectively. This tool is also able to send an alert when some abnormal value appears.

This article is divided in four sections. The first one shows the evolution of technology in health care and the work goals. The next chapter discusses and presents important aspects directly related to the development of this work. The third chapter presents the logical structure of the intelligent system developed. Then section four presents the main conclusions of the work and some guidelines for future work.

2   Background

2.1   Ambient Intelligence, Intensive Care and Critic Events

The Ambient Intelligence (AMI) corresponds to a future vision of intelligent computing in order to support people in various environments [5]. The primary focus behind the AMI environment is to enrich a technology particularly with the use of sensors and devices capable of communicating with database systems. Thus, you can build systems able to provide solutions to the user benefit based on the actual perception and historical information, habits and even emotions [6, 7]. AMI promotes successful interpretation of contextual information from sensors and can adapts it to user needs in a transparently and proactively way. Due AIM features the ICU of CHP [17] is an example of AMI.

Patients who are in an ICU are continuous monitored, in weak health condition and in a serious life-threatening [8]. The patient care in this unit has several adverse events. The respective events can be factors of great impact in the clinical condition of the patient in the future [9]. These events can occur several times a day. The possibility of having the ability to identify events automatically and in real-time represents an important help to the decision process [10]. Patient condition can modify several times for hour. To an Intensivist is very difficult to analyze and compare all the values in real-time. The system developed take off this concern from the intensivist giving to them more time to care the patient. The system is able to analyze all the values received and in real-time notify when some abnormal situation appears. Several studies have been conducted showing that the most common adverse errors are related to the mechanical or human error [11]. However, there are other problems that are difficult to analyse, for example clinical events. Usually these events are identified from some guidelines supplied by bedside monitors [12] and data streaming (e.g. vital signs and ventilation).

The identification of a critic event is recognized when an attribute values is out of the normal range for a certain period of time [13]. An earlier study was made in order to track vital signs critic events based in the value collected and the time event [10].

The results achieved in the past were the first step to develop a universal and most complete system by giving the possibility to the user configure it.

2.2 INTCare

This work was carried out under the research project INTCare. INTCare is an Intelligent Decision Support System (IDSS) [14] designed to ICUs. INTCare allows continuously monitoring of the data collected by the sensors connected to the patient. At same time this IDSS is able to predict clinical events in real-time by using data mining and the data collected. One of its goals is to make their job in a pervasive way [15, 16]. INTCare [18] was an important trigger to develop an intelligent environment. The environment is now prepared to identify critic events and support the system developed in real-time.

3 Tracking System

This is an intelligent and autonomous system, where the decision makers can use it to track patient values in two ways: analyze if a value is too low or too higher to be considered critic; analyze if the value variance is significant and if it has some clinical significance. In the first case (Algorithm 1) an intelligent agent is used to categorize all the values collected in real-time. The agent categorizes the value received as 0 (not critic) or 1 (critic) using the table containing the ranges. For example if the SPO2 value is critic when the value is lower than 80, always a value lower than 80 arises, the system identifies it as critic. Then the critic events concept already used in intensive medicine [10] is applied. In the second case (Algorithm 2) an agent is used to monitoring the variation of values by variable. The user can define a clinical significance in order to better understand the curve values. For example if the user defines a Blood Pressure with a variation from the last value upper than 20, it should be considered to future analysis. In this case the system indicates when the defined variance is verified. Additionally the user also can define a time. For example if the values collected had those variation for a time duration of 10 min, it can be considered as a clinical event.

3.1 Acquisition Process and Data Selection

The system can be adopted to different fields of study. In this case it was used for looking by critic values in several patient ventilation and vital signs atributes. In both cases the data inserted into the database are uninformative and difficult to understand. In this case it was necessary to carry out actions in order to demonstrate their value to doctors or nurses. This tracking system is designed to answer in real-time to the user needs or to alert when some abnormal value is collected. During the acquisition process a trigger is executed to assess if the value is valid and how critic is it. Then the second part of the system is executed by an intelligent agent. This agent is executed periodically. First it analyses the variation and then in accordance to the user indications it can analyze the clinical significance of the values collected.

The system developed is mainly concerned with the identification of critic events and to identify their significance. In the first case the table with the ranges is used to identify if a value is critic. In the second case critic events are identified only due to a changing of value. The table containing the range of values must be determined based on scientific and clinical knowledge by the hospital service/unit. Attributes can have several changes in values, however it is chosen the variations that best meets the end-user needs. In both cases the identification of the attributes and their underlying changes in the value are fundamental to a properly identification of the events.

3.2   Data Processing

The system automatically categorize a value as critic or not, covering patient streaming data. These records are used to determine their criticity, just in case if they have not been previously used. The number of rows is depending from the number of admitted patients in the service. After a patient be discharged all the data is transferred to other table. Periodically it is executed another agent to verify if all the records were processed. In fact there is a temporal spectrum to view critic events. The time range may be, for example, corresponding to records up to the last two hours.

Algorithm 1 presents the trigger to identify if a value collected is valid and then if it is critic or not. Critic value table contains the range of possible values and the normal values. If a patient has a valid value (inside of the normal range) and a value is lower than a minimum or it is higher than a maximum, the value collected is considered critic. The critic table is defined by the clinical staff according to their environment and type of patients. By default a table defined by some experts in the field [10] is used. In this case and according to the critic table, a value can be normal (0), critic (1) or too critic (2). This process is executed always some new value arrives.

Algorithm 1. Identify a value as critic or not

Requires: criticValueTable, attributeCategory and attributeValue

```
 1:  Function Type of Value (attribute Category, attribute Value)
 2:      For attributeCategory in criticValueTable.Category
 3:          If (attributeValue >= criticValueTable.MinimumPossibleValue and attributeValue <=
             criticValueTable.MaximumPossibleValue) then validValue = 1
 4:              IF (attributeValue >= criticValueTable.MinimumValue2 and attributeValue <=
                 criticValueTable.MaximumValue2) then criticValue = 2
 5:              Elseif   (attributeValue >= criticValueTable.MinimumValue and attributeValue <=
                 criticValueTable.MaximumValue) then criticValue = 1
 6:              Else criticValue = 0
 7:              End If
 8:          Else validValue = 0
 9:          End If
10:      End for
11:  End Function
```

Algorithm 2 is used to identify possible changes in the values collected, i.e., if the value now received is different than the value earlier received. The procedure responsible for carrying out the identification of critic events is capable of performing two more operations: changing the count values of the attributes and performing a magnitude analysis of the values difference.

The two next steps are made following the records timeline using an ascending order by attribute and patient identification. The counting process changes gives to the health professional the possibility to follow the patient and the number of value changes of a particular attribute monitored during a certain period of time. This information is useful to the health professionals because it extends their capability in identifying the patient condition and stability.

The ability to identify the difference of values allows the professionals to identify how sharp are being the values variations. Professionals also can identify how long a value is keeping stable. This information can be useful to for example modifying a ventilation parameter or to define a new therapeutic. In order to understanding these operations, the following algorithmic representation presents the system operations.

Algorithm 2. Identify value changes

Requires: matrix of patients to validate mtrPatientesNValid() and the matrix variation values mtrArangeValues()

```
 1:    Function Tracking of Patients (mtrPatientesNValid(), mtrArangeValues())
 2:       valueOne ← -1; idPatiente ← 0; theCounter ← 0
 3:       For attribute in mtrArangeValues() Do
 4:          For patiente in mtrPatientesNValid() Do
 5:             If idPatiente == patiente.idPatiente Then
 6:                If ((valueOne != patiente.value ) and valueOne != -1) Then
 7:                   theDifference ← module(valueOne – patiente.value); theCounter ← theCounter + 1
 8:                   If (((patiente.value + attribute.value) >= valueOne) or ((patiente.value –
 9:                      Updates Hits: critic event, module and changing count values
10:                      idPatiente ← patiente.idPatiente; valueOne ← patiente.value
11:                   Else idPatiente ← patiente.idPatiente; valueOne ← patiente.value
12:                   End If
13:                Else idPatiente ← patiente.idPatiente; valueOne ← patiente.value
14:                End If
15:             Else idPatiente ← 0; valueOne ← -1
16:             End If
17:          End For
18:       End For
19:    End function
```

Being the system responsible for feeding the main repository, it performs various operations on the data collected. If this operation is not implemented the time responses to professional requests would sequentially increase. Thus the information presented is always timely and focused on patients who are admitted in the service. If a professionals wants to consult earlier data, the system will use the historical repository.

3.3   Clinical Benefits

The system developed enables determining value changes and identifying critic events. The changes made by the system about the events allows the health professionals knowing how long a patient is having a critic event and how much the values varies. For example and using the ventilation system, this solution can be used to support the patient weaning process by analyzing the evolution of the associated variables. This system also gives the possibility to send alerts to the professionals with the most relevant results. The system is always running in background and when some of the conditions above mentioned appears the professional receives a message with the values and their changes. It allows to have a pervasive system, where the user did not need to be concerned with the system because it is prepared to always alert/inform when some abnormal situation is verified.

4 Conclusion and Future Work

Once completed the development of this intelligent system, their implementation in real environment (ICU of CHP) was important to identify the strengths and weakness of the system. During this process it was easy to understand their utility to health professionals in order to provide better patient care. As strengths they mentioned that the system is able to quickly identify critic events for all patients who are monitored by vital signs monitor or ventilator. It is easy to change system parameters, respectively the ranges of values that represent the critic events. Thus health professionals have the freedom to make their independent research. As a possible aspect of evolution it is the using of these data to predict critic values and curve variations. Although this system been designed inside a specific unit (ICU), it also can be transposed to other services/units and can be used in telemedicine and Ambient Intelligence without any changes.

For future work should be taken into consideration the following aspects: complementing the system with DM models to predict critic events and patient diseases; predecting future values by analyzing the curve; addressing and anticipating significant features in intelligent environment and apply the system to other services.

Acknowledgments. This work has been supported by FCT - Fundação para a Ciência e Tecnologia within the Project UID/CEC/00319/2013 and PTDC/EEI-SII/1302/2012.

References

1. Santos, M., Azevedo, C.: Data Mining Descoberta do conhecimento em base de dados. FCA - Editora de Informática, Lda (2005)
2. Portela, F., Santos, M.F., Gago, P., Silva, Á., Rua, F., Abelha, A.,. Neves, J.: Enabling real-time intelligent decision support in intensive care. In: ESM 2011 (2011)
3. Marins, F.A.S., Rodrigues, R., Portela, F., Santos, M.F., Abelha, A., Machado, J.M.: Extending a patient monitoring system with identification and localisation. In: 2013 IEEM (2013)
4. Koh, H., Tan, G.: Data mining applications in healthcare. J. Healthc. Inf. Manage. **19**(2), 64–72 (2005)
5. Acampora, G., Cook, D.J., Rashidi, P., Vasilakos, A.V.: A survey on ambient intelligence in healthcare. Proc. IEEE **101**(12), 2470–2494 (2013)

6. Augusto, J.C.: Ambient intelligence: basic concepts and applications. In: Filipe, J., Shishkov, B., Helfert, M. (eds.) Software and Data Technologies, pp. 16–26. Springer, Berlinl, Heidelberg (2008)

7. Machado, J.M., Abelha, A., Neves, J., Santos, M.: Ambient intelligence in medicine. In: IEEE BioCAS 2006, Art. No. 4600316, pp. 1–4 (2006)

8. Bricon-Souf, N., Newman, C.R.: Context awareness in health care: a review. Int. J. Med. Inform. **76**(1), 2–12 (2007)

9. Rothschild, J.M., Landrigan, C.P., Cronin, J.W., Kaushal, R., Lockley, S.W., Burdick, E., et al.: The critic care safety study: the incidence and nature of adverse events and serious medical errors in intensive care. Crit. Care Med. **33**(8), 1694–1700 (2005)

10. Portela, F., Gago, P., Santos, M.F., Machado, J.M., Abelha, A., Silva, Á., Rua, F.: Implementing a pervasive real-time intelligent system for tracking critic events in intensive care patients. In: IJHISI (2013)

11. Kaur, M., Pawar, M., Kohli, J.K., Mishra, S.: Critic events in intensive care unit. Indian J. Crit. Care Med. **12**(1), 28–31 (2008)

12. Keegan, M.T., Gajic, O., Afessa, B.: Severity of illness scoring systems in the intensive care unit. Crit. Care Med. **39**(1), 163–169 (2011)

13. Silva, A., Cortez, P., Santos, M.F., Gomes, L., Neves, J.: Rating organ failure via adverse events using data mining in the intensive care unit. Artif. Intell. Med. **43**(3), 179–193 (2008)

14. Portela, F., Santos, M.F., Machado, J., Abelha, A., Silva, Á., Rua, F.: Pervasive and intelligent decision support in intensive medicine – the complete picture. In: Bursa, M., Khuri, S., Renda, M.E. (eds.) ITBAM 2014. LNCS, vol. 8649, pp. 87–102. Springer, Heidelberg (2014)

15. Portela, F., Santos, M.F., Vilas-Boas, M.: A pervasive approach to a real-time intelligent decision support system in intensive medicine. In: Fred, A., Dietz, J.L.G., Liu, K., Filipe, J. (eds.) IC3 K 2010. CCIS, vol. 272, pp. 368–381. Springer, Heidelberg (2013)

16. Portela, F., Gago, P., Santos, M.F., Silva, A., Rua, F., Machado, J., Abelha, A., Neves, J.: Knowledge discovery for pervasive and real-time intelligent decision support in intensive care medicine. In: KMIS 2011, p. 12. Paris, France (2011)

17. Santos, M.F., Portela, F., Vilas-Boas, M., Machado, J., Abelha, A., Neves, J.: Information architecture for intelligent decision support in intensive medicine. Trans. Comput. **8**(5), 810–819 (2009). (World Scientific and Engi)

18. Portela, F., Aguiar, J., Santos, M.F., Silva, Á., Rua, F.: Pervasive Intelligent Decision Support System - Technology Acceptance in Intensive Care Units. In: AISC, Springer, Berlin (2013)

Detecting State Anxiety When Caring for People with Dementia

Darien Miranda[✉], Jesus Favela, and Catalina Ibarra

Computer Science Department, CICESE, Ensenada, Mexico
{dmirnada,cibarra}@cicese.edu.mx, favela@cicese.mx

Abstract. The care of people who suffer from dementia imposes significant stress on family members and caregivers. Often, these informal caregivers have no coping strategy to deal with these behaviours. Anxiety and stress episodes are often triggered by problematic behaviours exhibited by the person who suffers from dementia. Helping caregivers understand these behaviours could assist them to better deal with them and reduce caregiver burden. We report an experiment, using the naturalistic enactment technique, in which 10 subjects were asked to care for an older adult who acts as if she experiences dementia. We record physiological signals from the participants (GSR, IBI, EEG) during the sessions, that last for approximately 30 min. A preliminary analysis of the data provides evidence that state anxiety can be detected using wearable sensors. Furthermore, if episodes of problematic behaviours can also be detected, the recognition of anxiety in the caregiver can be improved, leading to the enactment of appropriate interventions to help caregivers cope with anxiety episodes.

Keywords: Behaviour recognition · Anxiety detection · Dementia care · Physiological signals

1 Introduction

It has been estimated that between 5 to 7 % of those 60 and older suffer from dementia, with the total number of persons with dementia (PwD) expected to double every 20 years worldwide [8]. Dementia is characterized by changes in personality and behavioural functions that can be very challenging for caregivers. Informal caregivers, mostly family members and friends, can be affected from the loss of intellectual functions and inability of the PwD to perform activities of daily living. In addition, PwD presents behavioural and psychological symptoms of dementia (BPSD) that impose additional burden on caregivers. These symptoms, which are estimated to be present in 90 % of PwDs [9], could include aggression, agitation, wandering, verbal aggression or psychosis, affect caregivers and eventually undermine their health and capacity to care for the PwD.

In a recent study 60 % of caregivers develop anxiety or depressive disorders in the first 24 months of caring for a person with dementia [3]. In addition,

© Springer International Publishing Switzerland 2015
J. Bravo et al. (Eds.): AmIHEALTH 2015, LNCS 9456, pp. 98–109, 2015.
DOI: 10.1007/978-3-319-26508-7_10

almost 25 % of caregivers of people with dementia have a significant clinically anxiety level [2]. Moreover, dementia care is particularly stressful, demanding more hours and complications on informal caregivers, than the care of non-dementia patients [7]. In another study, caregivers suffering anxiety reported a 63 % death rate greater than non-caregivers of the same age [10].

Numerous strategies have been proposed to deal with caregiver anxiety. These can be classified as: Focused on emotions; Based on problem resolution; and dysfunctional strategies [2]. Caregiver burden increases when dysfunctional strategies are used more frequently while problem solving strategies decrease. Monitoring coping strategies can help predict caregiver anxiety and burden [12].

In this work we focus on State Anxiety, which is experienced when the subject is confronted with a specific situation [4]. While caregivers can be subject of continuous stress that could lead them to experience long-term anxiety, detecting and dealing with anxiety episodes triggered by specific events, such as problematic behaviours by the person with dementia (for instance verbal abuse), can help in instrumenting adequate coping strategies improving the caregiver-PwD relation. The next section presents the Ambient-assisted Interventions Systems to deal with problematic behaviours, and an extension we are proposing to focus on the caregiver. Section 3 describes the experiment conducted to gather physiological data from informal caregivers facing problematic situations, which is based on the naturalistic enactment technique. The aim of this experiment is to gather data that could be used in future works to detect state anxiety on caregivers. In Sect. 4 we present the initial results from the experiment. Section 5 explains the limitations of this work and Sect. 6 presents our conclusions and proposals for future work.

2 Extending the Framework of Ambient-Assisted Interventions Systems (AaIS) for Dementia

An Ambient-assisted Intervention System (AaIS) focuses on suggesting or enacting strategies aimed at addressing problematic behaviours exhibited by PwD (see Fig. 1) [6].

An AaIS uses ambient intelligence to improve PwDs quality of life by identifying the presence of BPSDs, deciding on an appropriate intervention, and either modifying the environment or persuading the PwD or the caregiver to act on the system's advice. Both, inappropriate environments and upsetting personal interactions combine with unmet needs to trigger problematic behaviours. For instance, a PwD might exhibit apathy after being scolded by her caregiver or might undergo wandering triggered initially by her need to move after a long period of rest.

These BPSDs can be observed and reported by the caregiver or, alternatively, BPSDs can be inferred from information obtained from sensors located in the environment or worn by the PwD. Agitation, for instance, is manifested via repetitive movement and verbal expressions such as shouting or continuous talk. These behaviours can be inferred from data obtained from accelerometers and micro-phones. Finally, once there is evidence that the PwD is exhibiting a BPSD, a deci-sion model is used to decide on an intervention, which will be enacted in one of these three ways: (a) Intervene directly to change the configuration of the physical environment; (b) Communicate with the caregiver to recommend an action to per-form; or, (c) Communicate with the PwD to suggest an activity or provide him/her with information that could change his/her current behaviour. The planning and enactment of an intervention by the AaIS requires a representation of the factors influencing the PwD's behaviour. The decision model uses an ontological model of problematic behaviours to personalize non-pharmacological interventions pro-vided through AaIS services [6].

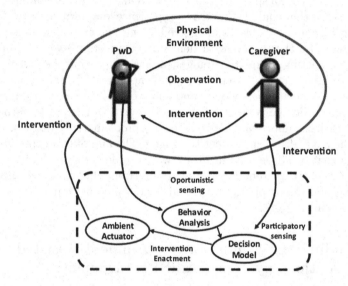

Fig. 1. An ambient-assisted intervention system monitors a person with dementia and the physical and social environment for problematic behaviours to select an appropriate intervention [6]

By detecting problematic behaviours and inferring probable causes, behaviour-aware applications could provide tailored and opportune interventions, notifying caregivers, offering assurances to the patient, or directly modifying the physical environment. For example, as daylight decreases at nightfall, a person with demen-tia might experience confusion and anxiety and not recognize his or her surround-ings. This could lead to a desire to wander, a phenomena known as sundowning syndrome. If this behaviour is detected, increasing the lighting conditions could eliminate the problematic behaviour.

We propose to extend the AaIS framework to analyse the behaviour of care-givers and enact coping strategies that would assist them in dealing with situa-tions that cause them stress or anxiety. Thus, the extended framework includes the monitoring of the caregiver, an analysis of his/her behaviour and the enact-ment or suggestion of coping strategies, as illustrated in Fig. 2.

An important aspect of the extended AaIS framework is the detection of negative behaviours in the caregiver, such as anxiety or stress. Behaviours that might also trigger problematic behaviours in the PwD, since emotional contagion has been found to grow stronger in PwDs. That is, the PwD might sense anxiety on the caregiver, and unconsciously mimic that behaviour [11].

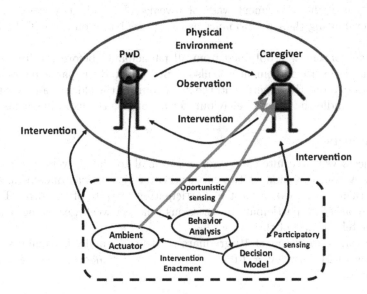

Fig. 2. Extended AaIS framework which includes assisting the caregiver in dealing with stress and anxiety.

In this paper we describe an experiment aimed at collecting physiological data from caregivers under stressful conditions and an initial attempt at inferring stress. The next section describes the experiment conducted.

3   An Experiment to Induce Anxiety on Informal Caregivers

We designed an intervention to induce anxiety on informal caregivers under controlled and naturalistic conditions. To achieve this we applied a technique known as Naturalistic Enactment (NE) [1]. NE was originally proposed to evaluate pervasive healthcare technologies, where having high ecological validity and direct user involvement is important, yet using actual patients can be risky. NE consists of a naturalistic enactment of tasks (i.e. the exposure to situations and tasks in natural conditions) to simulate the experience of the user under normal conditions, and thus unearth issues and behaviours that would otherwise have been difficult to capture.

In order to "expose" our subjects to a realistic and stressful caregiving situation under controlled conditions, we conceived an exercise that consisted of a naturalistic enactment of a therapy session with a person acting as being a PwD. An elder of 75 years old acted as if she suffered from mild dementia. She was trained with typical behaviours such as: mumbling, screaming, wandering, repetitive questioning, among others. She was already familiar with these behaviours from acquaintances that suffer from dementia. The participants were told that they would be working with a person who actually suffers from dementia. Also, the real goal of the experiment was not revealed. Instead, they were told that we were evaluating their performance as caregivers based on the initial training provided.

Written consent was obtained from all participants before the first session and a non disclosure agreement was also signed to avoid the participants to talk to each other about the experiment, the behaviours of the elder or any techniques on how to handle the elder's behaviour, for as long as the experiment lasted.

3.1 Subjects

The subjects were recruited by sending an email to the University's graduate students. A compensation of two movie theater tickets was offered, although many of them expressed interest in participating in spite of the prize. Participants were asked to participate in 3 sessions (one per week), each one requiring approximately 90 min of their time.

Participants consisted of 10 graduate students (5 male, 5 female) with an average age of 24.7 (st dev. = 1.0593). Table 1 shows demographic data from the participants.

Table 1. Participants in the study.

Subject	Gender	Age	Caring experience
S1	Male	24	No
S2	Male	25	No
S3	Female	24	No
S4	Female	26	No
S5	Female	24	No
S6	Male	26	No
S7	Male	23	No
S8	Male	25	Yes
S9	Female	26	No
S10	Female	24	Yes

3.2 Training

All subjects participated in training session to familiarize them with the cognitive therapies they were going to be asked to apply in the sessions with the older adult. The training session lasted approximately 90 min, and all participants practised the therapies and had a chance to ask questions. They were not given any strategies on how to cope with problematic behaviours from the older adult. Participants were told that the older adult had mild cognitive decline and could exhibit some behavioural problems such as forgetting recent instructions, apathy, unwillingness to complete the task, etc. They were told that the tasks did not have to be completed if the older adult was not cooperating, but that they should try to complete the therapy if possible. They were told that they were able to withdraw at any time of the session. None of the participants stopped the session. We also show them how to fill the auto report form. Finally we asked them to sign the consent form.

3.3   Therapy Tasks

Before beginning the task, we equipped participants with an electrical pulse reader (Zephyr Hxm) on the chest to monitor heart rate/Inter-beat Interval, an Empatica E3 wristband to get Galvanic Skin Response data and a Muse band EEG monitor. All sessions were videotaped for further analysis.

For five minutes, and once instrumented, the subjects relaxed by concentrating on their own breathing with eyes closed to obtain baseline physiological data. Participants were asked to guide the older adult through a therapy session which involved two of the 8 tasks that were explained during the training session. Table 2 presents these tasks performed by each participant in the three sessions of the study.

Table 2. Therapies performed with the older adult by each participant.

Participant	Therapy 1	Therapy 2	Therapy 3
S1	Lace tying	Memory puzzle	Image classification
S2	Image classification	Lace tying	Words puzzle
S3	Words formation	Words puzzle	Memory puzzle
S4	Lace tying	Image classification	Memory puzzle
S5	Image classification	Lace tying	Words puzzle
S6	Objects separation	Memory puzzle	Lace tying
S7	Objects separation	Lace tying	Words puzzle
S8	Words puzzle	Lace tying	Image classification
S9	Words formation	Image classification	Memory puzzle
S10	Memory puzzle	Words formation	Lace tying

The whole intervention lasted 15 days, each participant conducted a therapy with the older adult lasting approximately 30 min. Each day two participants assisted to the site.

Each participant assisted to three sessions. For each session, one or two tasks were made, with several iterations in each task. To avoid acclimatization none of the therapies were repeated by participants. Also, none of the participants assisted with the same partner more than once.

We divided the experiment in three weeks. Each subject participated once every week. We couched the older adult to enact different anxiety events. First week, she acted levels from 0 to 2. In the second and third week, she acted levels from 0 to 3. In the last week, we trained the participants to use coping strategies such as breathing exercises and task disengagement. However, none of the participants used them.

3.4   Setup

We setted a room inside a real house to make it look as if a person with dementia lived there. The customs included: old furniture, low illumination, old pictures and paper hint tags over the hand washer. A wooden table was used to install the equipment: A Macbook, a Video Camera, and a smartphone to monitor the experiment.

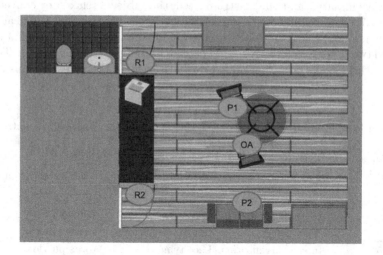

Fig. 3. Experimental setup. The therapy activities were conducted on a table, with the PwD (OA) and the participant (P1) sitting facing each other. The second participant (P2) observed from the coach, while two researchers (R1,R2) monitored the session from a nearby table.

Two researchers stood at the wooden table to operate the equipment and take notes. We sat both the participant and the elder face to face in a circular table. We asked the participants to use the bathroom to wear the Zephyr band since it is worn under the clothes. A second participant sat on a couch and we asked him to observe the session. This participant was also being monitored with a single empatica e3 wristband.

3.5   Data Gathering

We developed two separate applications for the Empatica E3 sensor and the Zephyr HxM band. For the first device, we developed the "Care Me Too" application for Android which connects to the E3 device via Bluetooth Low Energy, displays the data in real time and saves it in .csv format. This application also can help to tag the events with user input, making it useful for naturalistic studies.

For the Zephyr HxM program, we used the anxiLogger command line program (https://github.com/panzerfausten/anxiLogger) developed for an earlier study [5]. The output .csv file was then appended to the Care Me Too session data for timestamp synchronization via a python library called "maxiProcesser". (https://github.com/panzerfausten/maxiProcesser)

For the Muse band we used the provided Muse lab desktop application. The data was saved in a .muse binary file and then exported to .csv plain text for further analysis.

We used a macbook laptop in site to connect the Zephyr and muse devices, and a Samsung galaxy S4 for the E3 wristband to collect the data. Additional data of the observer participant was also gathered. We did this by using a second Empatica E3 device in record mode which requires no additional bluetooth connection.

4   Data Analysis and Initial Results

All videos from the sessions were analysed to segment the events of interest, namely, when the older adult enacted a behaviour that could induce anxiety on the subject. For instance, in one case the older adult, while engaged in the therapy asks the subject: *"Where is my mother?"*. These segments where classified as one of three possible levels meeting our criteria (See Table 3). Then,

Table 3. Event tagging criteria.

Level	Criteria	Event example
0	PwD is passive, PwD is willing to participate, Participant and PwD engaged with the task.	The PwD performs the activity as requested
1	Reluctant behaviours, Unwilling to participate, Complaining about the task.	"I don t like this game" "This is too hard" "Do it your self"
2	Mumbling, Talking nonsense, Unpredictable behaviour.	"Where is my mother?" "Who are you?"
3	Shouting. Threatening the participant, Paranoia, Urge to leave	"MOTHER, WHERE ARE YOU!!??" "I WANT TO LEAVE NOW!" "WHO ARE YOU? LET ME GO!"

we took a window of the corresponding GSR and IBI data and processed them individually.

4.1 GSR Pre-processing

We developed a python library to process all the physiological data, including export, feature extraction, timestamp synchronization, and plotting anxiety data from all the devices. We started by down-sampling the GSR data from 4.0 Hz to 1.0 Hz by calculating the average value of all the data falling into each 1 s window. This due we expected the anxiety spans to last seconds. Then, we applied a Gaussian filter to smooth the signal and reduce noise. Finally, we used a python scipy method to detect peaks and filtered all the peaks greater to a threshold (t >= 0.04 for not normalized data). We also calculated the "Half Recovery Time" of the signal. That is, the point where the signals fall into the exact half of the peak value. This library also plots the data and can export the GSR signal attributes (peaks, half recovery time, amplitude...) into .csv and .json files which can be used for application purposes.

4.2 HR and IBI Pre-processing

Heart rate and Inter-beat Interval (IBI) data was not necessary to down sample because of the nature of the signal. The sensor only reports data when the heart beat happens. However, we did group it in windows of one seconds to compare it with the rest of the signals. The data noise was very low and it required no extra pre processing.

4.3 Video Processing

All the videos were transcribed with the f4 transcription program for Mac Os X. Then, we generated video subtitles by taking the transcript timings and exporting them with a custom python script to a SubRip format (.srt) for ease of analysis.

4.4 Data Segmentation

In order to obtain ground truth, two researchers coded the sessions live, by taking note of time, level of perceived anxiety, and a description of the event. This description was noted by either what the participant and/or the elder said or did at the moment. The participants also had a paper form to indicate their anxiety level after completing each iteration of the task, they were also asked to report the time when an iteration was initiated and completed. However, many of them found it difficult to report it, mainly because they were engaged with the activity.

Finally, we segmented each session in 30 s segments and labelled them as "No anxiety" and "Anxiety". A third label "ambiguous" was used when the data was not enough to discriminate the presence of anxiety. To determinate the label we used the observation data, auto report and the recorded video. For the video we used an heuristic of the subject movements, voice tone and eye gaze. Once we tagged the segments with a perceived level of anxiety, we plotted the corresponding segment of all the signals for visual interpretation and feature extraction.

4.5   Initial Results

One of the main reasons in this paper was to induce anxiety and obtain an physiological response. Taking as example the GSR data of the second session of the participant 7 (Fig. 4) we can see an initial relaxation span from the seconds 0–200. During this period, the participant did not receive any stimulation from the person with dementia.

[h!]

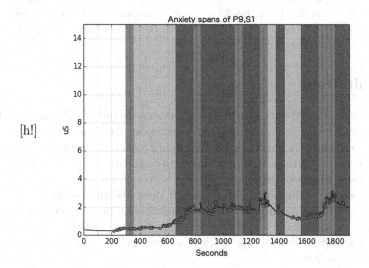

Fig. 4. Obtained anxiety spans. Red sections indicate the anxious spans, green not anxious spans, and gray ambiguous spans.

Some seconds later, the PwD enters the room and is introduced to the participant. During this period (seconds 200–300) we can see slight changes in his/her GSR level. From second 350 until 650 the signal increases within a moderate range. One reason to this might be that the person did not receive any strong stimulation which matches with the reported anxiety levels and labelled as non anxious. We can see some immediately increases when the anxiety periods start as recorded around seconds 620 and 830. If we see the observation data, a level 2 PwD action is reported around second 602. The portion of the correspondent transcript says: *"PwD: Hey.. Do you know where is my mother?" "Participant: Huh.. no." "PwD: I want to go with her now"*. This gives us hints that there is a relation between the stimulation we used and the physiological response.

We also conducted a preliminary classification test using SVM with the "python-scikit" tool. We used data only from subjects 1,6,8,9 and 7. For each subject we used his/her data as testing and the remaining 4 participants as training. We used the maximum, minimum, variance, averages and half-recovery times of the peaks amplitudes in the 30 s segment for the GSR signal and the maximum, minimum, average and standard deviation in the IBI signal as input features. A total of 212 positives and 212 negatives samples was available. We obtained an average of 71.81 % and 66.71 % of precision and recall respectively using a polynomial kernel.

One of the main differences with this experiment is the way the participant is exposed to the stimulation. In the laboratory experiments, the participant is in a controlled environment. The stimulation is controlled by exact frequencies and intensities. This gives a cleaner, easier to interpret physiological signals. In this experiment, by having a naturalistic enactment situation, we obtain a noisier, harder to interpret signal. For example, in a laboratory experiment, the GSR signals starts at a low level, peaks at an stimulation and then decreases to the original level by having a relaxation span. In this experiment, the signal almost never decreases to the original value.

5   Limitations

Although we gathered data from different devices, we only used two physiological signals to conduct tests and visual interpretation. Anxiety detection is a hard problem, and becomes harder in naturalistic situations. Ground truth gathering is a time consuming task when working with cognitive states. It took us 10 h of work for each 30 min of data.

The relationship between caregiver and person with dementia is also complex. In this paper we conducted an experiment with persons with no emotional attachment or long history to the person with dementia. Although the real situations might differ from the results exposed, we showed an initial way to gather data from caregivers.

Further anxiety detection methods are also needed. Although we obtained a considerable precision and recall score, more adequate methods shall be explored to obtain a more precise detection. A test with the complete dataset should consider similarities among the subjects to obtain a higher score.

6   Conclusions

Caregivers needs are usually ignored and not well understood. Although anxiety problems are generally suffered in the long term, caregivers could benefit from detection and remedial actions, lowering the emotional burden and improving their quality live.

In this study, we conducted a naturalistic enactment experiment to induce and detect anxiety states making use of wearable technology. We proposed a method for obtaining ground truth in a NE environment trough self-report, observation and video codification. Our initial results indicate that the analysis of physiological signals can be used to detect increased anxiety on the caregiver by using a machine learning approach. Once these anxiety episodes are detected, the caregiver can be made aware of them and appropriate actions can be recommended to deal with this, such as deep breathing or making the caregiver aware of the condition of the PwD.

References

1. Castro, L.A., Favela, J., García-Peña, C.: Naturalistic enactment to stimulate user experience for the evaluation of a mobile elderly care application. In: Proceedings of the 13th International Conference on Human Computer Interaction with Mobile Devices and Services, MobileHCI 2011, pp. 371–380. ACM, New York (2011)
2. Cooper, C., Katona, C., Orrell, M., Livingston, G.: Coping strategies and anxiety in caregivers of people with alzheimer's disease: the laser-ad study. J. Affect. Disord. **90**(1), 15–20 (2006). http://www.sciencedirect.com/science/article/pii/S0165032705003034
3. Joling, K.J., van Marwijk, H.W., Veldhuijzen, A.E., van der Horst, H.E., Scheltens, P., Smit, F., van Hout, H.P.: The two-year incidence of depression and anxiety disorders in spousal caregivers of persons with dementia: who is at the greatest risk? Am. J. Geriatr. Psychiatry **23**(3), 293–303 (2015)
4. Julian, L.J.: Measures of anxiety. Arthritis Care Res. **63**(0 11), S467–S472 (2011). doi:10.1002/acr.20561
5. Miranda, D., Calderón, M., Favela, J.: Anxiety detection using wearable monitoring. In: Proceedings of the 5th Mexican Conference on Human-Computer Interaction, MexIHC 2014, pp. 34:34–34:41. ACM, New York (2014). http://doi.acm.org/10.1145/2676690.2676694
6. Navarro, R., Rodriguez, M., Favela, J.: Intervention tailoring in augmented cognition systems for elders with dementia. IEEE J. Biomed. Health Inf. **18**(1), 361–367 (2014)
7. Ory, M.G., Hoffman, R.R., Yee, J.L., Tennstedt, S., Schulz, R.: Prevalence and impact of caregiving: a detailed comparison between dementia and nondementia caregivers. Gerontologist **39**(2), 177–186 (1999)
8. Prince, M., Bryce, R., Albanese, E., Wimo, A., Ribeiro, W., Ferri, C.P.: The global prevalence of dementia: a systematic review and metaanalysis. Alzheimer's Dement. J. Alzheimer's Assoc. **9**(1), 63–75.e2 (2015)
9. Sadowsky, C.H., Galvin, J.E.: Guidelines for the management of cognitive and behavioral problems in dementia. J. Am. Board Fam. Med. **25**(3), 350–366 (2012)
10. Schulz, R., Beach, S.R.: Caregiving as a risk factor for mortality: the caregiver health effects study. Jama **282**(23), 2215–2219 (1999)
11. Sturm, V.E., Yokoyama, J.S., Seeley, W.W., Kramer, J.H., Miller, B.L., Rankin, K.P.: Heightened emotional contagion in mild cognitive impairment and alzheimer's disease is associated with temporal lobe degeneration. Proc. Nat. Acad. Sci. **110**(24), 9944–9949 (2013)
12. Tutar, H., Cankurtaran, E., Tekin, P., Caykoylu, A.: The relationship between coping strategies and caregiver burden in caregivers of people with alzheimer's dementia. Alzheimer's and Dementia 9(4, Supplement), P484 (2013). http://www.sciencedirect.com/science/article/pii/S1552526013016452, alzheimers Association International Conference 2013 Alzheimers Association International Conference 2013

Mass Segmentation in Digital Mammograms

María Victoria Carreras-Cruz[(✉)],
María de Lourdes Martínez-Villaseñor,
and Kevin Nataniel Rosas-Pérez

Universidad Panamericana Campus México, Augusto Rodin 498,
Col. Insurgentes-Mixcoac, México, DF, Mexico
{mvcruz,lmartine}@up.edu.mx

Abstract. Digital mammograms are among the most difficult medical images to read, because of the differences in the types of tissues and their low contrasts. This paper proposes a computer aided diagnostic system for mammographic mass detection that can distinguish between tumorous and healthy tissue among various parenchymal tissue patterns. This method consists in extraction of regions of interest, noise elimination, global contrast improvement, combined segmentation, and rule-based classification. The evaluation of the proposed methodology is carried out on Mammography Image Analysis Society (MIAS) dataset. The achieved results increased the detection accuracy of the lesions and reduced the number of false diagnoses of mammograms.

Keywords: Mammogram enhancement · Mammogram segmentation · Breast mass detection · Image classification

1 Introduction

Breast cancer appears more frequently and in increasingly earlier stages of life. Early detection is the most effective way to face breast cancer, and mammogram (breast X-ray) is considered the most reliable method to achieve it [1]. Unfortunately, breast cancer is frequently missed on mammograms due to the difficulty of interpretation and inconsistency in reading. Statistics shows that only 20–30 % of breast biopsies are proved cancerous [2], and 10 % of all cases of breast cancer go undetected by mammography [3]. Moreover, digital mammograms are among the most difficult medical images to read, because of the differences in types of tissues and their low contrasts. Among the various types of breast abnormalities that are visible in mammograms, clustered microcalcifications, mass lesions, distortion in breast architecture and asymmetry between breasts are the most important ones [4]. The mass lesions associated with early breast cancer can be circumscribed or spiculated (stellate) [4]. Circumscribed mass lesions are round with smooth, sharply defined margin, while the spiculated masses have the shape of a star with undefined and irregular borders. At the early stages of breast cancer, these signs are difficult for specialists. Computer-aided diagnoses (CAD) that analyze mammograms assists medical staffs to achieve high efficiency and accuracy, avoiding high costs of double reading by experts [5]. Conventional enhancement techniques, region-based enhancement techniques, feature-based enhancement techniques, and fuzzy enhancement techniques are used to enhance mammogram images. The mammograms image

© Springer International Publishing Switzerland 2015
J. Bravo et al. (Eds.): AmIHEALTH 2015, LNCS 9456, pp. 110–115, 2015.
DOI: 10.1007/978-3-319-26508-7_11

segmentation includes breast regions segmentations, and regions of interest segmentation using single and multiple views [3].

This paper presents a computer aided diagnostic process for mammographic mass detection which is part of an on-going project [6–8]. This method can classify between tumours and healthy tissue among various parenchymal tissue patterns. The major contribution of process is the preservation of the original grey levels, shape, size and localization of possible tumours mass. Algorithms currently used only edge the region of interest with a triangle or rectangle without highlighting the shape, size and texture of the possible tumor mass. The preservation of these characteristics transmits relevant information for the radiologist and pathologist improving the accuracy of clinical diagnosis. It also helps the oncologist and surgeon to apply more effective and specific treatment that improves the patient's prognosis.

In the next section, a detailed description of the proposed method is given. In Sect. 3 data set and our experimental results are presented. Finally, in the last section, we draw our conclusions.

2 Process for Mammographic Mass Detection

The proposed process is divided in five stages: extraction of regions of interest, noise elimination, global contrast improvement, combined segmentation, and rule-based classification.

Regions of Interest Extraction Stage. Mammograms contain unnecessary information that should be removed before proceeding with the image processing. This stage consists of two main phases. The first phase involves the removal of background information and unwanted parts from the image, like the occluded tissue by the arm. The second phase is about detecting and eliminating microcalcifications using a well-known method [10].

- **Removal of background information.** The images of the MIAS datasets are 1024 × 1024 pixels, and almost 50 % of the whole image comprised a noisy background, (Fig. 1(a)). The automatic cut starts calculating a global threshold to convert a grayscale image into a binarized image using Otsu's method [11] (Fig. 1 (b)).
- **Elimination of tissue occluded by the arm**. Points which delimit the area to be removed are detected in order to determine an equation to describe a borderline using least square regression method obtaining a linear polynomial, (Fig. 1(c)).
- **Detection and removal of microcalcifications**. A well-known method is used to detect and eliminate microcalcifications [10]. It includes the Top-Hat morphological process [12] and code for Sobel [13] and Canny edge detection [14] (Fig. 1(d)).

Noise Elimination. The noise is eliminated using a 3 × 3 median filter [15] (Fig. 1(e)).

Improvement of Global Contrast. Mammograms are difficult images to interpret, so in order to improve the quality of images, it is necessary to enhance the contrast of the image. The gray scale is modified based on the cubic function, Eq. 2, where: P (i, j)

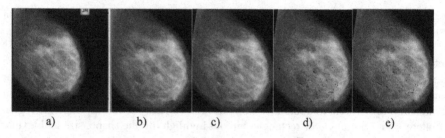

Fig. 1. Mammogram with mass, (a) Original (b) Removal of background information, (c) Elimination of tissue occluded by the arm, (d) Elimination of microcalcifications (e) Noise elimination.

corresponds to the pixels of the original image, P1(i, j) is the transformed image, M is the maximum gray value of the pixels of noise-eliminated image, and f is the brightener factor which varies depending on the average of gray intensity of the same image:

$$M = \max(P(i,j)) \tag{1}$$

$$P1(i,j) = round(\frac{P(i,j)^3}{f * M^2}) \tag{2}$$

This process is made with the purpose of increasing the difference between the darkness and brightness pixels, giving more relevance to the skylights, (Fig. 2(a)).

Combined Segmentation. A new image is generated combining the resulting image of thresholding process using the maximum of the image without noise (Fig. 2(b)), with the resulting image of the application of Sobel edge detector operator (Fig. 2(c)). Any pixel that appears in either of the two images is taken into account (Fig. 2(d)). Next, preservation of the form is done by iteratively filling the shape (Fig. 2(e)). In this process, if a pixel exists in correspondence to the detected edges of Sobel mask that is in the neighborhood V8 of a matching pixel in the binarized image, it is added to the image. Finally, a process of global thresholding is performed to remove spurious pixels.

$$circularity = \frac{I}{A} \tag{3}$$

Where I = number of pixels at a distance less or equal to the radio from the centroid.

Rule-Based Classification First of all, feature extraction is done. The extracted features from each of the resultant regions are: area (A), proportional area (A/total area of mammary tissue), eccentricity (the ratio of the distance between the two foci of the ellipses and the length of the major axis), circularity (Eq. 3) [16]. These rules were generated based on the experience of mammographic interpretation.

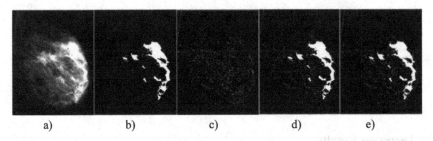

a)   b)   c)   d)   e)

Fig. 2. (a) Improvement of global contrast (b) thresholding image, (c) Sobel edge detector operator (d) combined image (e) iteratively filling.

Next, the suspicious mass candidates are determined with the following IF-THEN rules:

1. if A > 150 pixels and A < 69000 pixels and
   eccentricity > 0.2 and eccentricity < 0.9 and
   circularity >=0.81 and
   proportional area > 0.00075 and proportional area < 0.04
   then it is a region of interest
2. if more than two possible regions of interest appear, then two
   with greater circularity are chosen

The labeled elements, (Fig. 3(a)), are superimposed over the original image extracted candidates for tumorous masses segmentation, maintaining its original grey levels, and also the shape, size and localization, (Fig. 3(b)).

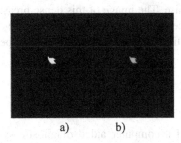

a)   b)

Fig. 3. (a) Labeled elements, (b) Original image extraction of candidates for tumorous masses segmentation.

3 Experimental Results and Discussion

The MIAS Database [9] provided by the Mammography Image Analysis Society was used in our experiments. Data were divided in three sets for our experiments: training set, test set and validation set (Table 1).

Table 1. Distribution of selected cases

Tipo	Training set	Test set	Validation set	Total
Circumscribed	11	11	0	22
Spiculated	9	9	0	18
Normal	0	0	209	209
Total	20	20	209	249

3.1   Detection Results

Rule-based classification was applied to the images of the database MIAS. Table 2 shows the detection results: number of tumorous masses, true positives (TP), true negatives (TN), false positives (FP), false negatives (FN), sensitivity, and specificity.

Table 2. Detection results

Type	Mammograms	Mass	TP	TN	FP	F N	Sensitivity	Specificity
Circumscribed	22	23	21	0	4	2	**0.91**	
Spiculated	18	18	13	0	6	5	**0.88**	
Normal	209	0	0	144	85	0		**0.63**

Two medium benign circumscribed masses were missed over adipose tissue; two medium benign spiculated masses went unnoticed over adipose tissue; one medium benign spiculated mass was ignored as it was standing over adipose and glandular tissue; one medium benign spiculated mass was missed over dense tissue, and a big malign spiculated mass went unnoticed over dense tissue.

In summary, a malign mass was missed because it was located in the breast with the densest tissue of the data base. The image of this dense breast tissue does not meet the minimum contrast difference required by our algorithm. The other missed masses were benign. The resulting sensitivity was of 0.91 for circumscribed masses and of 0.88 for spiculated masses.

4   Conclusions

In this paper we presented a computer aided diagnostic system for mammographic mass detection. This method can distinguish between tumours and healthy tissue among various parenchymal tissue patterns. It involves extraction of regions of interest, noise elimination, and improvement of global contrast, combined segmentation, and rule-based classification. Image segmentation, filtering, contrast enhanced and gray level thresholding techniques are applied for enhancing the image. Features are extracted from the resultant image. The evaluation of the system is carried out on Mammography Image Analysis Society (MIAS) dataset.

The achieved results are promising, so we continue working towards increasing the detection accuracy of the lesions and reducing the number of false diagnoses of mammograms. In our ongoing project, we are experimenting with an image database of mammograms provided by a Mexican private institution dedicated to mammographic study.

References

1. National Cancer Institute: National Cancer Institute FactSheet. http://www.cancer.gov/cancertopics/factsheet/detection/mammograms. Accessed 25 May 2015 (2014)
2. Zaïane, O.R., Antonie, M-L., Coman, A.: Mammography classification by an association rule-based classifier. In: Third International Workshop on Multimedia Data Mining and ACM SIGKDD Conference, pp. 62–69. Edmonton, Alberta, Canada (2002)
3. Kumar, N.H., Amutha, S., Babu, D.R.R.: Enhancement of mammographic images using morphology and wavelet transform. Int. J. Comput. Technol. Appl. **3**, 192–198 (2013)
4. Tabar, L., Dean, P.: Teaching Atlas of Mammography, 4th edn., p. 326. Thieme, Stuttgart (2012)
5. Onega, T., Smith, M., Miglioretti, D.L., et al.: Radiologist agreement for mammographic recall by case difficulty and finding type. J. Am. Coll. Radiol. **9**, 788–794 (2012). doi:10.1016/j.jacr.2012.05.020
6. Carreras-Cruz, M.V.: Segmentación automática de masas tumorales sobre tejido blando en imágenes radiológicas (SATBIR) utilizando técnicas de análisis de imágenes. Una aplicación para mamografías. Ph.D. Dissertation. Intituto Tecnológico y de Estudios Superiores de Monterrey (2007)
7. Carreras-Cruz, M.V.: Procesamiento e interpretación automatizada de imágenes, apoyada en la segmentación y equipo para llevar a cabo este procedimiento. Mexican Patent MX/a/2008/007657. Instituto Mexicano de la Propiedad Industrial (IMPI), filed 12 June 2008, issued March 2013 (2013)
8. Carreras-Cruz, M.V, Rayón-Vilella, P.: Circumscribed mass detection in digital mammograms. In: Proceeding CERMA 2006, Proceedings of the Electronics, Robotics and Automotive Mechanics Conference, vol. 1, pp. 19–24. IEEE Computer Society, Washington, DC, USA (2006)
9. Suckling, J., Parker, J., Dance, D., et al.: The mammographic image analysis society digital mammogram database. In: 2nd International Workshop on Digital Mammography (1994)
10. Fu, J.C., Lee, S.K., Wong, S.T.C., et al.: Image segmentation feature selection and pattern classification for mammographic microcalcifications. Comput. Med. Imaging Graph. **29**, 419–429 (2005)
11. Otsu, N.: A threshold selection method from gray-level histograms. IEEE Trans. Syst. Man Cybern. **9**, 62–66 (1979)
12. Beuche, S.: Segmentation d'images et morphologie mathématique, vol. 294 (1991)
13. Umbaugh, S.E.: Digital Imaging Processing and Analysis: Human and Computer Vision Applications With CVIPtools, 2nd edn., p. 956. CRC Press, Taylor & Francis Group, Boca Raton, FL (2011)
14. Canny, J.: A computational approach to edge detection. IEEE Trans. Pattern Anal. Mach. Intell. **PAMI-8**, 679–698 (1986)
15. Jain, R., Kasturi, R., Schunck, B.G.: Machine Vision. McGraw Hill Higher Education, p 549 (1995). ISBN-10: 00070320187
16. Miller, V.C.: A quantitative geomorphic study of drainage basin characteristics in Clinch Mt area Virginia and Tennessee. New York, USA (1953)

Comparison of a Vision-Based System and a Wearable Inertial-Based System for a Quantitative Analysis and Calculation of Spatio-Temporal Parameters

Irvin Hussein López-Nava[1] (✉), Iván González[2], Angélica Muñoz-Meléndez[2], and José Bravo[2]

[1] Instituto Nacional de Astrofísica, Óptica y Electrónica, 72840 Puebla, Mexico
hussein@ccc.inaoep.mx
[2] Universidad Castilla La Mancha, 13071 Ciudad Real, Spain

Abstract. Clinical gait analysis provides an evaluation tool that allows clinicians to assess the abnormality of gait in patients. There are currently specialized systems to detect gait events and calculate spatio-temporal parameters of human gait, which are accurate and redundant. These systems are expensive and are limited to very controlled settings. As alternative, a wearable inertial system and a single depth-camera system are proposed in order to detect gait events, and then, estimate spatial and temporal gait parameters. An experimental protocol is detailed in this paper using both systems in order to compare their performance with respect to a specialized human gait system for two age groups, elder and youth. This research attempts to contribute to the development of clinical decision support technologies by combining vision systems and wearable sensors.

Keywords: Gait analysis · Gait events · Spatio-temporal gait parameters · Vision system · Inertial sensors

1 Introduction

Clinical gait analysis involves the measurement, description, and assessment of quantities that characterize human locomotion [1]. This type of analysis provides an evaluation tool that allows the clinician to assess the abnormality of gait in patients with movement disorders [2]. Gait disorder is a typical symptom of Parkinson's disease which usually leads to immobility, and may reflect early warning signs of dementia, Alzheimer's disease, pathological changes and fear of falling [3]. Patients' gait patterns with gait disorder are characterized by a short-step gait, reduced velocity, asymmetry gait, and an increase of cadence [4].

Gait is defined as a cyclic movement of the feet in which one or the other alternate in contact with the ground [5], and it can be decomposed into gait cycles, see Fig. 1(a). In normal symmetrical gait, toe-off (TO) occurs at about

© Springer International Publishing Switzerland 2015
J. Bravo et al. (Eds.): AmIHEALTH 2015, LNCS 9456, pp. 116–122, 2015.
DOI: 10.1007/978-3-319-26508-7_12

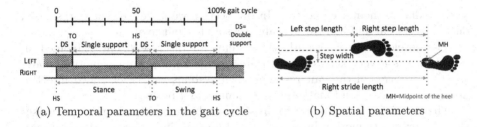

(a) Temporal parameters in the gait cycle   (b) Spatial parameters

Fig. 1. Spatio-temporal gait parameters

60–62% of gait cycle, dividing the cycle into stance (when the foot is on the ground) and swing phases (when the foot leaves the ground) [6]. The stance phase begins with a heel strike (HS), and can be subdivided into the single support and double support phases. TO and HS events, referred to as gait events (GEs) determine the gait phases. The correct timing of the GEs must be measured for the estimation of spatio-temporal gait parameters (S-TGPs) as shown in Fig. 1.

Measurements of the S-TGPs are particularly used to identify gait deviations, make diagnoses, determine appropriate therapy and monitor patient progress. [7]. Traditional diagnosis of many gait disorders involves human observation of the posture and movement of the gait. These human observations tend to be subjective and depend on the experience and judgement of the clinician, which can vary from person to person [8]. Gait analysis technology, that includes specialized systems for 2D or 3D motion capture and tracking, tactile ground surface indicators, and magnetic/inertial sensors, can help to the clinician to get objective measures.

In this work, two systems for estimation of GEs and S-TGPs are presented and compared. Also, an experimental protocol and measures to evaluate the performance of both systems, depth camera system and wearable inertial system, with respect to a reference system is detailed. Unfortunately and as far as we know, the accuracy and performance between these types of technologies, and of these technologies with respect to reference instruments are issues that have been poorly investigated. This research aims at contributing to this analysis.

The rest of the paper is organized as follows. Section 2 addresses related work. Sections 3 and 4 present the proposed systems to measure GEs and S-TGPs. Section 5 gives details about the experimental protocol. Finally, Sect. 6 closes with concluding remarks about the challenges and opportunities of the study.

2   Related Work

Gait analysis is performed using technology such as video cameras, electromagnetic or inertial sensors, force platforms, among others. It is worth to mention that there exist highly specialized systems for estimating GEs and S-TGPs of human gait, such as Vicon motion capture system (Vicon Motion Systems Ltd., Oxford, UK). However, these systems are not typically available in clinical settings due to their size and cost. In this section we review recent works based on vision system and inertial wearable sensors for gait analysis.

The development of vision-based systems for the assessment of biomedical parameters is a very active research area in the field of human motion analysis [10]. In terms of the gait research, such systems can be classified into two approaches: marker and markerless, as summarized below.

The use of markers attached to the subject's body boosts accuracy and makes the measurements more robust during motion tracking, however these systems are more invasive than the markerless ones. Regarding marker-less video-based systems for the estimation of S-TGPs, in [11,12] several feature extraction procedures from human silhouettes have been used for gait recognition. These studies combine different techniques over two-dimensional contours to compute dissimilarity scores with respect to a set of reference human gait phase silhouettes, such as Fourier descriptor extraction, histogram matching, and dynamic time warping (DTW), among others. Furthermore, markerless systems can adopt a tridimensional approach by extracting silhouettes of the subject from multiple calibrated cameras [13] or from a single depth camera [14], and projecting them to a discretized volume space to compose a 3-D point cloud, which is useful for fitting a skeletal model [13] or for extracting footfalls [15] from the low part of the body.

The works based on wearable inertial systems can be divided according to the anatomical reference used to set the sensors since this configuration determines the set of parameters that can be calculated. The more significant works of this family are summarized below.

In [16] a single-accelerometer sensor was placed on the lower back at the level of vertebra L2-L4 in order to estimate step length of older persons. The authors use an inverted pendulum model of human walking to estimate the spatial gait parameter. In [9] two inertial sensors were attached at the midpoint of each shank to measure angular velocity of subjects with stroke. The authors detect gait events based on a pendulum walking model. In [17] an inertial measurement unit (IMU) was installed on the forefoot over the bases of first and second metatarsals. GEs of healthy subjects and patients with different degrees of ankle disease were detected based on kinematic features. In [18] eight IMUs, 3D accelerometers and 2D gyroscopes were placed on the arms, forearms, thighs and shanks of youth subjects for detecting gait parameters. The authors introduced a method for temporal gait parameter extraction based on hidden Markov models.

Two low-cost systems are presented and compared in this study. A vision-based markerless system composed by a single depth camera, and a wearable inertial system comprising two inertial sensors. The proposed systems will be used to estimate GEs and S-TPs of elder and youth subjects under controlled conditions, and will be compared with respect to a specialized system used as ground truth.

3   Depth Camera System

For the experiment conducted the depth sensor of a Kinect device (Microsoft Corporation, WA, USA) will be used. The Kinect will be specifically positioned

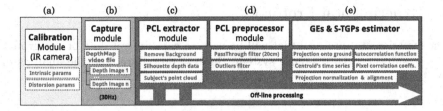

Fig. 2. Overview vision system.

in the laboratory environment to capture the test subjects' frontal view during the gait trials. An overview of the proposed algorithm for extracting GEs and S-TPs is shown in Fig. 2. First, to get accurate real-world distances from the Kinect depth data a calibration process is required. Then, the `Capture` module (Fig. 2(b)) is ready for recording depth images of walking sequences at 30 Hz. All subsequent processing from depthmaps to subject's point clouds (PCLs) is made off-line by the `PCL extractor` module to avoid frame rate slowdown (Fig. 2(c)). The `PCL extractor` performs background subtraction to get subject's silhouette directly from depth images in each frame. Then, subject's PCL can be reconstructed using the silhouette's depth data. In the next stage the `PCL preprocessor` (Fig. 2(d)) applies some filtering procedures to cut off points from the subject's PCL that are below 20 cm and correspond to shanks and feet (PassThrough filtering) and remove noisy measurements (Outliers filtering) from the segmented PCL. The preprocessed PCL feeds the `GEs & S-TGPs estimator` (Fig. 2(e)) where it is projected onto de ground plane, and its centroid is calculated. Additionally, the projected PCL from each frame is normalized and aligned using an estimation of the gait direction. The autocorrelation function of normalized centroids' time series and a pixel correlation coefficient from the normalized projections over frames are used to compute GEs and S-TPs.

4   Wearable Inertial System

The second approach for measuring human gait is based on a wearable inertial system. Two IMUs to be placed on the lower limbs, as is explained in Sect. 5 are used in this part. Periodic temporal patterns that occur in typical human gait can be captured by accelerometers. Raw acceleration signals are processed in order to obtain gait patterns from characteristic peaks related to steps. The characteristic peaks detection is based on a probabilistic method, `Bayesian models`, and are implemented to classify the characteristic peaks into steps or non-steps. The `models` can be trained previously using gait data from real people during controlled tests, such as elders. The acceleration signals, X-axis and Z-axis, are segmented based on GEs of actual steps correctly classified, see Fig. 3 for explanation of coordinated system of the inertial sensors. Finally, temporal gait parameters are estimated from `segmented acceleration signals`. In [19] a complete description of this approach is detailed.

5   Experimental Protocol

The experimental protocol that will be used to capture gait data of two groups of test subjects, the reference system, the test procedure, and the analysis of results, are presented below.

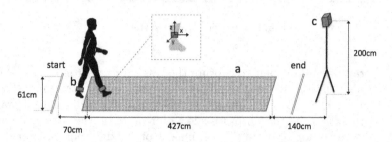

Fig. 3. General scheme for the tests: (a) GAITRite system, (b) Wearable inertial system, and (c) Depth camera system.

Test Subjects. Proposed systems will be evaluated with test subjects of two groups of age, elders (60–80 years) and youths (20–35 years). Participants do not have gait disorders or known limitation that prevents comply with the protocol.

Reference System. The GAITRite (CIR Systems Inc., PA, USA) is a gait analysis tool for automated measurement of S-TGPs. The GAITRite system contains seven sensor pads encapsulated in a roll up carpet to produce an active area 61 cm wide and 427 cm long. This system provides the gait parameters that have been detailed in Fig. 1. The setup of the reference system, with respect to the proposed systems, is showed in Fig. 3.

Procedure. Prior to the tests, participants will be asked to complete an informed consent form. Then, height, weight and length of legs of each participant will be registered. The tests will be carried out without shoes to record the direct contact of the foot during walking. The Kinect will be located at 140 cm past the GAITRite with a height of 200 cm. The sensor units will be placed 10 cm above the external (lateral) malleolus of both lower limbs of the participants, and must to be aligned with the sagittal plane of the participants body according the standard anatomical position. "Start" and "stop" lines will be placed 70 cm in front of and past the GAITRite to ensure the participants will walk at their comfortable speed when they will reach the electronic walkway and they did not decelerate before the recording area. Participants will be asked to look at a visual target placed at eye level in front of the gait direction to minimize distractions that might affect the natural gait. Each participant will walk across the GAITRite with the sensors placed on their ankles five times; the first and last will be trials with no data collected. Each repetition will be referred as a single session.

Analysis of Results. After data processing of both approaches, the results will be compared with respect to the reference values of the output reports of the GAITRite. The assessment will be divided into two phases. The first one consists in evaluating the number of gait events (GEs) detected by each approach. The second consists in evaluating the spatio-temporal gait parameters estimated by each approach. Then, a statistical analysis will be applied to compare both approaches. The number of GEs detected by each method will be counted. Any falsely detected GE will be labeled as *extra event*, while a true undetected GE will be labeled as *missed event*. The sensitivity, or true positive rate, of each approach in detecting GEs, and the precision, or positive predictive values, will be calculated. Sensitivity and precision provide an evaluation of the performance of both approaches [20]. For each approach, the differences between the estimations of each gait parameter p and the reference value r will be calculated. For every parameter p, as estimated by both approaches, the absolute and relative error will be determined, applying Formulas 1 and 2.

$$absolute\ error = |p - r| \tag{1}$$

$$relative\ error = \frac{|p - r|}{|r|} * 100 \tag{2}$$

Statistical Analysis. First, a statistical test will be conducted to determine systematic differences between test sessions for each gait parameter of each approach. Then, descriptive statistics will be conducted for calculating the absolute errors to verify if there exist a significance difference between both approaches.

6   Discussion

A depth camera system and a wearable inertial system to automatically detect GEs and S-TGPs are presented and compared. The research described in this paper is in progress. The experimental protocol will be applied under controlled conditions and the results will be compared with respect to a specialized system used as reference or ground truth. The study is oriented to support the design of ambulatory, low-cost, and ubiquitous technologies for gait monitoring.

Acknowledgements. This work is supported by the FRASE MINECO project (TIN2013-47152-C3-1-R) and the Mexican National Council for Science and Technology, CONACYT (grant number 271539/224405). Also, we appreciate the support of UBIHEALTH project under International Research Staff Exchange Schema (MC-IRSES 316337).

References

1. Ghoussayni, S., Stevens, C., Durham, S., Ewins, D.: Assessment and validation of a simple automated method for the detection of gait events and intervals. Gait Posture **20**(3), 266–272 (2004)

2. Davis, R.B., DeLuca, P.A., Õunpuu, S.: Analysis of gait. In: Biomechanics: Principles and Applications, vol. 20, p. 131 (2002)
3. Haworth, J.M.: Gait, aging and dementia. Rev. Clin. Gerontol. **18**, 39–52 (2008)
4. Hesse, S.: Rehabilitation of gait after stroke: evaluation, principles of therapy, novel treatment approaches, and assistive devices. Top. Geriatr. Rehabil. **19**(2), 109–126 (2003)
5. Trew, M., Everett, T.: Human Movement: An Introductory Text. Churchill Livingston, London (2001)
6. Kirtley, C.: Clinical Gait Analysis: Theory and Practice. Elsevier Health Sciences, USA (2006)
7. Bilney, B., Morris, M., Webster, K.: Concurrent related validity of the GAITRite walkway system for quantification of the spatial and temporal parameters of gait. Gait Posture **17**(1), 68–74 (2003)
8. Lee, H., Guan, L., Burne, J.A.: Human gait and posture analysis for diagnosing neurological disorders. Proc. IEEE Int. Conf. Image Process. **2**, 435–438 (2000)
9. Yang, S., Zhang, J.T., Novak, A.C., Brouwer, B., Li, Q.: Estimation of spatio-temporal parameters for post-stroke hemiparetic gait using inertial sensors. Gait Posture **37**(3), 354–358 (2013)
10. Rafi, M., Hamid, M.E., Khan, M.S., Wahidabanu, R.S.D.: A parametric approach to gait signature extraction for human motion identification. Int. J. Image Process. **5**(2), 185–198 (2011)
11. Choudhury, S.D., Tjahjadi, T.: Gait recognition based on shape and motion analysis of silhouette contours. Comput. Vis. Image Underst. **117**(12), 1770–1785 (2013)
12. Choudhury, S.D., Tjahjadi, T.: Silhoutte-based gait recognition using procrustes shape analysis and elliptic fourier descriptors. Pattern Recogn. **45**(9), 3414–3426 (2012)
13. Caillette, F., Howard, T.: Real-time markerless human body tracking with multi-view 3-D voxel reconstruction. Proc. Br. Mach. Vis. Conf. **2**, 597–606 (2004)
14. Stone, E., Skubic, M.: Passive in-home measurement of stride-to-stride gait variability comparing vision and kinect sensing. In: Proceedings IEEE Engineering in Medicine and Biology Society, pp. 6491–6494 (2011)
15. Stone, E., Anderson, D., Skubic, M., Keller, J.M.: Extracting footfalls from voxel data. In: Proceedings IEEE Engineering in Medicine and Biology Society, pp. 1119–1122 (2010)
16. Zijlstra, A., Zijlstra, W.: Trunk-acceleration based assessment of gait parameters in older persons: a comparison of reliability and validity of four inverted pendulum based estimations. Gait Posture **38**(4), 940–944 (2013)
17. Mariani, B., Rouhani, H., Crevoisier, X., Aminian, K.: Quantitative estimation of foot-flat and stance phase of gait using foot-worn inertial sensors. Gait Posture **37**(2), 229–234 (2013)
18. Guenterberg, E., Yang, A.Y., Ghasemzadeh, H., Jafari, R., Bajcsy, R., Sastry, S.S.: A method for extracting temporal parameters based on hidden markov models in body sensor networks with inertial sensors. Trans. IEEE Inf. Technol. Biomed. **13**(6), 1019–1030 (2009)
19. López-Nava, I.H., Muñoz-Meléndez, A., Pérez Sanpablo, A.I., Alessi Montero, A., Quiñones Urióstegui, I., Núñez Carrera, L.: Estimation of temporal gait parameters using bayesian models on acceleration signals. Comput. Methods Biomech. Biomed. Eng. 1–8 (2015)
20. Banker, R.D., Datar, S.M.: Sensitivity, precision, and linear aggregation of signals for performance evaluation. J. Account. Res. **27**(1), 21–39 (1989)

Interactions within the AmIHealth Environments

Arm Muscular Effort Estimation from Images Using Computer Vision and Machine Learning

Leandro Abraham[1,2,3]([✉]), Facundo Bromberg[1,3], and Raymundo Forradellas[2]

[1] Laboratorio DHARMa, DeSI,
Universidad Tecnológica Nacional, FRM, Mendoza, Argentina
{leandro.abraham,fbromberg}@frm.utn.edu.ar
[2] CEAL, Universidad Nacional de Cuyo, Facultad de Ingeniería, Mendoza, Argentina
[3] Consejo Nacional de Investigaciones Científicas y Técnicas (CONICET),
Buenos Aires, Argentina

Abstract. A problem of great interest in disciplines like occupational medicine, ergonomics, and sports, is the measurement of biomechanical variables involved in human movement and balance such as internal muscle forces and joint torques. This problem is solved by a two-step process: data capturing using impractical, intrusive and expensive devices that is then used as input in complex models for obtaining the biomechanical variables of interest. In this work we present a first step towards capturing input data through a more automated, non-intrusive and economic process, specifically weight held by an arm subject to isometric contraction as a measure of muscular effort. We do so, by processing RGB images of the arm with computer vision (Local Binary Patterns and Color Histograms) and estimating the effort with machine learning algorithms (SVM and Random Forests). In the best case we obtained an FMeasure = 70.68 %, an Accuracy = 71.66 % and a mean absolute error in the predicted weights of 554.16 grs (over 3 possible levels of effort). Considering the difficulty of the problem, it is enlightening to achieve over random results indicating that, despite the simplicity of the approach, it is possible to extract meaningful information for the predictive task. Moreover, the simplicity of the approach suggests many lines of further improvements: on the image capturing side with other kind of images; on the feature extraction side with more sophisticated algorithms and features; and on the knowledge extraction side with more sophisticated learning algorithms.

Keywords: Muscle arm effort · SVM · Random forests · LBP · Color histograms

1 Introduction

Musculoskeletal system biomechanics is a scientific discipline that aims to study the mechanical structures, laws, models and phenomenons that are important to the balance and movement of humans. The biomechanical variables most studied

© Springer International Publishing Switzerland 2015
J. Bravo et al. (Eds.): AmIHEALTH 2015, LNCS 9456, pp. 125–137, 2015.
DOI: 10.1007/978-3-319-26508-7_13

when analyzing balance and movement are internal and external muscles forces, and joint torques. The analysis of these variables allows the identification of harmful movements, overexertions, awkward postures, musculoskeletal disorders, optimal movements, among other states of the human body that have high impact in its health and performance. This results in its application in disciplines like occupational medicine [4], ergonomics [28], and sports [16], among others.

The estimation of internal muscular forces and joint torques is not made through direct measurement, but indirectly through dynamical models. These are: inverse dynamics, forward dynamics, and electromyography guided models [21,22,30]. Possible inputs for these models are the level of activation of the muscle, obtained by processing the electric signal (electric activity) produced by the muscles when contracting; the kinematic variables of joint positions at each instant; and the external forces involved in the movement or posture. After a computer process they return as output, among other variables, the internal forces, the joint torques or the muscular activation level. Nowadays, the measurement of electric muscular activity during muscle contractions is performed by an expensive device called electromyograph (EMG). The use of this device requires the adherence of wired electrodes to the skin or the introduction of wired needles in the muscles. Although there exists as well the wireless EMGs, these are considerably more expensive and therefore rarely used in practice. To capture the kinematic variables, commonly used devices are: goniometers to measure angles between body parts (require fixing sensors on the body) and motion capture systems that visually measure the positions of body parts (require adherence of markers and using expensive multi-camera systems), among others. The mentioned technologies are expensive, they limit the body movements through electrodes, needles, marker suites, and goniometers; and require special mounting devices; all of which makes them unsuitable for use outside a laboratory environment. In recent years, automatic measurement of kinematic information using inexpensive cameras has achieved a significant level of maturity because of the appearance on the market of low cost depth sensors (Microsoft Kinect [2], Asus Xtion [1], among others). With these devices it has been made possible to measure the joints position [10] with acceptable precision. However, to the best of the author's knowledge, there is still no convincing image-processing technology for estimating the level of muscular activation. This paper presents an approach that aims to take the first steps to solve this problem.

The objective of the authors research line is to solve the problem of estimating the electric muscular activity by the indirect estimation of highly correlated variables, in particular for this paper, the weight of objects held in a static posture of isometric contraction. The correlation is justified by considering that the greater the weight, the greater will be the force needed to hold it, and greater the electrical activity produced to contract the muscle. We refer to these measures now on under the name of *muscular effort* or *muscular activity*. This line of research has practical applications in situations where it is necessary to estimate the muscular effort wirelessly. For example, it could be used to estimate the muscular activation patterns of an athlete during the execution of some movement. Another application could be to estimate the effort that a worker is performing during a task in order to detect harmful movements in an occupational environment. It's worth to clarify that these applications will be possible when this research line has reached maturity and when the framework has been tested in real conditions. This work presents the first experimentation for the research line, lacking of a practical application in the immediate future.

The main contribution of the present work is the application of computer vision and supervised machine learning for solving the problem of estimating the weight of object held by the arm of humans through postures of isometric contraction, from RGB images of the arm taken in uniform scenes, with the same conditions of illumination, scale and point of view for each one.

For shading some light on the originality of our contributions, its impact, and feasibility we present related works in Sect. 2. We present our approach for solving the problem in Sect. 3. Section 4 presents the experimental setup used for proving the effectiveness of our approach, followed by its results in Sect. 5. We end with discussions in Sect. 6, and conclusions in Sect. 7.

2   Related Work

As far as the authors have been able to investigate, there are no contributions in the literature that solve the specific problem of estimating muscular effort, exclusively from skin images. However, it is possible to find work related to the general problem of characterizing muscle contraction from body images but these either use extra information such as kinematic variables obtained through other capturing devices or EMG measurements, or rather aims to model the skin features for different underneath contractions. In this section we compare our contribution with the problems and techniques considered by these works, highlighting the differences that justify the originality of our proposal.

We start by the paper [5], whose main contribution is the interactive presentation of the approximated level of muscular activation that is produced in inferior extremities muscles when executing different movements. This information is presented in an augmented reality interface and the level is obtained from a database generated from EMG measurement and its respective kinematic information. This database is a straightforward indexing mapping between kinematic information and EMG measurements, with no model learning that maps them, and therefore prone to errors when used for estimation of muscle activity. When compared to our approach, it is based on kinematic information obtained by skeleton tracking from an RGBD sensor, and not on skin RGB images.

Another related problem is the one discussed by [26], consisting in the identification and classification of walking patterns between examples of healthy and injured subjects. Here, they use skin deformation information, together with EMG measurements of the subjects, as input to a neural network for the classification. Although this paper focuses on computer vision for extracting skin deformation information from RGB images, they don't use this skin information for estimating muscular activity, but rather use it with such information, obtained by direct measurements of EMGs.

Another group of works have been dedicated to solve the problem of modeling the deformation of the skin due to underlying muscle activity [11,12,18,23,24,29, 34], but with applications in computer graphics for animating virtual characters. The problem solved by these papers differ from the one that we plan to solve in that they don't attempt to estimate the muscular activity, but rather seeks to model the deformation due to muscle contraction, without prediction. Another difference is that they obtain the visual information from motion capture systems by marker tracking and depth information from RGBD sensors, instead of from RGB images as it is done in this work.

There is also a group that have used computer vision techniques to evaluate and measure the deformation and movement produced in the skin due to muscular contraction mainly using pixel movement information form RGB images [6,9,17,35]. The latest work of Carli et al., as asserted by the authors, is an improvement of the former, and both [6,17] aims at modeling skin deformation when the biceps is under isometric contraction. Although clearly related to our present work, their goal is on the opposite direction, being our goal the modeling of the underneath contraction from skin features, and not the other way around. It is worth to clarify that [9,35] work over an insect instead of over human skin.

Finally there is a group of works that pretend to solve the problem of prediction of electric muscular activity from kinematic information, most of them validating with EMG captures [3,8,13,25,31,32] or by muscular activation obtained from an inverse dynamic model [15]. Their approaches consider methods as neural networks [3,8,15,25], probabilistic Bayesian reasoning [3,31], curve fitting methods [3], regression models [32] and biomechanical models [13]. While these works solve the same problem we want to solve, they do so with kinematic information obtained from motion capture systems instead of visual skin information obtained from RGB images.

From the survey of the state of the art, we can argue that there is no previous work that performs estimation of muscular effort from external images of the skin using Computer Vision and Machine Learning, as we propose in this paper.

3   Our Approach

Our approach is an autonomous modeling of the relationship between skin characteristics and weights lifted by an arm in conditions of isometric contraction. This modeling is constructed by a supervised learning procedure outlined in Fig. 1. This general approach can be instantiated differently for the different components and we discuss these variations in this section. The input of the procedure are images of the arm region, corresponding to different conditions of weight lifting. Input images are cropped to the biceps region and segmented from the blue background ((A), detailed in Sub-sect. 3.1). By a feature extraction process, each image is characterized in a vector of numeric values ((B), detailed in Sub-sect. 3.2). Optionally these vectors could be complemented with anthropometric data of the subject ((C), detailed in Sub-sect. 3.3). These vectors could be also normalized in relation to minimum effort cases for the corresponding

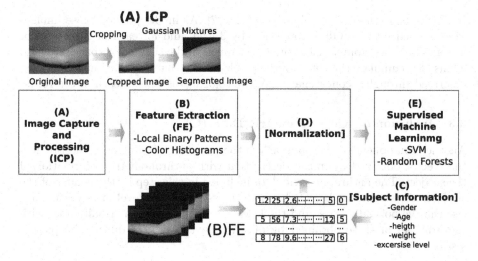

Fig. 1. Outline of the approach (Color figure online)

subject ((D), detailed in Sub-sect. 3.4). The resulting vectors are labeled with the corresponding weights and supplied as input to a machine learning algorithm during the learning stage ((E), detailed in Sub-sect. 3.5).

3.1 Capture and Segmentation (A)

The process starts by capturing static RGB images, with blue background, of subjects arms holding one of five possible objects of differing weights. Then, the images are cropped to the region of the biceps. After that, the blue background is removed by automatic segmentation process using the Gaussian Mixtures algorithm [33], pre-trained with some manually segmented images.

3.2 Feature Extraction (B)

Each segmented and cropped image is processed for feature extraction producing a vector of a fixed number of quantities (i.e., dimensions) that describes the image. The feature vector of training images is extended with a label indicating the actual weight sustained. In this work we evaluated our approach building the feature vector with information of texture and/or color.

For texture we used the Local Binary Patterns [19] feature extraction algorithm. Briefly, it proceeds by dividing the image into 9 regions of interest (ROI) through a 3 by 3 grid. Then, local binary patterns are computed for each of these ROI, generating for each of its pixels a binary code of 8 bits, one for each of its 8 nearest neighbors, deciding 0 if the pixel is greater than its neighbor or 1 otherwise. For each ROI the binary codes are accumulated in a histogram according to their decimal value, and these histograms are later concatenated in a vector that describes the whole image. We used 59 bins for each ROI histogram.

For color we used color histograms [20, 27]. As in the previous case, images were divided into 9 ROIs through a 3 by 3 grid, and for each of these a color histogram was computed using the HS channels of the HSV color space. We used 5 bins to accumulate the colors of the pixels of each channel. The image was then described through a concatenation of the color histograms of each of the ROIs.

3.3 Inclusion of Anthropometric Data (C)

Another component of the approach is the possibility to augment the raw feature vector obtained by image description with anthropometric information of the subject. The anthropometric data included in this step is: the gender of the subject, his weight, his height, his body mass index, the level of physical exercise that he normally does, and the level of exercise that he normally does with the arm (all of these obtained by questioning the subject during the picture session).

3.4 Feature Vector Normalization (D)

It is quite clear that generalizing among subjects is a difficult task, as their arms may differ in so many aspects that has no relation whatsoever with the muscle contraction, adding a lot of noise. Moreover, their arms may produce quite different skin patterns for the same muscle contraction. We propose here a first step to tackle these issues that could be thought as a calibration process, where the feature vector of some subject is normalized by subtracting from it the feature vector of the case of effort zero. This procedure breaks the standard supervised learning protocol, as for new subjects as input to the framework, it is provided not only the input data, but the output data of the zero effort cases. In practice, however this is a simple request for the subjects.

3.5 Estimation of Muscular Effort by Machine Learning (E)

The final component of our approach consists in running a supervised learning algorithm for predicting the weight lifted by a biceps muscle, when given images of the arm. In this work we evaluate the performance of radial basis Support Vector Machine [7] (SVM) and Random Forests [14]. In a first stage the algorithms are trained using a corpus of labeled subjects images through a dataset whose data-points consists of the feature vector produced as explained above, that may be normalized or not and may contain anthropometric data or not, and labeled with the actual weight lifted in that image.

During training we tuned the user-given parameters of the learning algorithms over a grid of possible values using a 10 fold cross-validation over the training set, choosing the parameters with overall better performance over the 10 cases. Radial SVM has two given parameters: C (the soft margin), and σ (the standard deviation of the kernel parameter), both tuned over the set of values $\{0.002, 0.02, 2.20, 200\}$. Random Forests was tuned over the number of random variables used for constructing each of its trees, considering different proportions over the total number of variables (of the input feature vectors): {2 %, 6 %, 12 %, 25 %, 50 %, 75 %, 100 %}. At the moment of the estimation of the effort level of a new image, the trained model is used.

As there have not been found previous work that estimate the muscular effort from images using a similar approach, we decided to include a third learning algorithm, the random classifier, as our competitor.

4   Experimental Setup

The current and following sections presents our experimental setup. With these experiments we intend to answer empirically the main question of this work: whether computer vision and supervised-learning techniques are capable of extracting enough information from arm images for inferring the weight they are lifting. For that, we start presenting in the next Sub-sect. 4.1 the process followed for capturing the image corpus, followed by Sub-sect. 4.2 that explains the process followed for generating the training and testing datasets, and conclude with the Sub-sect. 4.3 that describes the performance measures used for evaluating the outputs of the machine learning algorithms.

4.1   Capture of Raw Image Data

For this work we captured images from 100 human subjects. The group of subjects presents variability in their characteristics. It is conformed by both women and men of white to latin dark skin that exercise with differing levels of intensity from low to moderate, with ages ranging between 17 and 54 years old, weights ranging between 47 and 113 kgs, their heights varying between 1.6 mts to 1.9 mts, and their body mass index varying from 19.32 and 34.16. For each subject, 3 photos holding 5 objects of different weights were captured using a Canon EOS 1000D camera with Zoom Lens of 75–300 mm, without flash and manual focus. The same set of objects were used for each subject: object $O0$ of 0 grs, the object $O500$ of 500 grs, the object $O1$ k of 1300 grs, the object $O2$ k of 1900 grs, and the object $O4$ k of 3800 grs. The photos were captured as close as possible of the biceps, using a blue background (to ease the autonomous segmentation of the biceps). Each subject was told to exert an isometric contraction effort, holding in front of the camera a posture where the segment of the arm from the shoulder to the elbow was separated approximately 45° from the torso and the segment of the arm from the elbow to the hand was horizontal. All the photos were captured over this posture in order to control this variability for the experiments. The scene was artificially illuminated with a little searchlight of 60 W, located in front of the subject, but from the right side, elevated about 1.5 m from the subject, and aiming to the arm. As mentioned earlier, each image was then cropped to the biceps zone in order to remove clutter from the image, and then segmented from the background.

4.2 Datasets Generation

Our approach is tested in the standard training/testing approach, where the model is learned over the training set, and evaluated over the test set. We generated 10 pairs of training/testing datasets, each pair generated by first selecting randomly 8 out of the 100 subjects (8 %), and producing as testing set the 120 images corresponding to 8 subjects times 5 weights times 3 (repetitions) images; and as training set the images of the remaining 92 subjects (92 %). The experimental results shown in the following section are over different instances of the approach, and for each case it is reported the *mean* and *standard deviation* over the 10 datasets pairs.

4.3 Performance Measures

In this section we present the performance measures used for the evaluation of each instance of the proposed framework. As the problem is solved as one of image classification, we report the classical performance measures for classification tasks: accuracy over all the confusion matrix, named as Overall Accuracy and computed as OvA = sum of the diagonal values/sum of the whole matrix values, also Precision (P), Recall (R), FMeasure (FM), and Accuracy (A); computed for each class independently, resulting in n of them (n = number of classes), and grouped by reporting their means over all the classes. For each class i, they are computed as follows: P_i = number of correctly classified examples of class i/total number of examples classified as class i; R_i = number of correctly classified objects of class i/total of examples that truly are of class i, $FM_i = 2 \times ((P_i \times R_i)/(P_i + R_i))$, and finally A_i = sum of the quantities of the diagonal + the sum of the quantities not belonging neither to the row i nor to the column i/total number of examples. We also report the *mean absolute error* (MAE) by transforming the object class label to its corresponding value in grams. This measure tells us how is the error made at estimating the weight of the held out object. It is calculated as the mean of the absolute values of the differences between the predicted weight minus the true weight. Therefore, the smaller the MAE, the better the result of the estimation.

5 Experimental Results

To conclude the validation of our hypothesis and the contribution of this paper, we present in this section the results of the experiments over all instantiations resulting from selecting the learning algorithm, the feature extraction algorithm, whether it is used anthropometric data or not, and whether a normalization is conducted over the dataset or not. Each case is ran over all 10 training datasets, and the mean and standard deviation (subindex and parenthesis numbers) of the performance measures over the corresponding test sets are reported. The results are shown in Tables 1 (classification over 3 levels) and 2 (classification over 5 levels). The first column labeled 'Desc' describes the feature extraction

Table 1. Estimation results for 3 levels of effort. Cases with normalization were grayed out. Best performance measure obtained results are in bold.

Desc.	SI	N	MLAlg.	$\hat{P}$	$\hat{R}$	FM	$\hat{A}$	OvA	MAE
RDM				$34.7_{(5.81)}$	$34.72_{(6.03)}$	$34.36_{(5.92)}$	$56.48_{(4.02)}$	$34.72_{(6.03)}$	$1657.22_{(147.08)}$
LBP	NO	NO	RF	$49.38_{(9.85)}$	$49.58_{(7.52)}$	$48.39_{(8.2)}$	$66.38_{(5)}$	$49.58_{(7.52)}$	$1095.13_{(219.46)}$
LBP	YES	NO	RF	$49.3_{(7.32)}$	$49.44_{(6.52)}$	$48.48_{(6.65)}$	$66.29_{(4.34)}$	$49.44_{(6.52)}$	$1137.36_{(182.17)}$
LBP	YES	YES	RF	$71_{(6.43)}$	$69.86_{(5.36)}$	$69.77_{(5.32)}$	$79.9_{(3.57)}$	$69.86_{(5.36)}$	$572.63_{(101.86)}$
LBP	NO	YES	RF	$71.21_{(7.65)}$	$70.69_{(7.24)}$	$70.55_{(7.22)}$	$80.46_{(4.83)}$	$70.69_{(7.24)}$	$556.8_{(137.65)}$
LBP	NO	NO	SVM	$46.87_{(8.02)}$	$43.61_{(6.58)}$	$40.32_{(7.54)}$	$62.4_{(4.39)}$	$43.61_{(6.58)}$	$1369.58_{(216.69)}$
LBP	YES	NO	SVM	$48.74_{(12.77)}$	$48.05_{(11.86)}$	$45.36_{(14.05)}$	$65.37_{(7.9)}$	$48.05_{(11.86)}$	$1184.86_{(379.45)}$
LBP	NO	YES	SVM	$67.96_{(5.75)}$	$68.61_{(4.73)}$	$65.91_{(6.74)}$	$79.07_{(3.15)}$	$68.61_{(4.73)}$	$606.94_{(97.95)}$
LBP	YES	YES	SVM	$69.13_{(13.56)}$	$66.94_{(3.57)}$	$60.06_{(4.87)}$	$77.96_{(2.38)}$	$66.94_{(3.57)}$	$641.25_{(72.58)}$
HSCH	NO	NO	RF	$48.02_{(9.87)}$	$48.47_{(8.62)}$	$47.27_{(9.17)}$	$65.64_{(5.74)}$	$48.47_{(8.62)}$	$1169.02_{(265.65)}$
HSCH	YES	NO	RF	$53.32_{(10.19)}$	$53.33_{(8.61)}$	$52.06_{(9.07)}$	$68.88_{(5.74)}$	$53.33_{(8.61)}$	$1081.94_{(207.04)}$
HSCH	YES	YES	RF	$71.18_{(6.29)}$	$\mathbf{71.66}_{(5.82)}$	$70.4_{(6.37)}$	$\mathbf{81.11}_{(3.88)}$	$\mathbf{71.66}_{(5.82)}$	$572.63_{(136.86)}$
HSCH	NO	YES	RF	$70.31_{(4.68)}$	$69.72_{(4.57)}$	$69.14_{(4.46)}$	$79.81_{(3.04)}$	$69.72_{(4.57)}$	$606.94_{(86.18)}$
HSCH	NO	NO	SVM	$47.05_{(8.35)}$	$45.97_{(8.11)}$	$44.02_{(8.55)}$	$63.98_{(5.4)}$	$45.97_{(8.11)}$	$1377.5_{(284.97)}$
HSCH	YES	NO	SVM	$48.34_{(9.65)}$	$46.38_{(6.9)}$	$44.22_{(7.43)}$	$64.25_{(4.6)}$	$46.38_{(6.9)}$	$1385.41_{(172.03)}$
HSCH	NO	YES	SVM	$67.24_{(6.62)}$	$66.11_{(5.32)}$	$64.02_{(6.07)}$	$77.4_{(3.55)}$	$66.11_{(5.32)}$	$691.38_{(106.14)}$
HSCH&LBP	NO	YES	RF	$69.52_{(5.21)}$	$68.47_{(5.03)}$	$68.12_{(4.73)}$	$78.98_{(3.35)}$	$68.47_{(5.03)}$	$599.02_{(95.59)}$
HSCH&LBP	YES	YES	RF	$71.3_{(5.46)}$	$70.83_{(5.27)}$	$\mathbf{70.68}_{(5.21)}$	$80.55_{(3.51)}$	$70.83_{(5.27)}$	$\mathbf{554.16}_{(100.29)}$
HSCH&LBP	NO	YES	SVM	$\mathbf{71.74}_{(7.98)}$	$71.52_{(7.11)}$	$70.35_{(7.84)}$	$81.01_{(4.74)}$	$71.52_{(7.11)}$	$556.8_{(149.51)}$

technique used, with LBP for Local Binary Patterns and HSCH for Color Histograms. The second column labeled 'SI' indicates whether anthropometric subject information is appended to the input dataset set or not. The third column labeled 'N' indicates whether normalization was applied or not. The fourth column 'MLAlg' describes the machine learning algorithm used, with SVM for Support Vector Machine, RF for Random Forests and RDM for the Random classifier. The remaining columns report each of the 6 performance measures.

We start with a simpler setup where we tried to predict only over 3 levels of effort, considering only the examples of $O0$, $O2$ k and $O4$ k. These results are shown in Table 1. As it can be seen in the Table, the prediction made with the proposed descriptors when normalization is not performed (not grayed out) were better than the random prediction. Despite of this, they present low classification measures and relatively high MAE. In those cases where normalization was applied (grayed out), the results became substantially better. In the best cases we obtain classification measures over 70 % and a MAE down to 554 grs. We also tested the performance of an instance of the approach that use as descriptor the combination of the two descriptors (HSCH&LBP), showing only minor improvements over the overall best cases, but large improvements for the SVM classifier. With this first experiment it is possible to prove that the normalization of the raw feature vectors proposed improves the performance of the framework, leading to acceptable values of classification measures and weight prediction.

In Table 2 we show the results of a second experiment. In order to improve the impact of our solution, we decided to evaluate the approach in the task of classification over the 5 levels of effort. As it is possible to see, when increasing the number of classes, the performance measures decreased. This happens because five different levels of effort are less discriminable visually than three. Here we can see also that the normalization step improves significantly the performance of the framework. Also in this case, the combined descriptors got

Table 2. Estimation results for 5 levels of effort. Cases with normalization were grayed out. Best performance measure obtained results are in bold.

Desc.	SI	N	MLAlg.	$\hat{P}$	$\hat{R}$	FM	$\hat{A}$	OvA	MAE
RDM				$20.7_{(3.76)}$	$20.41_{(3.17)}$	$20.39_{(3.39)}$	$68.16_{(1.26)}$	$20.41_{(3.17)}$	$1413.66_{(95.94)}$
LBP	NO	NO	RF	$34.62_{(7.34)}$	$32.51_{(5.81)}$	$31.61_{(6.03)}$	$73.01_{(2.33)}$	$32.52_{(5.82)}$	$1122.72_{(195.39)}$
LBP	YES	NO	RF	$26.12_{(5.71)}$	$27.25_{(4.23)}$	$25.51_{(4.85)}$	$70.9_{(1.69)}$	$27.25_{(4.23)}$	$1176.08_{(150.4)}$
LBP	YES	YES	RF	$45.48_{(6.84)}$	$46.33_{(5.48)}$	$45.14_{(5.82)}$	$78.53_{(2.19)}$	$46.33_{(5.48)}$	$826.16_{(130.32)}$
LBP	NO	YES	RF	$47.38_{(5.93)}$	$46.52_{(5.9)}$	$45.54_{(5.75)}$	$78.61_{(2.35)}$	$46.53_{(5.89)}$	$878.88_{(143.88)}$
LBP	NO	NO	SVM	$33.44_{(9.13)}$	$28.83_{(3.89)}$	$25.32_{(3.45)}$	$71.53_{(1.55)}$	$28.83_{(3.89)}$	$1499.75_{(203.72)}$
LBP	YES	NO	SVM	$26.89_{(7.03)}$	$28.01_{(3.75)}$	$24.96_{(4.4)}$	$71.21_{(1.49)}$	$28.04_{(3.74)}$	$1388.68_{(190.97)}$
LBP	NO	YES	SVM	$45.31_{(5.23)}$	$46.73_{(4.63)}$	$44.09_{(5.17)}$	$78.72_{(1.84)}$	$46.81_{(4.62)}$	$825.05_{(212.92)}$
LBP	YES	YES	SVM	$42.97_{(11.3)}$	$43.33_{(4.23)}$	$36.17_{(5.52)}$	$77.33_{(1.69)}$	$43.33_{(4.23)}$	$1267.75_{(123.59)}$
HSCH	NO	NO	RF	$30.91_{(4.86)}$	$30.7_{(5.1)}$	$29.1_{(4.69)}$	$72.31_{(2.04)}$	$30.77_{(5.11)}$	$1068.86_{(120.98)}$
HSCH	YES	NO	RF	$29.58_{(5.36)}$	$29.91_{(4.31)}$	$28.87_{(4.95)}$	$71.96_{(1.72)}$	$29.91_{(4.31)}$	$1098.75_{(129.61)}$
HSCH	YES	YES	RF	$45.6_{(4.45)}$	$46.61_{(5.29)}$	$44.94_{(4.73)}$	$78.65_{(2.12)}$	$46.62_{(5.3)}$	$825.43_{(109.69)}$
HSCH	NO	YES	RF	$46.52_{(5.77)}$	$47.44_{(4.1)}$	$45.13_{(4.98)}$	$78.98_{(1.64)}$	$47.95_{(4.11)}$	$890.3_{(103.48)}$
HSCH	NO	NO	SVM	$26.25_{(6.54)}$	$27.08_{(5.73)}$	$25.24_{(5.77)}$	$70.83_{(2.29)}$	$25.58_{(5.73)}$	$1380.58_{(198.27)}$
HSCH	YES	NO	SVM	$23_{(3.81)}$	$25.58_{(3.49)}$	$22.64_{(3.42)}$	$70.23_{(1.39)}$	$25.58_{(3.49)}$	$1418.75_{(136.12)}$
HSCH	NO	YES	SVM	$45.21_{(3.37)}$	$45.41_{(2.29)}$	$41.79_{(2.39)}$	$78.16_{(0.91)}$	$45.41_{(2.29)}$	$1076.41_{(65.72)}$
HSCH&LBP	NO	YES	RF	$45.32_{(5.59)}$	$45.66_{(5.39)}$	$44.23_{(5.13)}$	$78.26_{(2.15)}$	$45.66_{(5.39)}$	$857.83_{(107.03)}$
HSCH&LBP	YES	YES	RF	$45.54_{(5.15)}$	$46.1_{(6.38)}$	$45.01_{(5.55)}$	$78.44_{(2.54)}$	$46.11_{(6.36)}$	$824.43_{(151.76)}$
HSCH&LBP	NO	YES	SVM	$\mathbf{51.67}_{(5.47)}$	$\mathbf{51}_{(4.09)}$	$\mathbf{48.33}_{(4.79)}$	$\mathbf{80.4}_{(1.63)}$	$\mathbf{51}_{(4.09)}$	$842.66_{(151.74)}$

good results but they aren't significantly better than those obtained by the single descriptors. In these experiments also the case that got the best measures (HSCH&LBP+NO+YES+SVM) shows that combining the two descriptors make possible to get better results for the SVM classifier. It is possible to see that the classification measures obtained with normalization almost duplicate the values of the random classifier. Besides, in the better case, the MAE decreases significantly leading to an error of 825 grs which to the authors criterion is a good value considering that the minimum difference between two different examples could be 500 grs and the maximum difference could be up to 3800 grs.

From the results we can affirm that it is possible to differentiate the level of muscular effort that a person is performing from a photo of a biceps: between 5 levels with FMeasure $\approx 48\%$ and Accuracy $\approx 80\%$; and between 3 levels with FMeasure $\approx 70\%$ and Accuracy $\approx 81\%$. Besides, it is possible to estimate the weight that a person is holding with his arm from a photo of his biceps: over 5 different weights (0 grs, 500 grs, 1300 grs, 1900 grs and 3800 grs) with a mean absolute error ≈ 825 grs; and over 3 different weights (0 grs, 1900 grs and 3800 grs) with a mean absolute error ≈ 554 grs.

6 Discussions

From the experimental results analysis showing improvements over the random classifier, we can conclude that our approach performs acceptably in finding visual patterns of biceps images and their correlations with muscle effort. This is clearly an important and solid step for achieving in the future a practical application. Despite this positive result, the framework of feature extraction followed by supervised learning presented in this work is proven by our experiments insufficient for successfully estimating muscular effort with enough precision for practical use for several limitations. One that we believe is the most limiting factor is the amount of training samples that, although considerably large, is still insufficient when compared with the great variability among the human subjects, resulting in an under represented underlying distribution. Another limitation is the simplistic approach considered, specially the use, over the shelf, of general purpose feature extraction algorithms that uses only color information to infer the latent, more informative 3D contour information. The practicality of the approach is also limited for the cases that uses the normalization step, where the prediction stage over unseen subjects requires labeled images for the case of zero effort, as well as by the requirement of exposed skin images on the area to be sensed. In conclusion, our approach shows an important and solid step toward a practical application in the future, and through the limitations described, it helps in highlighting the best possible future steps to follow.

7   Conclusions and Future Work

In this work we present the first steps towards estimation of muscular activity from skin images using Computer Vision and Machine Learning. The proposed approach consists in a framework that considers the capture of images of the area of the muscle, the generation of a raw feature vector for the images using image descriptors, the optional inclusion of anthropometric subject information to the raw feature vector, an also optional step of normalization of the feature vector, and finally the training of a model and estimating of level of new examples using supervised machine learning techniques. The first contribution of this work is the experimentation of this framework over an image dataset of 100 subjects performing 5 and 3 different levels of effort in static posture of isometric contraction, being this the first steps in this line of research. In this work we propose to use HS Color Histograms and Local Binary Patterns as image descriptors. Regarding the machine learning techniques used in this work, they are Support Vector Machines and Random Forests. Another contribution is the proposal of feature vector normalization in relation to the feature vectors of minimum effort, in order to improve the estimation results helping the framework to better generalize over previously unseen subjects.

As future work we plan to try other ways of improving the performance of the approach. As the exploration of description techniques and parameters of the machine learning algorithms has been very limited, we will extend the experimentation to other image description techniques to build the feature vector, and to other parameters for the machine learning algorithms. Another alternative is to use deep learning, a technology that combines feature extraction and model learning in one framework. As it is showed in this work, calibration is required to get good results, so we will design and experiment other ways of calibration. We also will extend the dataset with more subjects in order to find tendencies of improvement of the results as the number of train subjects increases.

Acknowledgements. We thank CONICET for the funding of the author Leandro Abraham through a doctoral grant under the supervision of Dr. Raymundo Forradellas and the thesis supervision of Dr. Facundo Bromberg.

References

1. Asus xtion. http://www.asus.com/latin/Multimedia/Xtion/
2. Microsoft kinect sensor. http://www.xbox.com/es-ES/Kinect
3. Johnson, L.A., Fuglevand, A.J.: Evaluation of probabilistic methods to predict muscle activity: implications for neuroprosthetics. J. Neural Eng. **6**(5), 055008 (2009)
4. Chaffin, D.B., Andersson, G.B.J., et al.: Occupational Biomechanics. Wiley, New York (1984)
5. Bauer, A., Paclet, F., Cahouet, V., Dicko, A.H., Palombi, O., Faure, F., Troccaz, J., et al.: Interactive visualization of muscle activity during limb movements: towards enhanced anatomy learning. In: Eurographics Workshop on VCBM (2014)
6. Carli, M., Goffredo, M., Schmid, M., Neri, A.: Study of muscular deformation based on surface slope estimation. In: Electronic Imaging, p. 60640U. International Society for Optics and Photonics (2006)
7. Cortes, C., Vapnik, V.: Support-vector networks. Mach. Learn. **20**(3), 273–297 (1995)
8. Matheson Rittenhouse, D., Abdullah, H.A., John Runciman, R., Basir, O.: A neural network model for reconstructing emg signals from eight shoulder muscles: consequences for rehabilitation robotics and biofeedback. J. Biomech. **39**(10), 1924–1932 (2006)
9. Davide, Z., Andrea, G., Vincent, T.: The use of optical flow to characterize muscle contraction. J. Neurosci. Methods **110**(1), 65–80 (2001)
10. Dutta, T.: Evaluation of the kinect^{TM} sensor for 3-d kinematic measurement in the workplace. Appl. Ergonomics **43**(4), 645–649 (2012)
11. Park, S.I., Hodgins, J.K.: Data-driven modeling of skin and muscle deformation. ACM TOG **27**(3), 96 (2008)
12. Assassi, L., Becker, M., Magnenat Thalmann, N.: Dynamic skin deformation based on biomechanical modeling. In: Proceedings of the 25th CASA, vol. 2 (2012)
13. Laursen, B., Søgaard, K., Sjøgaard, G.: Biomechanical model predicting electromyographic activity in three shoulder muscles from 3d kinematics and external forces during cleaning work. Clin. Biomech. **18**(4), 287–295 (2003)
14. Leo, B.: Random forests. Mach. Learn. **45**(1), 5–32 (2001)
15. Marzieh, M., Ling, W., Qin, L., Yaxiong, L., Jiankang, H., Dichen, L., Zhongmin, J.: Muscle activity prediction using wavelet neural network. In: ICWAPR 2013, pp. 241–246. IEEE (2013)
16. McGinnis, P.: Biomechanics of Sport and Exercise. Human Kinetics, USA (2013)
17. Michela, G., Marco, C., Silvia, C., Daniele, B., Alessandro, N., Tommaso, D.: Evaluation of skin and muscular deformations in a non-rigid motion analysis. In: Medical Imaging, pp. 535–541. International Society for Optics and Photonics (2005)
18. Neumann, T., Varanasi, K., Hasler, N., Wacker, M., Magnor, M., Theobalt, C.: Capture and statistical modeling of arm-muscle deformations. In: Computer Graphics Forum, vol. 32, pp. 285–294. Wiley Online Library (2013)
19. Ojala, T., Pietikäinen, M., Harwood, D.: A comparative study of texture measures with classification based on featured distributions. Pattern Recogn. **29**(1), 51–59 (1996)

20. Chapelle, O., Haffner, P., Vapnik, V.N.: Support vector machines for histogram-based image classification. IEEE Trans. Neural Netw. **10**(5), 1055–1064 (1999)
21. Pandy, M.G., Barr, R.E.: Biomechanics of the musculoskeletal system. In: Standard Handbook of Biomedical Engineering and Design (2004)
22. Qi, S., Buchanan, T.S.: Electromyography as a tool to estimate muscle forces. In: Standard Handbook of Biomedical Engineering & Design (2004)
23. Robertini, N., Neumann, T., Varanasi, K., Theobalt, C.: Capture of arm-muscle deformations using a depth-camera. In: Proceedings of the 10th European Conference on Visual Media Production, p. 12. ACM (2013)
24. Sand, P., McMillan, L., Popović, J.: Continuous capture of skin deformation. ACM Trans. Graph. (TOG) **22**(3), 578–586 (2003)
25. Sd, P., Ae, P., Da, S.: Artificial neural network model for the generation of muscle activation patterns for human locomotion. J. Electromyogr. Kinesiol. **11**(1), 19–30 (2001)
26. Senanayake, S., Triloka, J., Malik, O.A., Iskandar, M.: Artificial neural network based gait patterns identification using neuromuscular signals and soft tissue deformation analysis of lower limbs muscles. In: IJCNN, pp. 3503–3510. IEEE (2014)
27. Shamik, S., Gang, Q., Sakti, P.: Segmentation and histogram generation using the hsv color space for image retrieval. In: ICIP, vol. 2, p. II-589. IEEE (2002)
28. Shrawan, K.: Biomechanics in Ergonomics. CRC Press, Boca Raton (1999)
29. Sifakis, E., Neverov, I., Fedkiw, R.: Automatic determination of facial muscle activations from sparse motion capture marker data. In: ACM TOG, vol. 24, pp. 417–425. ACM (2005)
30. Manal, K., Buchanan, T.S.: Biomechanics of human movement. In: Standard handbook of biomedical engineering & design, p. 26 (2004)
31. Anderson, C.V., Fuglevand, A.J.: Probability-based prediction of activity in multiple arm muscles: implications for functional electrical stimulation. J. Neurophysiol. **100**(1), 482–494 (2008)
32. Xu, X., McGorry, R.W., Lin, J.-H.: A regression model predicting isometric shoulder muscle activities from arm postures and shoulder joint moments. J. Electromyogr. Kinesiol. **24**(3), 419–429 (2014)
33. Yang, M.H., Ahuja, N.: Gaussian mixture model for human skin color and its applications in image and video databases. In: Electronic Imaging'99, pp. 458–466. International Society for Optics and Photonics (1998)
34. Youn, H.Q., Park, S.I., Hodgins, J.K.: A data-driven segmentation for the shoulder complex. In: Computer Graphics Forum, vol. 29, pp. 537–544. Wiley Online Library (2010)
35. Zoccolan, D., Torre, V.: Using optical flow to characterize sensory-motor interactions in a segment of the medicinal leech. J. Neurosci. **22**(6), 2283–2298 (2002)

Ubiquitous and Ambient Assisted Living eHealth Platforms for the Republic of Panama: Two Cases of Study

Juan Jose Saldaña[1(✉)], Luis Mendoza[1], Edgardo Pitti[1], and Miguel Vargas Lombardo[2]

[1] Software Engineering Department, Technological University of Panama, Chiriqui, Panama
{juan.saldana,luis.mendozal,edgardo.pitti2}@utp.ac.pa
[2] GISES-Technological University of Panama, Penonome, Panama
miguel.vargas@utp.ac.pa

Abstract. Using ubiquitous computing and software engineering, two E-Health platforms have being designed, developed and implemented to improve the Down's Syndrome risk estimation process and, with ambient assisted living, enhance how palliative care is being provided to the elderly patients, improving the quality of life in the country of Panama.

Keywords: Ubiquitous computing · eHealth · Software engineering · Palliative care · Downs syndrome · Ambient assisted living · Cloud computing

1 Introduction

As mentioned in [1, 2], in Panama, a lot of medical information are still being record in paper. The information systems related with Health are not developed with standards that help to manage the patient's clinical information. Down's syndrome and Palliative Care are some examples of these affected areas.

Information provided by the finance and economic ministry [3] shows that one of every seven hundred births present Downs syndrome, and around fifteen thousand cases are registered bye 2012 in Panama.

Panama seniors population has more than 60 years and it is growing because advances in medicine have achieved an increase in life expectancy, but most people also arise likely to have advanced disease, involving prioritization attentions at the end of life. That is why providing control pain in patients with terminal disease takes more importance every day in the health sector as a humanitarian necessity is not a medical obligation.

Structuring a platforms capable of bringing the management of patients receiving palliative care in Panama is necessary to help achieve the main goal of palliative care, providing a better quality of life for patients and their families.

To research and improve the Downs syndrome risk estimation process and how palliative cares are provided in Panama, it is necessary to collect, organize and share information using ubiquitous computing. In this paper we present two case studies of ubiquitous eHealth platforms designed and developed based on ubiquity and interoperability.

© Springer International Publishing Switzerland 2015
J. Bravo et al. (Eds.): AmIHEALTH 2015, LNCS 9456, pp. 138–147, 2015.
DOI: 10.1007/978-3-319-26508-7_14

The rest of the document is organized as follow: Sect. 1 describes what ubiquitous is. Section 2 explains the origins of palliative care. Section 3 provides information of palliative care in the country of Panama. Section 4 resume what is Down's syndrome and the impact in the country of Panama. Section 5 explains the main point of the analysis, design, development and implementation of both platforms. Section 6 presents the conclusions and acknowledgment.

2 Ubiquity

Ubiquity is the quality of ubiquitous and it refers to the ability to have presence everywhere.

Mark Weiser describe in his work "The Computer for the Twenty-First Century" [4] the impact that would have the Communication and Information Technolgies in the el impacto que tendría las Tecnologías de la Información y de la Comunicación (TIC) in the everyday life of the human being developing at the lates 80 a program that he called Ubicomp (Ubiquitous Computing). In this model, the communications capacity were beyond what was expected at the time, so it open the next generation of computing with information technology accessible wherever and whenever.

Weiser thought that ubiquitous computing was opposite to virtual reality because virtual reality puts people on a computer-generated world while ubiquitous computing place computers at the service of people in the real world. Based on that Weiser expected to create an environment where devices regardless the size and functionality could interconnect and manage information, making it more accessible and consistently with the people's daily activities.

Ubiquitous computing has many areas of research and application being one of them health care [5], siendo una de estas el campo de la salud, which gives rise to the term ubiquitous computing in the area of health or pervasive healthcare. It aims to provide technology services to the health sector of ubiquitous computing allowing access to information inside and outside the medical facilities.

Ubiquitous computing has become notorious in recent years with several projects. The telemonitoring service offered by telemedicine, is the result of one such project, which allows specialists to perform remote and real-time monitoring to older patients or palliative care patients [6].

Ubiquitous System Patient Medical Records or SUHPC is another example ubiquitous projects created based on ubiquitous computing, which allow to manage the patient record remotely. The information can be accessed in real time in diverse institutions based on the health information requirements [7].

3 Origin of Palliative Care

Since the beginning of the fourth century BC in ancient Greece, terminal ill was not treated because it was regarded as a divine punishment, and if it were to be treated, it would be considered offenses Gods. Later through the spread of the

Christian doctrine [8], the need to help patients who have a near death is established, giving rise to the first "hospices or hospitals," appearing first in the Byzantine territory, then in Rome and finally it spreads throughout Europe.

In the Middle Ages, the term hospice is used to refer to the place where pilgrims and dying visited searching for shelter and food. Usually these people were sick and dying because the science of this time was not as advanced. As early as 1842 Madame Jeanne Garnier hospice uses the term to refer specifically to the care of pilgrims with advanced disease [9], founding the so-called Hospice or Calvarios.

In 1967 Dr. Cicely Saunders [10] began his movement "Modern Hospice", attributed to St. Christopher's Hospice Foundation, this movement promotes the care of patients with advanced disease, with to provide comfort and dignity, giving rise to what is today known as palliative care.

The World Health Organization (WHO) in 1990 defines Palliative Care (PC) as "total care of patients whose disease no longer responds to treatment. Priority is given to control pain and other symptoms and problems of psychological, social and spiritual order with the goal of providing the best quality of life for patients and their families" [11].

Later in 1998 the World Health Organization added palliative care for children and families, as it also applies for chronic pediatric disorders. Finally in 2002 the organization redefines care, emphasizing prevention of suffering.

4 Palliative Care in Panama

Studies conducted in 2012 indicated that 8 % of the world population has more than 65 years and it is estimated that within 20 years this percentage increased to 20 % [12]. This increase in older people is due to the great strides we have today medicine, as it provides improvements in the treatment of various infectious diseases, and other innovations. However this increase in life expectancy involves chronic degenerative diseases to the patient which also affect the family's patient.

According to the 2010 census of Panama, population adults 60 and olders its about 9.7 % and it is estimated that by 2020 this will be around 12.4 % [13], indicating that this increase will involve a great impact the health sector in the country, bringing with it the need to ensure greater emphasis these people.

These home care are given the emergence of HOSPES Association for Palliative Care in 1992, this being the first in the country to offer care in home mode. Three years later in 1995, the Program for Palliative Care and Pain Relief is created within the premises of the National Cancer Institute (ION), allowing it to provide the care in outpatient and inpatient mode. In 2003 arises the law 68, which requires all health facilities in the country to provide the PC with professionals who have within their facilities. In the years 2006–2007 it begins to provide the PC inside the country, covering every type of care. Finally on June 21, 2010 under Resolution 499, the National Palliative Care Program of Panama is created.

The hospice has been providing in Panama for over 20 years, which has evolved over time but still the information is not electronically saved and many times the palliative care is not applied to the patient when its necessary. Some cases the palliative care arrive to the patients home after the patient has die.

In order to cover all the steps in which the patient need to receive palliative care, it has been divide in tree types: Home Care, Ambulatory Care and Hospital Care

- Home Care: This attention mode is very important because the patient will not be in the health institutions. it lets the patient to share with his family at home in his last stage
- Ambulatory Care: This mode has two ways to perform. In the first case, the patient has with the ability to attend the institution for care. In the second case, it is necessary the presence of a person (family or friend) to ensure the care of the patient. This person is known as primary caregiver and he needs to receive ongoing training on how should give care to the sick.
- Hospital Care: This last method is applied when the patient can not remain at home or the caregiver no longer has the professional skills to care for the sick. The patient has increased their suffering caused by the disease, thus requiring more treatments onerous for each symptom and pain relieving suffering of the patient.

Evolution Notes: In palliative care, it is really important to record the current status of the patient in each stage to evaluate the evolution of the illness with each applied treatment. The evolutions notes are divided in four sections, called SOAP or Subjective, Objective, Assessment Plan.

- *S (Subjective):* This section records all the information provided by the patient, as symptoms and pains The subjective impressions of the specialist is also included.
- *O (Objective):* In this section, the vital signs, physical and complementary exams of the patients are recorded
- *A (Assessment):* In this section the specialist evaluate the status of the and its evolution.
- *P (Plan):* This section modify the plan applied previously according to the patient's new tests and evaluation.

5   Downs Syndrome

Trisomy 21 also know as Down's Syndrome is an Aneuploidy where the fetus shows a genetic alteration having 3 chromosomes 21 [14]. This trisomy is one of the major causes of deficiencies or physical disabilities in children, premature deaths that take place before birth, situation that many mothers are unaware. This chromosomal disorder causes various physical deformities, hearth defects, organ malformations, mental retardation, thyroid disorder and diseases like Alzheimer's. Trisomy 21 responsible for Down's syndrome is the most frequent aneuploidy. How is the Down's Syndrome Currently calculated? As mentioned in [15] screening is a probabilistic technique applied to a population to calculate the risk or probability that the fetus suffer a particular disease.

In the screening, first serum and biochemical markers are established and compared with historical medians references values of the population. When the test results of the patient and the MOM or Multiple of Median of the markers have different values, the test is considered positive.

The screening methods for Downs syndrome are performed in the second and first trimester being the first trimester the most difficult to execute. One of the main barriers of this test is the lack of sampling data to perform the test.

For the first trimester trisomy 21 screening, it is necessary to perform a more effective detection taking in consideration some mother's characteristics like her weight, her ethnicity, if she has diabetes or if is smoke. These factors could affect the result of the test so it needs to be corrected.

6   Ubiquitous eHealth Platforms Design, Development and Implementation

6.1   Ubiquitous Paleative Health Care Platform

The first step to realize was to make a state of the art of paleative care in Panama. All the requirements, resources, actors, process and current issues where gathered from specialist, current documents, final user interviews. All this information was analyzed and to develop an ubiquitous platform to provide improved health care in the country. In the Fig. 1 can be appreciate the general use cases and actors of the system.

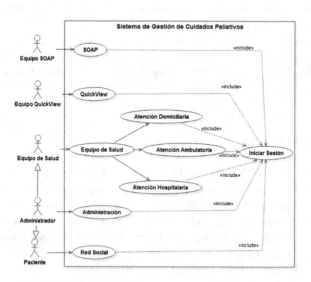

Fig. 1. Paleative care use case diagram

The main classes of the platforms are presented in Fig. 2. The usability was a very important factor in the design of the platform and it was based on Goal Oriented Design by Allan Cooper [16, 17].

The interaction with the platform was designed based on the usability and specifict goal that each type of user will have with the platform.

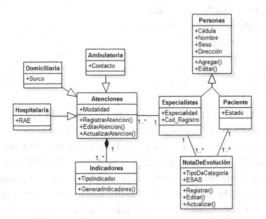

Fig. 2. Paleative health care class diagram

The production version of the Paleative Health Care platform can be appreciated in Fig. 3.

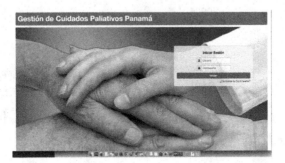

Fig. 3. Ubiquitous paleative health care platform in Panama

6.2 Ubiquitous Platform for Down's Syndrome Risk Estimation Process

The eHealth Management Platform PLAGETRI21 [1] is based on the calculation risk method of Likelihood, published in [18] combining the a priori risk for maternal age obtained from the meta-analysis by, with the likelihood obtained from combining the MoM of the different markers used in each profile. The MoM calculated using the multivariate normal distribution. This calculation follow a mathematical and statistical process:

- Risk estimation based in the maternal age.
- Markers standardization.
- Multiple of medians (MoM) calculation.
- Weight and correction factors adjustments.
- Maternal weight corrections.
- Covariates corrections.
- Likelihood ratio estimation.
- Risk estimation.

The architecture is based on the architecture presented in [19–21] which allow the interoperability between many hospital information systems.

PLAGETRI21 is able to interact using the HL7 standard with many data source of clinical information. It uses the Clinical Document Architecture CDA to save domain-sampling data from diverse sources around the country without the necessity of installing any software at the client side and using laptop and mobile devices. The CDA standard allow the interoperability of with other platforms that also implement this standard in their architecture. The message body structured HL7 CDA consists of two parts that are the header and message body as appreciated in Fig. 4.

```
<ClinicalDocument>
        <!-- CDA Header -->
        <!-- CDA Body -->
        <component>
            <structuredBody>
                <component>
                    <section>_</section>
                    <section>_</section>
                </component>
            </structuredBody>
        </component>
</ClinicalDocument>
```

Fig. 4. HL7 CDA structure

As an example, to send data about the height and weight of the patient the tag <entry> is used, and is structured as follows:

```
<entry>
<observation classCode="OBS" moodCode="EVN">
<code code="363808001" codeSystem="2.16.840.1.113883.6.96"
codeSystemName="SNOMED CT" displayName="Peso Corporal"/>
<effectiveTime value="201504071430"/>
<value xsi:type="PQ" value="71.6" unit="kg"/>
</observation>
</entry>
<entry>
<observation classCode="OBS" moodCode="EVN">
<code code="384627007" codeSystem="2.16.840.1.113883.6.96"
codeSystemName="SNOMED CT" displayName="Estatura"/>
<effectiveTime value="201504071430"/>
<value xsi:type="PQ" value="1.65" unit="m">
</observation>
</entry>
```

The interconnection with other data sources involves security and privacy of the information, like is presented by Geissbuhler. The data that is extracted from the different data sources include general information of the patient like age, sex, ethnic, blood type, place of birth, residence. Specific fields like name, last names, and personal id are not included in the sampling data source. The platform also implements the geospatial interoperability standard proposed in [22, 23]. The inclusion of geographical information to the platform enable the clinical information being georeferenced by birth place, residence place and location where the patient receives the medical care, allowing us to research how the location data affect the process. The production version of the ubiquitous platform can be observed in Fig. 5.

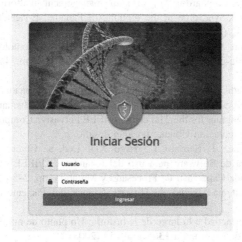

Fig. 5. Down syndrome risk estimation platform

The platform is running on a private cloud inside the Technological University of Panama and the Electronics Health and Supercomputing Research's Group developed it.

7 Conclusions

The Down's syndrome risk estimation process platform enhance the accuracy of the result because it not only use as a input data information based on the population sampling but also adding valuable and not before geographical information to the procedures.

Thanks to the information that is being captured organized and shared from diverse sources in the country, the first trimester screening test will be applied allowing to detect earlier any illness in order to provide the treatment in an timely manner.

The palliative care platform allows, thanks to its ubiquities properties, to record personal and medical information in real time. It also lets specialist of the field to have access to this information and apply adequated medicines and treatment. The platform is a tools that the patients family has to be in touch with the medical specialist.

Ubiquitous computing and ambient assisted living open to us a broad source of resources that can be applied to improve many areas of healthcare.

Acknowledgments. The Research Group Electronics Health and Supercomputing (GISES) of the Technological University of Panama support this research. As well as Dr. Miguel Vargas-Lombardo National Research Investigator award (SNI) from the SENACYT. Both projects are being presented as main topics looking for funds with SENACYT.

References

1. Saldaña, J., Vargas-Lombardo, M.: eHealth management platform for screening and prediction of down's syndrome in the republic of Panama. E-Health Telecommun. Syst. Netw. **03**(03), 33–42 (2014)
2. Tran, V.-A., Johnson, N., Redline, S., Zhang, G.-Q.: OnWARD: ontology-driven web-based framework for multi-center clinical studies. J. Biomed. Inform. **44**(Suppl 1), S48–S53 (2011)
3. Domínguez, Y.: Sindrome de Down Batalla Social. http://www.diaadia.com.pa/primerplano/s%C3%ADndrome-de-down-batalla-social-268675. Accessed 1 January 2015
4. Weiser, M.: The computer for the 21st century. IEEE Pervasive Comput. **1**(1), 19–25 (2002)
5. Pomares, E.S.: Computación Ubicua: un gran desafío, p. 2
6. Escayola, J., Martínez, I., Serrano, L., Trigo, J.D., Led, S., García, J.: Propuesta de una Nueva Arquitectura de Software para uso del Estándar ISO/IEEE 11073 en Dispositivos Médicos de Limitada Capacidad de Procesado y Memoria, pp. 2–5 (2008)
7. Robledo, G.R.: Sistema Ubicuo de Historia Clínica del Paciente. Instituto Politécnico Nacional (2006)
8. Tricas, G.: La Enfermedad a lo largo de la historia: Un punto de mira entre la biología y la simbología. Index de Enfermería **13**(47), 49–53 (2004)
9. Montes, G.: Historia de los Cuidados Paliativos, vol. 7, pp. 1–9 (2006)

10. Cook, M.: Cicely Saunders, la mujer que transformó el cuidado de los moribundos, vol. 11 (2005)
11. World Health Organization: Cancer pain reli. In: Cancer Pain Relief: With a Guide to Opiod Availability, 2nd edn., pp. 1–70. World Health Organization, Geneva (1996)
12. Valencia, M.I.B.: Envejecimiento de la población: un reto para la salud pública. Revista Colombiana de Anestesiología **40**(69), 192–194 (2012)
13. INEC Contraloría General de la República de Panamá: Estimaciones y proyecciones de la población en la republica, provincia, comarca indígena por distrito, según sexo y edad; 2010–20
14. Gyselaers, W., Vereecken, A., Van Herck, E., Straetmans, D., Martens, G., de Jonge, E., Ombelet, W., Nijhuis, J.: Screening for trisomy 21 in Flanders: a 10 years review of 40.490 pregnancies screened by maternal serum. Eur. J. Obstet. Gynecol. Reprod. Biol. **115**(2), 185–189 (2004)
15. Saldaña, J.J.B., Rovetto, C., Pitti, E., Vargas, M.: Modelado formal de la metodología para la predicción de pacientes con Síndrome de Down en Panamá (2015)
16. Guersenzvaig, A.: El usuario arquetípico: Creación y uso de personajes en el diseño de productos interactivos. Hum. Comput. Interact
17. Honduvilla, M., Bernabé Poveda, M.A., Manrique Sancho, M.T.: La usabilidad de los geoportales : Aplicación del Diseño Orientado a Metas (DOM), no. 1
18. Benn, P.A.: Advances in prenatal screening for down syndrome: I. general principles and second trimester testing. Clin. Chim. Acta **323**(1–2), 1–16 (2002)
19. Barbarito, F., Pinciroli, F., Mason, J., Marceglia, S., Mazzola, L., Bonacina, S.: Implementing standards for the interoperability among healthcare providers in the public regionalized healthcare information system of the lombardy region. J. Biomed. Inform. **45**(4), 736–745 (2012)
20. Esri, A.: HL7 and Spatial Interoperability Standards for Public Health and Health Care Delivery, January (2011)
21. Feldmann, R.L., Shull, F., Denger, C., Host, M., Lindholm, C.: A survey of software engineering techniques in medical device development. In: 2007 Joint Workshop High Confidence Medical Devices, Software, Systems Medical Device Plug-and-Play Interoperability (HCMDSS-MDPnP 2007), pp. 46–54, June 2007
22. Granell, C., Fernández, Ó.B., Díaz, L.: Geospatial information infrastructures to address spatial needs in health: collaboration, challenges and opportunities. Futur. Gener. Comput. Syst. **31**, 213–222 (2014)
23. Ahern, D.K.: Challenges and opportunities of eHealth research. Am. J. Prev. Med. **32**(5 Suppl), S75–S82 (2007)

Making the Physical Therapy Entertaining

An Application Based on Wearable Technology and Mobile Games

Andrea Torres[1](✉), Gustavo López[2], and Luis Guerrero[2,3]

[1] Posgrado en Computación e Informática, Universidad de Costa Rica,
San Pedro, Costa Rica
andrea.torres@ucr.ac.cr
[2] Centro de Investigaciones en Tecnologías de la Información y Comunicación,
UCR, San Pedro, Costa Rica
gustavo.lopez_h@ucr.ac.cr,
luis.guerrero@ecci.ucr.ac.cr
[3] Escuela de Ciencias de la Computación e Informática, Universidad de Costa
Rica, San Pedro, Costa Rica

Abstract. In physical therapy, goniometers are used to measure limb movement during restoration exercises. These devices aren't always readily available to therapists, and the exercises themselves are monotonous and offer little motivation for the patients. We have developed a low-cost device prototype we've tested in knee rehabilitation exercises, and developed a framework with which a mobile application can use gathered data from said device, such as is the case of an example game also addressed here, intended to increase patient motivation and commitment when exercising.

Keywords: Physical therapy · Wearable medical devices · Videogames

1 Introduction

Rehabilitation in Physical Therapy helps overcoming physical impairments in order to develop or restore maximum body movement. The main causes that lead people to require physical therapy are ageing, injuries, diseases, and other disorders. It is conducted by a physical therapist and includes: examination, evaluation, diagnosis, prognosis, treatment, and re-examination of a physical movement restriction.

In recent years, some research projects have been exploring the use of wearable technology to monitor physical movement for rehabilitation [1, 2]. Moreover, videogames have been incorporated into the physical therapy process to make it less monotonous [3].

This paper proposes a wearable device that allows physical therapy monitoring with a built in game which dynamics force the player to perform physical therapy exercises, called Funtherapy. Our goal is to provide an entertaining way to perform the tedious movements required in physical therapy, as well as real time monitoring of exercises, in order to prevent injuries while performing these.

© Springer International Publishing Switzerland 2015
J. Bravo et al. (Eds.): AmIHEALTH 2015, LNCS 9456, pp. 148–154, 2015.
DOI: 10.1007/978-3-319-26508-7_15

The main contribution of this research is the accurate measurement of movements that allow physical therapy monitoring, while using videogames to increase the interest on the daily exercises and the motivation of the patient on knee rehabilitation.

The research was done with expert supervision from the School of Physical Therapy at Universidad de Costa Rica (UCR), to assess the system's applicability to physical therapy for knee rehabilitation. Functional testing was also executed in real scenarios, performed by physical therapists. Results were promising, as the experts stated that the system could be applied for constant remote monitoring of patients and to help patients do the exercises as they should.

The rest of the paper is structured as follows: Sect. 2 presents the background and shows some related work. Section 3 describes the design and development of the prototype, to make physical therapy entertaining. Section 4 concludes the paper and points out potential future work.

2 Background

This section describes some examples of wearable technology applications in healthcare and physical therapy.

2.1 Wearable Technology Applications in Healthcare

Advances in technology have enabled the application of wearable technology into healthcare [4]. These applications use wearable medical devices, which can be described as an autonomous, non-invasive system that performs a specific medical function such as monitoring or support [5]. Wearable medical devices are composed of [5]:

- Sensors, either physiological or environmental to monitor health (e.g., body temperature, pulse rate, respiration rate, blood pressure) or surrounding conditions (e.g., temperature, humidity).
- Processing unit and all computational hardware required for input and output of computation of information.
- Customized clothing to attach all the components to the user.

Wearable medical devices include a wide range of sensors such as accelerometers and gyroscopes, smart fabrics, actuators, wireless communication networks, power supplies, and data capture and processing technologies [6]. Moreover, they allow movement that other types of systems restrain.

Alrige and Chatterjee [7] proposed a taxonomy of wearable technologies in healthcare with the goal to characterize the developments in this area. Their taxonomy divides the spectrum in three dimensions: functionality, application, and form. According to this taxonomy, Funtherapy is Single-Sensor, in the functionality dimension. In the application dimension, the system is for monitoring and assistance, so it offers more value for patient more than for therapists. Finally in the form dimension, Funtherapy is an accessory, however, if the mobile application is considered, it is also portable.

2.2   Related Work

Several researches have been conducted to create accurate devices that measure physical movement. For instance, Huang et al. [8] presented a wearable physical therapy support system that gathers patient exercise compliance and performance, and provides visual information for the therapist.

Yurtman and Barshan [9] developed an autonomous system that detects and evaluates physical therapy exercises using wearable motion sensors. They monitor exercises similar in the scope of Funtherpay; however, their algorithm uses a multi sensor approach to do it (we used a single one).

Kimel [10] designed a device to improve patient-therapist communication using a network-based monitoring system. Ananthanarayan et al. [11] presented a similar device. However, their knee support like device allows more than just monitoring, it has a haptic visualization of the knee angle, allowing the patient to measure in a more precise manner the knee angle and perform in a better way the therapy exercises.

Muñoz et al. [12] developed an Arduino based prototype that measures knee movement and angles, using a Led to allow the user to know when the exercise angle is reached.

Nerino et al. [13] developed an unassisted system for post-surgical knee rehabilitation, from which the patients get feedback about the correct positions and executions of the exercises in a mobile app. A similar system for rehabilitation at home was proposed by Ayoade and Baillie [14], where the movement visualizations are displayed in a computer, and the patients get feedback by a color-coded and repetition counter.

The main difference between these proposals and the one proposed by this research is that it provides the user's feedback integrated in the videogame, allowing constant monitoring, and not just some graphic notifications.

Moreover, the videogame follows the exercise dynamics according to the therapist recommendations. Finally, instead of a knee sleeve/support device, we use a small sensor in the ankle to measure knee angles.

3   Design and Development

FunTherapy consists of two main components: a wearable device that tracks the user movements and a mobile application (goniometer and videogame) that gathers information and utilizes the wearable device as an interaction mechanism.

3.1   The Wearable Device

As it was stated by Glaros and Fotiadis [5], every wearable system is usually composed of three main parts: sensors, processing unit, and clothing. This section describes these three components within the context of the Funtherapy system.

The sensor used for this system was one Adafruit's Flora Accelerometer/Compass/Gyroscope Sensor LSM9DS0. This sensor contains a 3-axis accelerometer, a 3 axis magnetometer, and a 3-axis gyroscope. For communication purposes between the wearable and the mobile, we use an HC-06 generic Bluetooth module. As for the processing unit, an Adafruit's wearable electronics platform Arduino Flora was used. And finally, a lithium battery with 2000 milliamps and 3.7 V was also used.

The software runs in a mobile phone and the input are Euler angles [15] in a three dimension system: roll (x-axis, Eq. 1), pitch (y-axis, Eq. 2), and heading (z-axis, Eq. 3). X, Y, and Z in these equations are data gathered from the accelerometer in the corresponding axis.

In the first version of the prototype we used a plastic case to fit all of the components together. However, the case's material is going to be changed in order to increase user comfort while using the device.

3.2   App Design

Since mobile devices have achieved considerable penetration within the general public in recent years, it was decided to develop the framework and test system as a mobile application, such that it could eventually be made available at little to no cost to therapists and their patients along with the corresponding hardware interface.

In the first phase, we worked with professional therapists of the School of Physical Therapy at UCR, simulating the operation of the goniometer, an instrument used for measuring angles on limbs. The app has an interface that shows the movement of the leg flexion and extension, derived from the information obtained through the wearable.

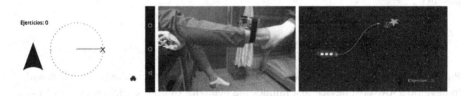

Fig. 1. Goniometer test at 90°

The first tests were carried out with an exercise to work knee flexion and extension: the patient is positioned in a sitting position and is tasked with stretching his leg towards the front, in a 90° (as shown in Fig. 1). The results showed that it was necessary to adjust the measurements, since the goniometer measures angles formed by the tibia and femur, and the wearable is over the tibia. Adjustment corresponds to 5 additional degrees, according to the measurements made by therapists. Wearable measurements were then repeated and compared with the goniometer results, resulting in completely matching results (Table 1).

The second exercise works with the knee flexion and extension in the rear part of the leg. The patient lies down and is instructed to move the leg in the direction of the coccyx, as closest as the muscles allow it. The results match between the wearable and the goniometer, adding the adjustment indicated by therapists.

Table 1. Goniometer vs wearable device test

Wearable	Goniometer	Wearable + adjust
85	90	90
65	70	70
60	65	65
80	85	85
75	80	80

Feedback was requested from the therapists who participated in the study, revealing several potential improvements in the way they interacted with the prototype device, such as being able to modify variables used for exercise measurement.

In the second phase, we designed a game based around classic sidescroller space shooters in which items that the player must catch move towards the player's avatar as he/she performs one of the exercises described previously (in the example, patient must catch the stars, as shown in Fig. 1).

Our decision to use this game was that most of the people that suffer an impairment that forces them to attend physical therapy had some type of interaction with this kind of games. Therefore, we hope that this similarity to a well-known game will engage people in the gameplay, providing the required concentration and immersion.

The game provides therapists with the same control over exercise variables as the developed prototype used in our trials, so that it can be adjusted to the needs of different patients.

4   Conclusions and Future Work

Preliminary results from trials performed with physical therapists indicate it is possible to develop a low-cost device that mimics the behavior of goniometers used for physical therapy applications, with the added benefit of integrating endpoints which other more complex applications can leverage for various purposes.

Due to the scope of the project, in this article we've focused on developing a simple videogame intended to be used for knee rehabilitation, however it should be evident that the project's framework is highly adaptable and allows for a wide variety of applications on physical therapy and other fields at a very low cost.

This could potentially lead to interest for this sort of devices and applications in places where professional tools aren't readily available, such as medical facilities in third world countries.

As for future work, despite the current prototype being in itself a work in progress, there are many projects this basework could spawn, such as determining whether physical improvement of patients can be improved by introducing motivation-inducing game design principles, introducing accessibility features so that therapists can also make use of the system through visual or audio cues, or explore more kind of game archetypes that could be applied to other exercise types.

Acknowledgments. This work was partially supported by CITIC-UCR (Centro de Investigaciones en Tecnologías de la Información y Comunicación) grand No. 834-B4-159 and by ECCI-UCR (Escuela de Ciencias de la Computación e Informatica at Universidad de Costa Rica). We thank professor Judith Umaña Cascante of Escuela de Terapia Física at Universidad de Costa Rica for her support.

References

1. Patel, S., Park, H., Bonato, P., Chan, L., Rodgers, M.: Wearable sensors and systems; home monitoring; telemedicine; smart home. J. NeuroEng. Rehabil. **9**(21), 1–17 (2012)
2. Appelboom, G., Camacho, E., Abraham, M., Bruce, S., Dumont, E., Zacharia, B., D'Amico, R., Slomian, J., Reginster, J., Bruyère, O., Connolly, E.S.: Smart wearable body sensors for patient self-assessment and monitoring. Arch. Public Health **72**(1), 1–9 (2014)
3. Geurts, L., Vanden Abeele, V., Husson, J., Windey, F., Van Overveldt, M., Annema, J.H., Desmet, S.: Digital games for physical therapy: fulfilling the need for calibration and adaptation. In: Conference on Tangible, Embedded, and Embodied Interaction (2011)
4. Raso, I., Hervás, R., & Bravo, J.: m-Physio: Personalized Accelerometer-based Physical Rehabilitation Platform (n.d.) (2010)
5. Glaros, C., Fotiadis, D.: Wearable devices in healthcare. In: Silverman, B.G., Jain, A., Ichalkaranje, A., Jain, L.C. (eds.) Intelligent Paradigms for Healthcare Enterprises. Studies in Fuzziness and Soft Computing, pp. 237–264. Springer, Berlin (2005)
6. Chan, M., Estève, D., Fourniols, J.-Y., Escriba, C., Campo, E.: Smart wearable systems: current status and future challenges. Artif. Intell. Med. **56**(3), 137–156 (2012)
7. Alrige, M., Chatterjee, S.: Toward a taxonomy of wearable technologies in healthcare. In: Donnellan, B., Helfert, M., Kenneally, J., VanderMeer, D., Rothenberger, M., Winter, R. (eds.). LNCS, vol. 9073, pp. 496–504Springer, Heidelberg (2015)
8. Huang, K., Sparto, P.J., Kiesler, S., Smailagic, A., Mankoff, J., Siewiorek, D.: A technology probe of wearable in-home computer-assisted physical therapy. In: ACM Conference on Human Factors in Computing Systems (2014)
9. Yurtman, A., Barshan, B.: detection and evaluation of physical therapy exercises by dynamic time warping using wearable motion sensor units. In: International Symposium on Computer and Information Sciences (2013)
10. Kimel, J.: Thera-Network: a wearable computing network to motivate exercise in patients undergoing physical therapy. In: International Conference on Distributed Computing Systems Workshops (2005)
11. Ananthanarayan, S., Sheh, M., Chien, A., Profita, H., Siek, K.: Pt Viz: Towards a wearable device for visualizing knee rehabilitation exercises. In: Proceedings of the SIGCHI Conference on Human Factors in Computing Systems (2013)
12. Muñoz, D., Pruett, A., Williams, G.: Knee: an everyday wearable goniometer for monitoring physical therapy adherence. In: CHI 2014 Extended Abstracts on Human Factors in Computing Systems (2014)
13. Nerino, R., Contin, L., da Silva Pinto, W.J.G., Massazza, G., Actis, M., Capacchione, P., Pettiti, G.: A BSN based service for post-surgical knee rehabilitation at home. In: Proceedings of the 8th International Conference on Body Area Networks, pp. 401–407. ICST (Institute for Computer Sciences, Social-Informatics and Telecommunications Engineering), Brussels, Belgium (2013)

14. Ayoade, M., Baillie, L.: A novel knee rehabilitation system for the home. In: Proceedings of the 32nd Annual ACM Conference on Human Factors in Computing Systems, pp. 2521–2530. ACM, New York, NY, USA (2014)
15. Pio, R.: Euler angle transformations. IEEE Trans. Autom. Control 11(4), 707–715 (1966)

Vision Based Extraction of Dynamic Gait Features Focused on Feet Movement Using RGB Camera

Mario Nieto-Hidalgo[✉], Francisco Javier Ferrández-Pastor,
Rafael J. Valdivieso-Sarabia, Jerónimo Mora-Pascual,
and Juan Manuel García-Chamizo

Department of Computing Technology, University of Alicante,
P.O. Box 90, 03080 San Vicente del Raspeig, Alicante, Spain
{mnieto, fjferran, rvaldivieso,
jeronimo, juanma}@dtic.ua.es

Abstract. Bipedal gait involves the entire body but some subsystems are decisive for gait while other parts of the body play complementary roles (dynamic balance, harmony of movement, etc.). We have proposed a functional specification of gait. It is based on logical expression format and takes into account only observational kinematic aspects. The specification is open enough that it can be used in other gait analysis problems (rehabilitation, sport, children, etc.).

We have developed a prototype of an extraction system of gait features by analysing image sequences. Prototype is restricted to the analysis of the movement of the feet and it allows to determine the dynamic parameters (heel strike, toe off, stride length and time, etc.) satisfactorily. Experiments have been performed on our own dataset of 17 cases.

Keywords: Gait analysis · Computer vision · RGB · Heel strike · Toe off · Frailty · Senility

1 Introduction

Traditionally, several branches of medicine such us orthopaedics, rheumatology, neurology and rehabilitation analyse the human walking to obtain helpful information (e.g. early diagnosis of diseases like frailty or dementia). One of the main techniques used to obtain this information is the gait analysis: quantification of measurable parameters of gait and its interpretation [1]. This process is based on subjective measurements carried out under clinical conditions by specialists.

Most of the relevant authors in this matter, remark the physical activity as the main component involved in frailty syndrome evaluation as well as other biological markers [2–4]. There are works that identify the gait as a high cognitive task [5]. In the gait cycle, attention, planning, memory and other cognitive process are involved [6]. Waite et al. [7] conclude in their study about gait slowdown that it is a predictor factor of dementia. Similar to this study are [8–11].

© Springer International Publishing Switzerland 2015
J. Bravo et al. (Eds.): AmIHEALTH 2015, LNCS 9456, pp. 155–166, 2015.
DOI: 10.1007/978-3-319-26508-7_16

Advances in new technologies have led to the proliferation of applications that study gait analysis (e.g. human identification, video surveillance or sports related). These new technologies provide, on one hand, techniques to measure parameters of human gait more precisely and, on the other hand, intelligent analysis systems. Non-wearable (e.g. video cameras, floor sensors, etc.) or wearable devices (e.g. accelerometers, gyroscopes, etc.) can measure and characterise human gait parameters (e.g. length, stride length, stride velocity, cadence, etc.). Intelligent analysis techniques (e.g. computer vision) provide new strategies to interpret and understand human walking.

This work proposes a new technique based in computer vision that is used to measure gait parameters and to characterise human walking using only video cameras. The development effort focuses on classification and inference algorithms specialised in the modelling of human walking. This proposal will allow designing intelligent and low-cost systems. The use of image sensors installed in digital cameras is also energy efficient because rely on visible light only.

Human walking is a specialized form of motion that it is obtained in video sequences from different recording devices (digital cameras). The human gait analysis is difficult due to the variability of poses and actions involved. To treat this problem, this research includes segmentation, tracking and pose analysis using low level algorithms to extract the main parameters of gait analysis.

This paper is organized as follows: Sect. 2 reviews related works. In Sect. 3, a general gait specification is proposed. Section 4, presents our algorithm for "heel strike" and "toe off" events extraction. Results of this algorithm are shown in Sect. 5. Finally, Sect. 6 provides a discussion and conclusions.

2 Related Work

Most of the relevant authors usually divide the vision gait analysis techniques in two types: model based techniques and shape based techniques. The first ones try to fit a mathematical model of the gait structure and movement. Some of them use a skeleton model, others divide the silhouette in elliptic or volumetric shapes, and then measure spatio-temporal features like stride length, steps per second, etc. The other techniques analyse the shape of the subject and its change over time.

A cascade fusion scheme defined in [12] represent links between gait images and its correspondent foot accumulative pressure image. These images are accumulative records of the reaction force of the ground against the pressure produced by a foot during a gait cycle. Although this is a high precision technique, the main disadvantage of this approach is that it requires the person to walk on barefoot because accumulative pressure images vary depending on the footwear. It also requires expensive sensors on the floor to obtain such images which is contrary to our objective of using low cost devices.

A novel representation of motion information in high resolution, Pose Energy Image (PEI), proposed in [13]. PEI, is the average image of all the silhouettes in a gait cycle which belongs to a particular pose state. The computation performance of PEI is slow. To resolve this, Pose Kinematic is proposed. It is defined as the percentage of time spent in each of the N key pose states.

Following with the PEI approach, [14] propose to use gait phase at the instant of entering and leaving from one camera to another for tracking a person in a multicamera system. As starting point, they use a sequence of the silhouette of a person's gait. From this sequence, they define some key poses using the K-means clustering algorithm. Each key pose is a PEI. Once key poses are obtained, each silhouette of the sequence is projected in eigenspace to calculate the feature vector. Following, a similarity score of the input and each key pose is calculated.

The shadow projected by a person is used in [16] to improve gait recognition using aerial cameras in which the person is shown from above. They use spherical harmonics to analyse gait features showing better results than other methods using Fourier, Gait Energy Image or Active Energy Image. They also propose the combined use of shadow and person silhouette to improve recognition using oblique camera where there is a good view of both. The main drawback of this approach is that it is dependant of the light to produce shadows.

A set of different gait features is analysed in [21] for person identification. They extract the silhouette and then obtain the contour using Canny. Then they extract 4 features: evolution of the width/height proportion, evolution of maximum and minimum width of the bounding box, evolution of the silhouette area and evolution of the centre of gravity. These 4 features follow a cyclic pattern that match the gait cycle and are used to identify a person through deterministic learning. The system is previously trained to learn the patterns of the 4 features for each person that are intended to be identified.

We first considered these shape based techniques because they do not need deep knowledge of gait. That is why these techniques are really good for person identification. However, what we need is a full characterization of gait which is better provided by model based techniques like the following.

The use of Kinect sensor to measure gait parameters during a treadmill walking with frontal view is examined in [15]. Heel strike and toe off events obtained with a Kinect sensor are compared with those obtained with a motion tracking system. The results show that heel strike has less error than toe off because heel strike is produced closer to Kinect sensor. The study shows that Kinect sensor may be used as an alternative device to measure some gait parameters for treadmill walking. However, we discard this approach for our problem since the use of a treadmill can alter the gait of the subject.

An approach for parkinsonian gait recognition is presented in [18]. They use the silhouette to obtain the bounding box and fit a human model to find head, torso and legs segments. The skeleton is obtained by computing the mean points of each body segment. Following, they obtain legs movement and the posture inclination while the person is walking to get a particular score that it is compared with a normal gait model in order to get a similarity score. Similarly we use the notion of fitting a human model to obtain the feet area in our algorithm.

A method called STM-SPP is proposed in [20]. This method is composed by three modules: extraction and post-process of the silhouette, subject classification using PSA and EFD, and combination of both results. Silhouette extraction module is carried out using background subtraction and morphologic operations to remove noise. PSA module analyses a group of shapes using matching of settings. A setting is defined as a set of geometrical location points of a figure. Those points are obtained from an anatomical analysis in which different key body points (head, torso, knee...) are considered as fraction of the subject's height. They calculate stride length using: the width of the bounding box of the zone defined as feet, the contraction and dilation bounding box period. EFD allows to characterize the contour of the subject in key points of a gait phase. From this approach we incorporate the idea of using the bounding box width in our algorithm to identify gait cycle.

Although we finally choose a model based technique, we do not discard using a shape based technique in the future to improve the characterization using a combined method such as the three phase gait recognition approach presented in [17]. They analyse the spatio-temporal shape and movement of a subject's silhouette to identify him. In first phase, they use the phase-weighted magnitude spectra of the Fourier descriptor of the silhouette contour in 10 phases of gait period to analyse the spatio-temporal changes in shape. In second phase, they perform an analysis of the body shape and movement by fitting ellipses in the segments of the contour for the 10 phases of gait using a histogram matching with the Bhattacharyya distance as a dissimilarity score. In the last phase, they use Dynamic Time Warping to analyse the angular rotation pattern of the front knee taking into account the arms swing. Finally, the scores obtained in each phase are fused using a score weight system to obtain a robust identification against occlusion or unavailable or distorted frames.

3 Gait Specification

Computer vision to characterize environment and human behaviour is part of our research area related to technological systems to ambient assisted living. In particular, we are working in early detection of frailty and dementia syndromes in elderly people through the analysis of gait using computer vision.

The main advantages of visible light based systems are: innocuousness to people and environmental sustainability.

The first fact is because it allows to extract information from the object of study without affecting the analysed phenomenon or system. This remark is more referred to be consequent with the postulates of physics, in the meaning of what Heisenberg established [22], than a practical context, because at a macroscopic level, the physic of capturing images doesn't affect gait. However, we consider appropriate this innocuousness, especially to remark that most of the sensors are intrusive, i.e., they are transducers that flood the environment and the subject of study with energy (infrared light, acoustic emissions, microwaves, etc.). Other systems requires the cooperation of the subject of study. In both cases, the subject of study might be affected by the direct effect of the physical phenomenology or by the subjective incidence derived from the cooperation of the subject.

The second fact is because the amount of energy that is thrown to the environment grows with the power of the devices and with the amount of them that are operating in a specific region of space and time. This accumulative effect can overflow the healthy limits. This is the reason why it is necessary to watch over the using of such systems in order to control the excessive accumulation in a certain place and time.

The relation between syndromes that affect elderly people and gait analysis are sufficiently justified by the state of the art. However, as part of the research area about people assistance, our interest embraces other activities in any range of age (sport, rehabilitation, children syndromes, etc.). The revision of the state of the art allow us to check that the parameters of gait analysed are related to the physiology of gait, which is causally coherent: characterization of a phenomenon based on the parameters that regulate the phenomenon. At such effect, we have been able to find several definitions of gait:

Gait is defined by [14] as a periodic activity in which each cycle is composed by two steps: right foot forward and left foot forward.

In [19] define gait as a kinematic problem, so it has static and dynamic aspects. Static components are related to physical construction of a person from the different gait phases. The dynamic components are related to the temporal changes of a person during a gait cycle.

Gait is also defined as a sequence of repetitive movements that varies over time and from one subject to another in [23].

These definitions involve some variables of the physical movement of a person and, perhaps, physiological parameters, and even from psychology.

The visual analysis of gait is focused on the study of the person's movement information extracted from a sequence of images. Although transduction is made from visible light, the analysis is an indirect measure of kinematic magnitudes (movement without considering its causes). Through computer vision, we unlink the results from the dynamic approach (movement considering its causes) of gait because the forces involved have a physiological and emotional influence that could compromise the objectivity of the analysis. It would be another system the responsible to infer the causes (characterize syndromes) from results of the computer vision analysis.

The absence of sufficiently objective and complete formal specification of gait definition to provide coverage to computer vision analysis has led us to propose a new kinematic specification of people gait using the method proposed in [24]. To do so, we build a simple syntactical structure formed by a transitive predicate to assign the model and another formal predicate to assign the objectives as conjunctions.

```
<problem> <to be verb> <article> <model> <preposition> <objective>
(<conjunction> <objective>)* "."
```

The process to obtain a formal specification of gait requires: decide a reference model and define the objectives that gait should satisfy.

To delimit the model, we have considered the cases shown in Table 1, cases we consider human gait as well as other cases we do not consider as human gait.

The composition of conditions of the examples and counterexamples produces the following definition:

"Gait is the anthropomorphic upright self-displacement, in an alternating stepping of two feet, with no additional fulcra, keeping at least a point of support at every time, on a horizontal or slightly inclined surface."

Therefore, the kinematic variables of gait are defined in Table 2.

Table 1. Cases of movement considered as gait and counterexamples.

Examples	Counterexamples
Gait of elderly people	Other robots
Gait of an adult person	Translation of other animals
Gait of a child	With more or less than two legs
Sport gait	Swim
Walking over a treadmill	Fly
Walking under psychotropic influence	Run
Upright translation of apes	Climb
Upright translation of bears	Triple jump
A bipedal robot walking	Up or down ramps or stairs
Walking with an exoskeleton	Stand on a mechanic stairs
"Moonwalker"	Crawl

Table 2. Human gait variables.

Shape variables	Movement variables
Silhouette shape	Step and stride length
Silhouette position	Step and stride time
Displacement plane	Cadence
Centroid	Single support time
Height and other body variables	Double support time
Arm angles and lengths	Speed
Leg variables	Acceleration
Foot variables	Foot maximum height

The proposed definition assumes that the whole body participates in gait, which is reasonable even if there are some body parts that have a greater effect than others and, therefore, it allows to characterize the gait easily, as is the case of feet. That is why in this work we have only considered the feet for characterizing the gait. However, future works might require additional information such as legs layout, full skeleton, the evolution of the centroid, or even the movement of the upper extremities and head.

4 Heel Strike and Toe off Extraction Algorithm

This algorithm detect both "heel strike" and "toe off" spatio-temporal events using a side view of a person walking. The algorithm can process sequences captured with a standard RGB camera. The sequences are processed following the phases shown in Fig. 1 flow chart.

The first step is to obtain the subject's silhouette, to do that we use "Mean of Gaussians" background subtractor. The next step is to locate toe and heel of each foot.

Our algorithm doesn't use any marker attached to the body, the reason why we use this approach is to be able to reduce the required infrastructure to a single mobile device in future versions.

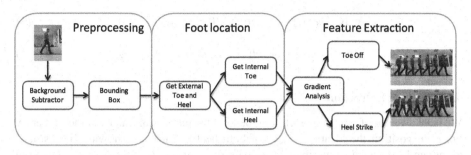

Fig. 1. Flow chart of heel strike and toe off extraction algorithm.

Without using visual markers, we do not have information that allow us to segment through colour. However, it is possible to get the shape of the silhouette and it is known that the feet are located in the lower part, so a first segmentation can be applied, removing the upper part of the silhouette (keeping around 20 % of the height of the silhouette). Also the width of the foot can be obtained from the bounding box of the silhouette. It is the minimum width of the bounding box (Eq. 4), which is achieved when feet are in parallel. Then, to obtain the forward foot toe and backward foot heel we have to obtain the maximum x of the silhouette for the toe (Eq. 1) and the minimum x for the heel (Eq. 2), assuming gait direction from left to right, as shown in Fig. 2a.

$$\arg\max_{x,y}(\forall_{x,y} \in silhouette : x) \tag{1}$$

$$\arg\min_{x,y}(\forall_{x,y} \in silhouette : x) \tag{2}$$

Once these two points are achieved, feet silhouette is cut in two from the heel plus foot width (blue square in Fig. 2b) and from the obtained toe minus foot width (Fig. 2c). These two cuts provide the bounding box corresponding to each foot. Then, for each bounding box, the lower right pixel (for toe, Fig. 2b) and the lower left pixel (for heel, Fig. 2c) are searched.

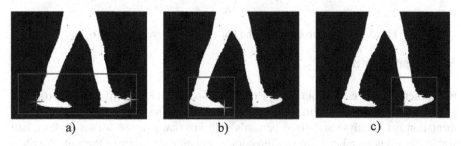

Fig. 2. (a) Output of get external toe and heel phase; (b) output of get internal toe phase; (c) output of get internal heel phase.

$$\max\_bbox(i) \rightarrow grad(x)_i < 0 \wedge grad(x)_{i-1} \geq 0 \tag{3}$$

$$\min\_bbox(i) \rightarrow grad(x)_i > 0 \bigwedge grad(x)_{i-1} \leq 0. \tag{4}$$

4.1 Feature Extraction

We have a vector of size n for each foot, being n the number of frames of the sequence. For each position the location "x, y" of both heel and toe are known. "Heel strike" event can be detected using gradient analysis on X, when the heel gradient goes from positive to zero (stops moving, Eq. 5), and the toe off event when the toe gradient goes from zero to positive (starts moving, Eq. 6).

$$heel\_strike(i) \rightarrow grad(x)_i \leq 0 \wedge grad(x)_{i-1} > 0 \tag{5}$$

$$toe\_off(i) \rightarrow grad(x)_i > 0 \wedge grad(x)_{i-1} = 0 \tag{6}$$

This approach may produce some false positives so we use the evolution of the bounding box to filter the results. The "heel strike" event is produced before the bounding box reaches its local maximum (Eq. 3) and the "toe off" event is done after reaching it. Only the closest results to the local maximum of the bounding box are taken into account to filter some of the false positives. Other false positives are produced during the first and last frames of the sequence when the silhouette is not completed. To filter these false positives we spatially limit the working area so we only keep the events produced inside that area.

Having now the events of heel strike and toe off, we can derive other variables such as step and stride length and time as well as single and double support times.

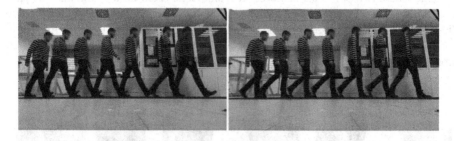

Fig. 3. Heel strike events on the left and toe off events on the right.

5 Experimentation

Experimentation is carried out using RGB data, because the objective of our project is to embed the proposed algorithm to a mobile device. The main objective of experimentation is to analyse stabilized person's gait. For that purpose we set an 8 m. hall with a camera perpendicular to gait direction to obtain a side view of the gait. We use a structure, Fig. 4b, designed to set different cameras allowing to capture footage from

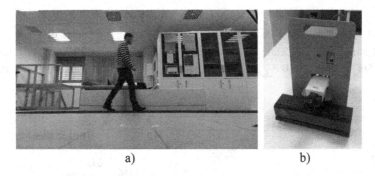

Fig. 4. (a) The recording setup, (b) multicamera structure.

different sources with a similar point of view. During the recording stage we have used Kinect 2, a surveillance Axis camera and a smartphone.

In order to have a reference of a pixel width, we set two markers located at 3 m. between them. This will allow us to calibrate the distance for step length and stride length variable calculations.

Using the described setup, we have recorded a total of 17 sequences of walking subjects. Manual marking is used with an error margin of ±1 frame of the "heel strike" and "toe off" events as ground truth. The difference in frames between the ground truth and our algorithm is analysed. For this test we use Kinect 2 which has a sampling frequency of 30 fps. We also assume an error of ±1 frame in the algorithm output. So our global error margin is ±2 frames, any difference equal or inferior to that value we considered as good.

Results related to Fig. 3 are shown in Table 3.

Table 3. Example of the results of a gait sequence.

Heel strike							
Ground truth	19	40	59	79	98	115	126
Algorithm	18	38	59	78	98	117	126
Diff	1	2	0	1	0	−2	0
Toe off							
Ground truth	26	46	66	85	105	119	129
Algorithm	25	46	66	85	105	119	129
Diff	1	0	0	0	0	0	0

As shown in Table 4 and Fig. 5, the standard deviation of both "heel strike" and "toe off" is below the error margin of 2 frames and the total number of samples inside the error margin are 94 % and 91 % respectively, so the results are very promising. However, we found an undetected case for "heel strike". In addition, there are 6 cases which difference is greater than the error margin in "heel strike" and 8 in "toe off".

Table 4. Results of all samples analysed.

Event	Total	False Positives	Not detected	Wrong	Standard deviation
Heel Strike	97	2 (2.06 %)	1 (1.03 %)	6(6.19 %)	1.49 frames (49.17 ms)
Toe Off	92	0 (0 %)	0 (0 %)	8(8.7 %)	1.73 frames (57.09 ms)

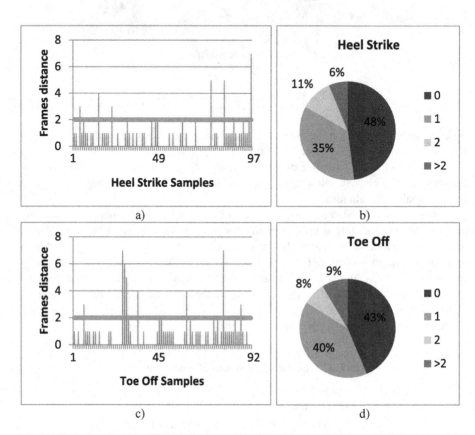

Fig. 5. Chart showing the difference in frames between the ground truth and our algorithm (not showing undetected nor false positive cases), (a) and (c) shows the difference in frames for each sample evaluated of heel strike and toe off respectively, (b) and (d) shows the percentage of samples for each difference for heel strike and toe off respectively.

6 Conclusion

In this paper, we propose a general gait specification and an algorithm that automatically extracts kinematic features involved in the human gait, using as input RGB image sequences. We have designed a "setup" to capture images of walking subjects in a controlled environment, placing the camera perpendicular to the direction of the gait. We have carried out a range of experiments using the dataset obtained on the gait recordings of different subjects. Experimentation is based on the proposed algorithm for determining the two key features in gait analysis: "heel strike" and "toe off" events. These events allow us to infer other ones as stride length, step frequency, step regularity, etc. The results are promising, due to "heel strike" and "toe off" events has been obtained with more than 90 % success rate without markers. The future work is to reduce the number of false positive through further data filtering and improvements taking into account other body parts and the relation between them and the gait. Obtained results are to be used consistently in the identification of frailty and senility syndromes.

Acknowledgement. This research is part of the FRASE MINECO project (TIN2013-47152-C3-2-R) funded by the Ministry of Economy and Competitiveness of Spain.

References

1. Mahoney, F.I., Barthel, D.W.: Functional evaluation: the Barthel Index. Md. State Med. J. **14**, 61–65 (1965)
2. Waltson, J., Fried, L.P.: Frailty and the old man. Med. Clin. North Am. **83**, 1173–1194 (1999)
3. Fried, L.P., Tangen, C.M., Waltson, J., Newman, A.B., et al.: Frailty in older adults: evidence for phenotype. J Gerontol. **56**, 146–156 (2001)
4. Van Lersel, M.: The interplay between gait and cognitive function in elderly people. Ph.D. thesis, Radboud University Nijmegen (2007)
5. Hausdorff, J.M., Yogev, G., Springer, S., Simon, E.S., Giladi, N.: Walking is more like catching than tapping: gait in the elderly as a complex cognitive task. Exp. Brain Res. **164**, 541–548 (2005)
6. Mulder, T., Zijlstra, W., Geurts, A.: Assessment of motor recovery and decline. Gait Posture **16**(2), 198–210 (2002)
7. Waite, L.M., Grayson, D.A., Piguet, O.: Gait slowing as a predictor of incident dementia: 6-year longitudinal data from the Sydney older persons study. J. Neurol. Sci. **229–230**, 89–93 (2005)
8. Camicioli, R., Howieson, D., Oken, B., et al.: Motor slowing precedes cognitive impairment in the oldest old. Neurology **50**, 1496–1498 (1998)
9. Verghese, J., Lipton, R.B., Hall, C.B., et al.: Abnormality of gait as a predictor of non-Alzheimer's dementia. N. Engl. J. Med. **347**, 1761–1768 (2002)
10. Verghese, J., Derby, C., Katz, M.J., et al.: High risk neurological gait syn-drome and vascular dementia. J. Neural Transm. **114**, 1249–1252 (2007)
11. Scarmeas, N., Albert, M., Brandt, J., et al.: Motor signs predict poor outcomes in Alzheimer disease. Neurology **64**, 1696–1703 (2005)
12. Zheng, S., Huang, K., Tan, T., Tao, D.: A cascade fusion scheme for gait and cumulative foot pressure image recognition. Pattern Recogn. **45**(10), 3603–3610 (2012)
13. Roy, A., Sural, S., Mukherjee, J.: Gait recognition using pose kinematics and pose energy image. Sig. Process. **92**(3), 780–792 (2012)
14. Roy, A., Sural, S., Mukherjee, J.: A hierarchical method combining gait and phase of motion with spatiotemporal model for person re-identification. Pattern Recogn. Lett. **33**(14), 1891–1901 (2012)

15. Xu, X., McGorry, R.W., Chou, L.-S., Lin, J.-H., Chang, C.-C.: Accuracy of the Microsoft Kinect™ for measuring gait parameters during treadmill walking. Gait Posture. http://dx.doi.org/10.1016/j.gaitpost.2015.05.002. Accessed 13 May 2015 ISSN 0966-6362
16. Iwashita, Y., Stoica, A., Kurazume, R.: Gait identification using shadow biometrics. Pattern Recogn. Lett. 33(16), 2148–2155 (2012)
17. Choudhury, S.D., Tjahjadi, T.: Gait recognition based on shape and motion analysis of silhouette contours. Comput. Vis. Image Underst. 117(12), 1770–1785 (2013)
18. Khan, T., Westin, J., Dougherty, M.: Motion cue analysis for parkinsonian gait recognition. Open Biomed. Eng. J. 7, 1 (2013)
19. Nixon, M.S., Carter, J.N.: Advances in automatic gait recognition. In: Sixth IEEE International Conference on Automatic Face and Gesture Recognition, 2004, Proceedings, pp. 139–144. IEEE (2004)
20. Choudhury, S.D., Tjahjadi, T.: Silhouette-based gait recognition using Procrustes shape analysis and elliptic Fourier descriptors. Pattern Recogn. 45(9), 3414–3426 (2012)
21. Zeng, W., Wang, C., Yang, F.: Silhouette-based gait recognition via deterministic learning. Pattern Recogn. 47(11), 3568–3584 (2014)
22. Heisenberg, W.: Über den anschaulichen Inhalt der quantentheoretischen Kinematik und Mechanik. Zeitschrift für Physik 43(3–4), 172–198 (1927)
23. Perry, J., Davids, J.R.: Gait analysis: normal and pathological function. J. Pediatr. Orthop. 12(6), 815 (1992)
24. García-Chamizo, J.M., Nieto-Hidalgo, M.: Formalización algebraica del método de arriba hacia abajo de diseño tecnológico. http://hdl.handle.net/10045/47233

Reflections from a Long-term Deployment Study to Design Novel Interactive Surfaces for Children with Autism

Franceli L. Cibrian[1], Deysi H. Ortega[1], Lizbeth Escobedo[2],
and Monica Tentori[1(✉)]

[1] Computer Science Department, CICESE, Ensenada, Mexico
{franceli,dortega}@cicese.edu.mx, mtentori@cicese.mx
[2] Tijuana Technological Institute, Tijuana, Mexico
Lizbeth.excobedo@gmail.com

Abstract. Designing interactive surfaces for children with autism is not trivial, and even more if intended for long-term use. In this paper, we reflect on the experiences and lessons learned from a 5-months deployment study conducted in a LivingLab where 6 classrooms of children with autism used an interactive surface as a multisensory therapy. We describe a set of design insights emerged from these study, and present how they could be used as a design principle to develop novel alternatives of the deployed interactive surface. First we present the design and development of SpaceHunters, an interactive floor exergame supporting the practicing of eye-foot coordination exercises; and then, we describe BendableSound, a fabric-based interactive surface enabling the improvisation of rhythmical sounds in an open-ended manner. We close discussing directions for future work.

Keywords: Interactive surfaces · Long-term deployment studies · LivingLabs · Children · Autism

1 Introduction

Children diagnosed with autism experience sensorimotor problems [1]: they have difficulties with visio-motor coordination [2] and sensorimotor synchronization [3], and are unable to coordinate or control their movements with a predictable external event like rhythm, specially when guided by vision [1]. Interactive surfaces, like tables, walls, and other surfaces augmented with multimedia information that can be manipulated with multi-touch and natural gestures, are promising to support therapies of children with autism [4, 5]. Interactive surfaces provide visual and auditory feedback to maintain the attention of children during the therapy session [4], and remove the complexity of the input interaction mechanism facilitating its use even by children with autism with motor impairments that might find difficult to interact with traditional input devices based on keyboard and mouse [5].

Current projects describing the design of interactive surfaces to support children with autism mainly mirror current practices and traditional therapies where ubiquitous

J. Bravo et al. (Eds.): AmIHEALTH 2015, LNCS 9456, pp. 167–176, 2015.
DOI: 10.1007/978-3-319-26508-7_17

technology is practically absent [4, 6]. Moreover, current interactions with the real world are saturated with manual processes and paper-based tools that are hardly representative of the new type of novel interactions, a new ubiquitous "engaging" world may empower. Long-term deployments of ubiquitous technologies are scarce [7], mainly because of the complexities associated with the deployment of ubiquitous technology to be used for long periods of time, and also with the challenging task of measuring and observing individuals interactions with a "ubiquitous world" in real situations.

In this paper, we argue that designing new and novel effective and efficient interactive surfaces needs to combine the benefits of participatory design sessions with the lessons learned and reflections obtained from long-term deployment studies of the use of ubiquitous technology We exemplify how LivingLabs[1] are appropriate environments to facilitate and enable researchers to conduct long-term deployments promoting iterative development and enabling empirical measurement [7]. We exemplify how the reflections of a long-term deployment study of the use of an interactive surface could be used as a driver to design better and newer alternative versions of interactive surfaces. Our contributions aim to inform the design and deployment of interactive surfaces aimed at augmenting current therapeutic practices of children with autism. First, we contribute with a set of design insights emerged from a deployment study of the long-term use of an interactive surface, and second, we describe how the design insights could be used to design new alternatives versions of a previously deployed interactive surface in a LivingLab of children with autism.

2 Related Work

Traditional methods for designing ubiquitous technology mainly leverage qualitative research demanding researchers to conduct contextual studies, interviewing and observing target users, to: first, understand current practices, users' needs, strategies, and problems faced; and second, envision specific vignettes as design scenarios where ubiquitous technology may have a positive impact in current practices [8]. For example, Join-In Suite [9], is a tabletop with a set of games that support collaboration to mimic Cognitive-Behavioral Therapy, is a was developed based on the qualitative evidence obtained from multiple interviews and observations. MEDIATE [4], an interactive environment designed to support multisensory therapies mimics the processes of traditional multisensory therapeutic interventions observed when administered to children with autism. However the interviews and observations resulted from these studies must be heavily interpreted by a group of researchers who try to "mimic current practices" balancing multiple design tradeoffs without much intervention of potential users when designing ubiquitous technology.

A recent design trend has emphasized the importance of involving potential users in the design decision-making process through participatory design sessions [10]. For

---

[1] Living Labs are highly interactive smart environments furnished with sensors, actuators, and novel displays that are seamlessly embedded and connected through advanced communication technologies where the activities conducted by users are measured and observed.

example, FroggyBobby [11], is an exergame to support children with autism during gross-motor therapies. The FroggyBobby design process involved 13 participatory design sessions with a multidisciplinary team with expertise in HCI, Ubicomp and medicine to supplement the understanding obtained from a contextual study and discuss issues around the design of the exergame and appropriate motor exercises. Most of these design studies used caregivers as "proxies" [12] to capture the needs and desires of children with autism that are commonly non-verbal and incapable of expressing their thoughts and feelings. Others have proposed methods using visual supports based on TEACCH[2] to enable non-verbal individuals communicate using laminated-cards, like IDEAS [13]. Despite, participatory design sessions have proved to be appropriate in involving end-users in the design decision-making, the majority of these design sessions still include low-tech prototypes and mockups that hamper the opportunities for users to imagine what is like to use the final prototype integrated into their everyday practices, and for long periods of time where the novelty effect will eventually wear off.

In this paper, we showcase a new design trend combining the benefits of participatory design sessions to build new "semi-working" prototypes that are deployed to enable users share new design insights that emerge from their own experiences in using ubiquitous technology integrated into their everyday lives, and envision more efficient and effective alternative prototypes.

3   SensoryPaint: Long-term Use of an Interactive Surface as a Multisensory Therapy for Children with Autism

For the past six years we have been creating a "Living Laboratory" in Pasitos[3] -a school-clinic located in Tijuana, Mexico where 15 physiologist-teachers serve approximately 60 low and mid functioning students[4] with autism aged 3 to 21. The technology available at this LivingLab supports several dimensions of the therapy cycle of students, including the use of augmented reality to support cognition [14], gestural displays to encourage positive behaviors [15], eye-gaze technology to support social interactions in real-life situations [16], and exergames to support sensorimotor therapeutic interventions [11, 17, 18]. The long-term use of such technology demonstrate that the deployed prototypes are easy to use and useful, supports sustained empirical measurement and iterative development, and offers numerous educational and therapeutic benefits to students [7].

SensoryPaint [17, 18] is an interactive surface deployed at this LivingLab and being used as a multisensory therapy. SensoryPaint is a painting tool that shows a superimposed reflection of the student projected onto a canvas wall. The color of the student's reflection changes from red to green to demonstrate proximity of the student to

---

[2] Treatment and Education of Autistic related Communication Handicapped Children (TEACCH), is a training program teaching individuals with autism how to use visual, attractive, structural and informative material to be more independent. http://teacch.com/.

[3] http://pasitos.org/home_i/index.asp.

[4] Individuals with autism attending to Pasitos, the majority children.

the surface (Fig. 1, left). The paintbrushes are rubber balls of various sizes, textures, and colors (Fig. 1). Students can either draw in a free form mode (*e.g.*, mimicking the open-ended interaction modality that is traditionally used during sensory integration therapies), use a coloring book (*e.g.*, predefined target activities) or splash color on the surface by throwing the rubber ball. Sounds are played in connection with ball movement to complete the multisensory experience.

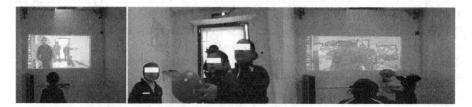

Fig. 1. A student in the mirror therapy using SensoryPaint (left). Students using SensoryPaint (center). Two students using SensoryPaint in a free form (right).

3.1 Deployment Study Methods

Teachers modified the school schedule to include SensoryPaint into their daily school curriculum. Each student attending to Pasitos used SensoryPaint for 15 min twice a week during 5 months. All six classrooms in Pasitos alternated the time of usage of Sensorypaint per month[5]. In every session, two students collectively used SensoryPaint. Teachers paired-up a mid-functioning student with a low-functioning student to promote imitation. During this time, students played with SensoryPaint in a free form and with the coloring book. Cloud cameras available in the room of the LivingLab video recorded the SensoryPaint sessions using two angles: capturing students' faces and body movements, and capturing on-screen interactions. The total time of observation was around 25 h. Researchers conducted monthly interviews with teachers, all the interviews were recorded (avg = 36 min, sd = 4 min). We also conducted a participatory design session (t = 36 min) with teachers to understand the impact of SensoryPaint on students and to figure out how can we improve the SensoryPaint design to better support teachers and students therapeutic goals. All the observations, reports, and audio from interviews and sessions were analyzed using grounded theory techniques and arranged in an affinity diagram.

3.2 Results: Design Implications for Sensorimotor Interactive Surface

The results of the long-term deployment study of the use of SensoryPaint, unveiled three design insights that were used to design and develop new interactive surfaces supporting sensorimotor therapeutic interventions.

---

[5] Pasitos' classroom has approximately 8–10 students, so around 60 students used SensoryPaint.

Balancing Sensory and Motor Stimuli. All teachers found SensoryPaint more valuable to support the development of age-appropriate motor skills, and less confident with the potential sensory benefits and stimulation obtained from using SensoryPaint in long-term – even though the results of a previous short deployment study of the use SensoryPaint showed multiple benefits around sensory stimulation for students [7].

Our qualitative analysis indicated SensoryPaint enabled students to re-direct their eye gaze and attention to their own body and supported the practicing of eye-hand coordination exercises, in an open-ended manner. Specifically, students increased the number of arm repetitions and were better in performing some motor exercises: *"One child that has difficulties when bending over begin to master such movement [referring to a child's motor performance after using SensoyPaint]"*[6] (Teacher classroom A).

All teachers explained that when students used SensorPaint, they enjoyed watching their movements' reflection in the mirror of SensoryPaint. In one classroom, 57 % of students were capable of recognizing their own movements, even those that were "atypical": *"For example, I asked children to look themselves in the mirror when exhibiting atypical movements, like hand flapping, and [a student] stopped their movements after noticing them in the mirror of SensoryPaint"* (Teacher classroom B).

In contrast, benefits around sensory stimulation, beyond those related to the tactile stimulation offered by the interaction with balls, were almost absent. Teachers expressed the visual and audio stimulation available in SensoryPaint were barely noticeable and not attractive to students: *"Maybe adding [to SensoryPaint] other kind of sounds, flashier to students, not just the bells, or maybe a song, or different type of songs."* (Teacher classroom A). Adding more appealing and attractive sounds could highly improve students' ability to re-direct their attention to another stimulus not just the tactile.

In the current version of SensoryPaint both sensory and motor stimuli compete for students' attention instead of complementing each other. Interactive surfaces to support sensorimotor interventions should be able to balance this competition enabling students to obtain a natural and seamless multisensory experience. Using the appropriate sound, visual and tactile stimulation could also provide appropriate guidance to the task at hand enabling teachers to easily go back and forth between an open-ended interaction modality and following a more task-oriented instruction.

Gameplay Dynamic. Feedback, prompts, and rewards are crucial elements to maintain students' engagement in any therapeutic intervention. Teachers spend a considerable amount of the time of the therapy prompting students and physically redirecting their attention to help them meet the goals of the therapy for the day. Therapeutic interventions of students must mimic these interactions to reduce the burden and workload of teachers that constantly prompt students during therapies, and provide the necessary guidance students need to successfully meet the goals of the therapy.

The current design of SensoryPaint does not give away prompts or model interactions when appropriate. The lack of a "tutorial-like" mode has made more challenging the use of the system for novel users, even though after several weeks students

---

[6] Participants' quotes were translated form Spanish to English.

get used to use SensoryPaint and needed less prompting: *"Now [students] are not requiring a lot of help, some students needed so much help in the beginning [of the use of SensoryPaint] but now they grab the balls by themselves [and start playing with SensoryPaint]"* (Teacher classroom A). Not having the appropriate prompting mechanism in place might reduce the chances of the early-adoption of any prototype supporting therapeutic interventions.

A similar trend was present with the rewarding and feedback mechanisms available in SensoryPaint. Teachers constantly had to verbally reward students saying congratulation messages after students mastered a movement or when they appeared more willing to meet the goals of the day: *"At the end of each therapy session [using SensoryPaint] I congratulate them!, I think they need a lot of [reinforcement] whenever they successfully and accurately did the movement [when using SensoryPaint]. And reinforcement is very good for them! For example, I said [Marley] you are doing very good!, and keep motivating him by verbally rewarding him."* (Teacher classroom A). All teachers suggested therapeutic interactive surfaces must provide positive feedback like claps sounds, congratulation messages, or noticeable visual feedback to maintain students motivated and incentivized. *"For example, a reward when the student finishes coloring the strawberry".* (Teacher classroom B).

An interactive surface should incorporate a gameplay dynamic rewarding and prompting students when appropriate. Having appropriate dynamic gameplay will help students to first explore the surface and uncover new features and functionalities, and then solve challenges more directed to improving their own sensorimotor skills.

Envisioning Novel and Natural Interactive Gestures. One of the best advantages of SensoryPaint is the combination of movement and tangible-based interaction gestures – using physical balls to paint with natural gestures. This interaction model has a dual functionality, is engaging and is appropriate for enable students practice motor skills, while they have fun. Uncovering novel interactive gestures is an important feature to maintain engagement while offering multiple benefits around motor development. Teachers found benefits besides attention in concentration. Teachers found that students were engaged for longer periods in predefined activities besides the free form activities, for example when coloring a specific form.

Even in the fourth week, and after using SensoryPaint for a long-time, students were still discovering new ways to play with SensoryPaint. New interaction modalities can emerge from different ways of observing students interacting with different input and output devices, or using their own senses inspired by the affordances offered by the technology.

4   Designing and Developing Sensorimotor Interactive Surfaces

Using the above mentioned design principles we designed and developed two prototypes as alternative versions of SensoryPaint: SpaceHunters and BendableSound. Both prototypes also support sensorimotor interventions.

4.1   SpaceHunters: An Eye-Foot Coordination Interactive Floor

SpaceHunters is an interactive floor exergame were students practice different eye-foot coordination exercises to help two astronauts when hunting space gems available in different planets of the Solar System [19]. On each planet, students must collaborate taking turns and working at the same to practice different eye-foot coordination exercises (Table 1, Fig. 2) adapting the amount of sensory stimulation on each level.

The objective of the game is to help two astronauts to retrieve hidden gems by navigating through the galaxy and exploring different planets in the universe (Table 1). For example, in planet earth, students take turns by walking in a straight line avoiding falling into the sea; while, in mars, students collaborate by stomping on hot rocks. Before each level, SpaceHunters provides a role-modeling tutorial about the exercises that students should practice and the way they must collaborate to get the gem. After students finish exploring each planet, SpaceHunters shows two astronauts saying a congratulation message and playing clapping sounds. Each time students play with SpaceHunters they uncover a different gem ensuring motivation and long-term engagement.

SpaceHunters uses the Kinect sensor and the TSPS[7] library to infer users' position, and all the multimedia interfaces were developed using Processing[8]. The effects are projected on the floor with a short-throw projector.

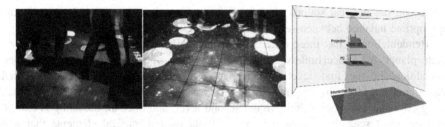

Fig. 2. SpaceHunter prototype. Screenshot from two differents levels of SpaceHunters, Mercury (right) and Mars (center); interactive floor mockup hardware (left).

4.2   BendableSound: A Fabric-Based Interactive Music Surface

"BendableSound" (Fig. 3) is a fabric-based interactive surface that enables students to manipulate musical elements appearing in a space-based theme to play rhythmical sounds. The fabric is a digital matrix storing sounds representing the pitch order of musical notes arranged in an ascending scale on the vertical axis, and in the horizontal axis, the musical tempo. Every time a student taps, grasps or touches an element on the surface it will play a sound according to its location pitch. The combination of appropriate fine-motor movements to navigate through the elements available in the

---

[7] http://www.tsps.cc/.
[8] https://processing.org/overview/.

Table 1. General structure of SpaceHunters.

Level	Gesture/Movement	Collaboration	Goal	Example
Mercury	Avoid objects	Work at the same time	Avoid a meteor shower	
Venus	Jump	Taking turns	Stomp in the correct order on stones	
Earth	Zigzag walking	Taking turns	Walking in a zigzag line avoiding falling into the sea	
Mars	Stomp	Work at the same time	Stomp the red hot rocks	
Jupiter	Jump	Work at the same time	Jump in every satellite of Jupiter	
Saturn	Track a line	Taking turns	Following the rings of Saturn	
Uranus	Walk	Work at the same time	Walk over the surface to coloring Uranus	
Neptune	Breathing	Work at the same time	Blow to the aircraft to arrive Neptune	

fabric and the musical sounds played when touching the fabric provide to users the appropriate balance between sensory and motor stimuli.

BendableSound has three different levels –similar to the variations available on each planet of SpaceHunters, and enabling both open-ended and task-oriented modalities. In the first level, students must discover sounds that are scattered throughout the fabric by tapping on the fabric canvas to erase a huge layer of black smog covering the space nebula. In the second level, and once all the smog is erased, students must seek throughout the space nebula hidden musical elements that will reproduce sounds if touched or moved. Both of these levels follow an open-ended interaction mode with no guided instruction. In the third level, an astronaut appears to give students step-by-step guidance to play a song by touching on the appearing and blinking elements. Song lists that students could play with the fabric include students' songs and nursery rhymes like "twinkle twinkle little star". BendableSound only reinforces positive actions and no penalty is provided if students do not appropriately follow the astronaut or follow the beat of the song.

The music sounds scattered in the fabric canvas change according to the way the user is touching the surface: a tap will play the sound of drums, ripping the fabric will play guitar sounds, and finger-tapping will imitate piano sounds (Table 2).

BendableSound uses an infrared camera and the CCV library to detect the fine motor-movements of tap and touch. Other movements are still under development but are available in the fabric through wizard of oz. BendableSound's multimedia interfaces were developed with QML and JavaScript (Fig. 3).

Table 2. Interaction gestures of BendableSound

Gesture	Effect	Instrument	Example
Tap	Bouncing	Piano/Drum	
Drag	Drag	Guitar/harp	
Rip	Follow	Guitar/Piano/harp	
Pinch	Create, disappear	harp/Guitar	

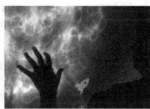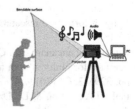

Fig. 3. The BendableSound prototype. A screenshot of the Level 1 of the BendableSound prototype (left). A user interacting with the fabric-based surface moving elements in the space (center). A mockup representation showing the hardware installation of the BendableSound prototype (right).

5 Conclusion and Future Work

In this work, we present how our reflections from the lessons learned of a long-term deployment study of the use of SensoryPaint can be used to design alternative versions of interactive surfaces to support sensorimotor interventions. Our results show that an interactive surface to support sensorimotor interventions should balance sensory and motor stimuli, mimic novel interaction gestures based on the practicing of fine and gross movements, support both open-ended and goal-oriented tasks, and promote a game dynamic play based on positive reinforcement and appropriate prompting. As future work, we plan to deploy both BendableSound and SpaceHunters in the LivingLab at Pasitos to study the long-term impact in supporting sensorimotor interventions and potentially aid motor and cognitive development for students.

References

1. Donnellan, A.M., Hill, D.A., Leary, M.R.: Rethinking autism: implications of sensory and movement differences for understanding and support. Front. Integr. Neurosci. **6**, 1–11 (2012)
2. Whyatt, C.P., Craig, C.M.: Motor skills in children aged 7–10 years, diagnosed with autism spectrum disorder. J. Autism Dev. Disord. **42**, 1799–1809 (2012)
3. LaGasse, A.B., Hardy, M.W.: Considering rhythm for sensorimotor regulation in children with autism spectrum disorders. Music Ther. Perspect. **31**, 67–77 (2013)

4. Parés, N., Soler, M., Sanjurjo, À., Carreras, A., Durany, J., Ferrer, J., Freixa, P., Gómez, D., Kruglanski, O., Parés, R., Ribas, J.I.: Promotion of creative activity in children with severe autism through visuals in an interactive multisensory environment. In: IDC 2005, pp. 110–116 (2005)
5. Putnam, C., Chong, L.: Software and technologies designed for people with autism: what do users want? In: Proceedings of the 10th International ACM SIGACCESS Conference on Computers and Accessibility (2008)
6. Villafuerte, L., Markova, M., Jorda, S.: Acquisition of social abilities through musical tangible user interface : children with autism spectrum condition and the reactable. In: CHI 2012 Extended Abstracts, pp. 745–760. ACM, New York, NY, USA (2012)
7. Tentori, M., Escobedo, L., Balderas, G.: A smart Environment for children with autism. IEEE Pervasive Comput. 2, 42–50 (2015)
8. DeSmet, A., Palmeira, A., Beltran, A., Brand, L., Davies, V.F., Thompson, D.: The Yin and Yang of formative research in designing serious (exer-)games. Games Health J. 4, 63–66 (2015)
9. Giusti, L., Zancanaro, M., Gal, E., Weiss, P.L.T.: Dimensions of collaboration on a tabletop interface for children with autism spectrum disorder. In: CHI 2011 Session, Wall Displays, pp. 3295–3304 (2011)
10. Fails, J.A., Guha, M.L., Druin, A.: Methods and techniques for involving children in the design of new technology for children. Found Trends® Hum. Comput. Interact. 6, 85–166 (2012)
11. Caro, K., Cibrian, F.L., Escobedo, L., Ramirez, C., Martínez-García, A.I., Tentori, M.: Diseño de un videojuego serio basado en movimiento para niños con el Trastorno del Desarrollo de la Coordinación. In: ENC 2013 (2013)
12. Tang, S.T., McCorkle, R.: Use of family proxies in quality of life research for cancer patients at the end of life: a literature review. Cancer Invest. 20, 1086–1104 (2002)
13. Benton, L., Johnson, H., Ashwin, E., Brosnan, M., Grawemeyer, B.: Developing IDEAS: supporting children with autism within a participatory design team. In: Proceedings of the SIGCHI Conference on Human Factors in Computing Systems. pp. 2599–2608. ACM (2012)
14. Escobedo, L., Tentori, M., Quintana, E., Favela, J., Garcia-Rosas, D.: Using augmented reality to help children with autism stay focused. IEEE Pervasive Comput. 13, 38–46 (2014)
15. Matic, A., Hayes, G.R., Tentori, M., Abdullah, M., Schuck, S.: Collective use of a situated display to encourage positive behaviors in children with behavioral challenges. In: Proceedings of the 2014 ACM International Joint Conference on Pervasive and Ubiquitous Computing, pp. 885–895. ACM (2014)
16. Escobedo, L., Nguyen, D.H., Boyd, L., Hirano, S., Rangel, A., Garcia-Rosas, D., Tentori, M., Hayes, G.: MOSOCO: a mobile assistive tool to support children with autism practicing social skills in real-life situations. In: CHI 2012, pp. 2589–2598 (2012)
17. Ringland, K.E., Zalapa, R., Neal, M., Escobedo, L., Tentori, M.E., Hayes, G.R.: SensoryPaint: a natural user interface supporting sensory integration in children with neurodevelmental disorders. In: CHI 2014 Extended Abstracts on Human Factors in Computing Systems, pp. 1681–1686. ACM, Toronto, Ontario, Canada (2014)
18. Ringland, K.E., Zalapa, R., Neal, M., Escobedo, L., Tentori, M., Hayes, G.R.: SensoryPaint: a multimodal sensory intervention for children with neurodevelopmental disorders. In: UbiComp 2014, pp. 873–884 (2014)
19. Cibrian, F.L., Martinez-Garcia, A.I., Tentori, M.: Hunting Relics: A collaborative exergame on an interactive floor for children. In: UbiComp 2014: Adjunct Publication, pp. 223–226. ACM (2014)

Low Complexity Neural Networks to Classify EEG Signals Associated to Emotional Stimuli

Adrian Rodriguez Aguiñaga[✉] and Miguel Angel Lopez Ramirez

Instituto Tecnológico de Tijuana, Calz Del Tecnológico S/N,
Tomas Aquino, 22414 Tijuana, B.C, México
{adrian.rodriguez,mlopez}@tectijuana.edu.mx
www.labcafe.org

Abstract. This paper presents a strategy to perform an emotional states recognition process by analyzing electroencephalography records; The recognition process were performed by a specific purpose neural network and the experimental criteria for it configuration are presented. Also a novelty electrode discriminant process were applied, which correlates electrodes to Brodmann regions, achieving a data reduction of 29.5 percent. The recognition rates average achieved up to 90.2 percent of recognition rate in the binary case and up to 82.51 percent in a multi-class scheme.

Keywords: EEG · Affective computing · Emotions · Neural networks · Brodmann · Arousal · Valence

1 Introduction

The development of technology that interacts in a more natural way with users, has been one of the biggest challenges in recent decades. Some of the most outstanding results are presented by Rosalind W. Picard in the Affective computing theory [1], that provide the basis to understand the impact of technology on the user emotional states.

To date several strategies has been intended the consolidation of Picard ideas (Table 1), however, those focused on the study of emotional responses has been stood out, due the importance of emotions in human communication rules. Although many of these proposals, implements intelligent techniques that recognize or/and classify the physiological responses of an emotional stimuli, most of the studied metrics could be easily manipulated by an average user and many authors suggest that bio-signal analysis are one of the most reliable information sources when are properly processed [2–5].

A wide range of bio-signal sources could be studied as the cardiac activity, galvanic skin resistance, muscle activity, respiration rate, temperature, brain activity and so on. However, due that the brain activity are considered as one of

A.R. Aguiñaga—Conacyt and Instituto Tecnológico de Tijuana.

J. Bravo et al. (Eds.): AmIHEALTH 2015, LNCS 9456, pp. 177–188, 2015.
DOI: 10.1007/978-3-319-26508-7_18

the most reliable information source and due some of the most remarkable results in the emotional states recognition are performed by the analysis of electroencephalography records (EEG), the feasibility to establish a relationship between the electrical activity in the cerebral cortex and emotional states is increasingly significant [2–4]. This paper presents then a strategy based in a neural network configuration strategy (NN), signal conditioning techniques and data reduction proposals to perform a multi-class emotion recognition process by EEG analysis, that achieves up to 90 % of recognition rate.

Table 1. Related work of classification and recognition techniques of emotional states.

Technique	Recognition Rate %	Reference
K-NN, LDA	81.25	[2]
Multilayer Perceptron Classifier	64	[6]
K-NN	82.27	[7]
Mahalanobis distance classifier	74.11	[8]
SVM	66.7	[9]
SVM	93.5	[10]
SVM	77.8	[11]
NN	43.14	[12]
NN	60	[13]
NN	93.3	[14]

2 Experimental Characterization

2.1 Data Sources

The lack of a standardized database is one of the major problems in the EEG emotion recognition process, since current standard databases as the International Affective Picture System digitized (IAPS) and the International Affective Digital Sounds (IADS) [15, 16], could be only implemented to perform the stimulation processes and dedicated databases as the bu-3DFE, PhysioNet, Ibug project and DEAP are not yet standardized.

- bu-3DFE [17]: are a data set that contains records of several physiological emotional expressions.
- PhysioNet [18]: are a collection of physiological signals, time series and images, constructed to perform behavior analysis.
- Ibug project [19]: are a wide range of bio-metric data associated to affective behaviors.
- Emotional physiological and video signals database (DEAP) [4]: are a very wide collection of Bio-signals, generated by several specialized experimental setups into an arousal and valence space.

Due that DEAP data-set are constituted by forty emotional stimuli responses of thirty-two persons is up to our best knowledge the most complete data collection are employed as data source for this paper.

2.2 Emotions

Despite the fact that *emotion* are a widely implemented concept, provide a clear definition of it results in a very complex endeavor and even the simple question of what are emotions?, hardly get the same answers [20].

Klaus R. Scherer, define emotions as *an episode of interrelated, synchronized changes in the states of all or most of the five[1] organismic subsystems[2] in response to the evaluation of an external or internal stimulus event as relevant to major concerns of the organism* [20].

2.3 Emotion Model

An unified representation generated by intertwining the Ekman, Friesen, Russell, Parrot, Plutchik and Geneva models [21–23] are presented in Fig. 1, implemented as a strategy to provide *"limits"* to the an expressed emotional state in a computational emotional recognition process as in [24].

The implementation of this strategy, provides a multi-class structure that describes a four emotional states model as: HA/LV (high arousal, low valence), HA/HL (high arousal, high valence), LA/LV (low arousal, low valence), LA/HV (low arousal, high valence) to associate each evoked potential (EP) to a certain class, according to it Geneva membership level as presented in Fig. 2.

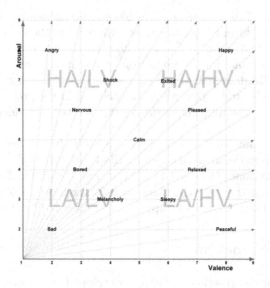

Fig. 1. Arousal-Valence emotion distribution.

---

[1] Information processing (CNS), Support (CNS, NES, ANS), Executive (CNS), Action (SNS), Monitor (CNS).

[2] (CNS), central nervous system; (NES), neuro-endocrine system; (ANS), autonomic nervous system; (SNS), somatic nervous system. The organismic subsystems are theoretically postulated functional units or networks.

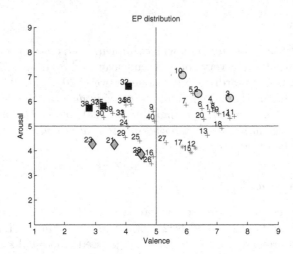

Fig. 2. Distribution of evoked potential trials in an arousal and valence space.

3   Signal Conditioning

3.1   Bounded Regions and Brain Rhythms

The large amount of data associated to bio-signal analysis are another important challenge to perform EEG pattern recognition, and the implementation of a technique that mitigates this problem are necessary. An electrode discrimination process based in a "*bounded region strategy*" were implemented as in [24]. This process identifies Brodmann with greater association[3] to emotional processes and defines the set of electrodes that would be included in the processing process as presented in Fig. 3. The implementation of this strategy provides a data reduction of 29.5 %.

Another important consideration is that a properly frequency analysis may reduces the computational burden, since EEG are subdivided into frequency bands or brain rhythms: *Delta 0.1 to 4* Hz, *Theta 4 to 8* Hz, *Alpha 8 to 12* Hz, *Mu 8 to 13* Hz, *Beta 12 to 25* Hz, *Gamma > 25* Hz and an adequate frequency delimitation could be performed by applying a band-pass filter from 0.1 to 47 Hz.

4   Feature Extraction

Most of the feature extraction techniques developed up to date carryout time series or frequency analysis; however, since we are working with biological signals, both resolutions most be considered.

---

[3] Visual activity are related to occipital region (Brodmann region 17), auditory activity are associated to temporal lobe (region 41), the limbic system as the main responsible to emotional processes are located in the temporal parietal areas and body sensations are located in the temporal and parietal regions [25–27].

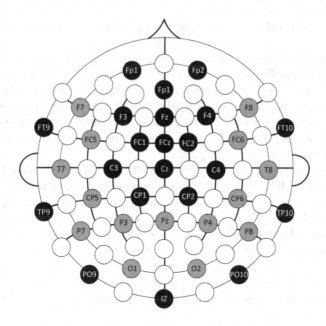

Fig. 3. Electrode association to a Brodmann bounded regions.

The Wavelet Transform (WT) are a widely implemented technique to analyze n-dimensional signals and due this technique satisfies the dual resolution constraint and further the transformation kernels can be employed directly as features in a pattern recognition process, it were selected as the feature extraction methodology [28]. WT as the Fourier transform (FT), provides spectral information of the signals. However, it didn't employs sine and cosine functions as transformation kernels, instead uses a function called *"Mother wavelet"* $\psi(t)$ and the discrete case can be described as

$$\psi_{j,k}(t) = \frac{1}{\sqrt{2^j}} \psi\left(\frac{(t-k)2^j}{2^j}\right), \tag{1}$$

where j and k are the scale and shift parameter respectively and both are integers.

Recall that wavelet coefficient γ of a signal $x(t)$ is the projection of $x(t)$ onto a wavelet and $x(t)$ be a signal of length 2^N, it can be expressed as

$$\gamma_{jk} = \int_{-\infty}^{\infty} x(t) \frac{1}{\sqrt{2^j}} \psi\left(\frac{(t-k)2^j}{2^j}\right) dt, \tag{2}$$

j are fixed at a particular scale, so that γ_{jk} is a function of k.

The above equation, γ_{jk} can be represented as a convolution of $x(t)$ with a dilated, reflected and the normalized version of the $\psi(t)$ as a sampled the points $1, 2^j, 2^{2j}, ..., 2^N$:

$$h(t) = \frac{1}{\sqrt{2^j}} \psi\left(\frac{-t}{2^j}\right), \tag{3}$$

this are the detail coefficients given at level j of the discrete wavelet transform (DWT).

Therefore, the choice of an appropriate $h[n]$ and $g[n]$, correspond exactly to a the wavelet coefficients of a discrete set of child wavelets for a given $\psi(t)$ and generally are not band-limited; it is necessary to suppress the values of the frequency components above half the sampling frequency to avoid aliasing (overlapping in frequency) effects, while the choice of the filters must be guided by the regularity of the scaling and the wavelet functions and its complexity is proportional to the signal length [28].

Select an appropriate $\psi(t)$, still are an heuristic task; however, due Daubechies wavelets presents the better performance in our experimental stage and some authors reported up to an 85 % of recognition rate by implementing this $\psi(t)$ [2,3], it were selected to perform this multi-resolution process analysis.

The embedded subsets also could be generated by the signal interpolations at different scales could be dilated and translated as

$$C_j(k) = \langle f(t), 2^{-j}\phi(2^{-j}t - k)\rangle, \tag{4}$$

to allows a directly computation of the wavelet coefficient $C_{j+1}(k)$ from $C_j(k)$.

4.1   Features Selection

Each levels for the DWT of a x signal are calculated by passing it, through a series of filters; first the samples are passed through a low pass filter with impulse response g resulting in a convolution of the two as

$$y[n] = (x * g)[n] = \sum_{k=-\infty}^{\infty} x[k]g[n - k], \tag{5}$$

the signal is also decomposed simultaneously using a high-pass filter h.

The outputs giving the detail coefficients (from the high-pass filter) and approximation coefficients (from the low-pass filter); it is important that the two filters are related to each other and they are known as a quadrature mirror filter.

Half of the samples can be discarded according to Nyquist's rule and it are filter out by the nominal sub-sampled of two at the DWT. This decomposition halved the time resolution, since only half of each filter output characterizes the signal. However, each output has half the frequency band of the input so the frequency resolution has been doubled.

The WT describes signal in terms of coefficients by representing their energy content in a specified frequency region and this signal $f(t)$ can be decomposed as

$$f(t) = \sum_{j}\sum_{k} d_{j,k}\psi_{j,k}(t) = \sum_{j} f_j(t), \tag{6}$$

where $j,k \in Z$ and $\psi(t)$ is a mother Wavelet and the Wavelet coefficients $d_{j,k}$ is the inner product

$$d_{j,k} = \langle f(t), \psi_{j,k}(t)\rangle = \frac{1}{\sqrt{2^j}} \int f(t)\psi(2^{-j}t - k)dt. \tag{7}$$

From the wavelet coefficients $d_{j,k}$, the energy of the details of f at level j can be expressed as

$$E_j = \sum_k d_{j,k}^2, \tag{8}$$

if the total energy of the details is denoted as $E_t = \sum_j E_j$, then the percentile energy corresponding at level j is

$$\varepsilon_j = \frac{E_j}{E_t} \times 100. \tag{9}$$

The level j is associated with frequency band ΔF, given by

$$2^{-j-1} F_s \leqslant \Delta F \leqslant 2^{-j} F_s, \tag{10}$$

where F_s is the sampling frequency.

4.2 Normalization

The EEG signal, were sub-sampled by the wavelet analysis process and normalized as in [28],

$$I_{(i,j)} = (I_{i,j} - \overline{I}_i)/(\sigma_i), \tag{11}$$

where $\overline{I}_i$ and σ_i are the average value and the standard deviation of the electrode i at the time j, this average and standard deviation are based on each individual pattern.

5 Recognition Process

A complex neural network (NN) architecture[4], were initially proposed as the recognition methodology; however, as can be observed in Fig. 4, the error rates are proportional to the neural network complexity at this particular case.

The implemented architecture were selected based on this experimental observations[5], as:

- Resilient back-propagation.
- Three layers topology, 2/3/4 units in the input layer, 14 hidden units in a single hidden layer and 2/3/4 on the output.
- 200 maximum epoch.
- Maximum square error (MSE), Goal = 0.002.
- 70 % for training data.
- 15 % to validate.
- 15 % to test.

---

[4] A neural network with up to fifty units per hidden layer and up to filthy hidden layers.
[5] Each performed under a 10-fold cross validation.

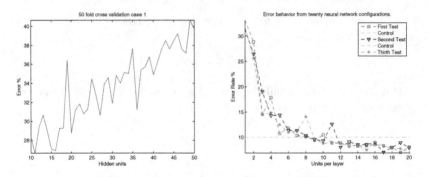

Fig. 4. Fifty performance level network configurations.

5.1 Experimental Setup

The four classes configuration described in Sect. 2, were employed to perform the pattern recognition process that only employs the three most significant experiments of each class as presented in Fig. 2, due the experimental configuration were designed to evaluate the recognition performance of each generated class, based in the presented clustering algorithm.

Algorithm 1. Feature input arrangement

---

input : Features $d_{j,k}$ arrays
output: Matrix arrangement E_k

Selecting features to provide input classes;
for $i \leftarrow 1$ **to** 3 **do**
 $\quad$ $e=$(electrodes array);
 $\quad$ **for** $j \leftarrow 1$ **to** 15 **do**
 $\quad\quad$ $\lfloor$ $C = [e(b); d_{j,k}]$;
 $\quad$ *"a" is the parameter that defines the number of emotional stated that would be analyzed;*
 $\quad$ **for** k **to** a **do**
 $\quad\quad$ **for** $l \leftarrow 1$ **to** 30 **do**
 $\quad\quad\quad$ $\lfloor$ $E_k = [l; C]$;
 $\quad$ E_k *is the arrangement of characteristics of the three case studies of each emotional state and all users;*

The neural network inputs depends on the number of classes to be sorted and are manipulated by the parameter a.

6 Results

The performance obtained by the application of the proposed strategies are presented in Figs. 5 and 6. Figure 5, presents the performance of a two class

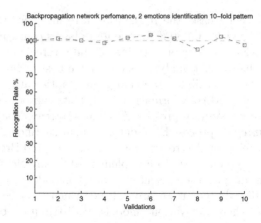

Fig. 5. Two class recognition performance

recognition process in a single trial setup, where the classes combinations are randomly selected from HA/HV -LA/LV or LA/HV -LA/LV, obtaining a 90.2 % of recognition rate.

Figure 6, presents the recognition performance for the three and four classes configurations that obtains a 84.2 % and 80.90 % of recognition rates, respectively.

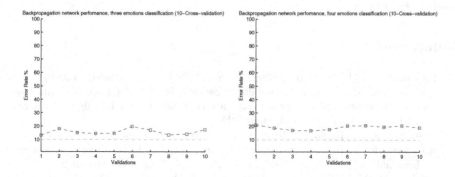

Fig. 6. Three and four class recognition performance

As can be observed, the performance in the process of classification obtained by the implemented techniques remain in acceptable ranges of classification, being remarkable the identification of a pattern in the behavior of the brain activity of four mental states between thirty-two study subjects.

7 Conclusions

As can be observed the binary case shows a uniform and stable performance of 90 % recognition, which are quite competitive with results presented in [2, 3, 29].

While for the multi-class case, the recognition rate mean for the three classes configuration were of 84 % and 80 % for the four classes configuration.

The obtained result by implementation of the strategies presented in this work, also ratifies the wavelet analysis as one of the best techniques to perform cognitive research, due it feasibility to manage the chaotic nature of the EEG signals and that the obtained transformation coefficients can be directly employed in a classification or recognition process. Also this strategy decrease the computational effort required to process EEG data, without sacrificing the recognition performance by correlating electrodes to a emotional related Brodmann regions. This electrode arrangements could be implemented in any electrodes and emotions configuration, in spite the presented strategy includes only four emotional states due it are distributed in an arousal and valence space represented by quadrants, however there are various models of distribution of emotions and this configuration could contemplate a greater amount of emotional states.

As future work this strategy is contemplated to be implemented in an emotional states recognition in people undergoing a rehabilitation process and despite the fact that one of the most important limitations to this type of research, is the lack of a standardized reference the increasing interest to provide experimental scenarios as the DEAP or the iBug projects, could provide an adequate generalization.

Acknowledgment. To the Instituto Tecnológico de Tijuana and Conacyt for making possible this project.

References

1. Picard, R.W.: Affective Computing, 1st edn. MIT Press, Cambridge (2000)
2. Murugappan, M.: Human emotion classification using wavelet transform and knn. In: 2011 International Conference on Pattern Analysis and Intelligent Robotics (ICPAIR), vol. 1, pp. 148–153, June 2011
3. Murugappan, M., Rizon, M., Nagarajan, R., Yaacob, S., Zunaidi, I., Hazry, D.: Lifting scheme for human emotion recognition using eeg. In: International Symposium on Information Technology, 2008, ITSim 2008, vol. 2, pp. 1–7, August 2008
4. Koelstra, S., Muhl, C., Soleymani, M., Lee, J.-S., Yazdani, A., Ebrahimi, T., Pun, T., Nijholt, A., Patras, I.: Deap: a database for emotion analysis; using physiological signals. IEEE Trans. Affect. Comput. **3**(1), 18–31 (2012)
5. Sanei, S., Chambers, J.A.: Eeg signal processing. In: Cardiff University (2007)
6. Lin, Y.-P., Wang, C.-H., Wu, T.-L., Jeng, S.-K., Chen, J.-H.: Multilayer perceptron for eeg signal classification during listening to emotional music. In: TENCON 2007–2007 IEEE Region 10 Conference, pp. 1–3, October 2007
7. Heraz, A., Razaki, R., Frasson, C.: Using machine learning to predict learner emotional state from brainwaves. In: Seventh IEEE International Conference on Advanced Learning Technologies, 2007, ICALT 2007, pp. 853–857, July 2007
8. Petrantonakis, P.C., Hadjileontiadis, L.J.: Eeg-based emotion recognition using hybrid filtering and higher order crossings. In: 3rd International Conference on Affective Computing and Intelligent Interaction and Workshops, 2009, ACII 2009, pp. 1–6, September 2009

9. Takahashi, K.: Remarks on svm-based emotion recognition from multi-modal bio-potential signals. In: 13th IEEE International Workshop on Robot and Human Interactive Communication, 2004, ROMAN 2004, pp. 95–100, September 2004
10. Li, M., Lu, B.-L.: Emotion classification based on gamma-band eeg. In: Annual International Conference of the IEEE Engineering in Medicine and Biology Society, 2009, EMBC 2009, pp. 1223–1226, September 2009
11. Rozgic, V., Ananthakrishnan, S., Saleem, S., Kumar, R., Prasad, R.: Ensemble of svm trees for multimodal emotion recognition. In: Signal Information Processing Association Annual Summit and Conference (APSIPA ASC), 2012 Asia-Pacific, pp. 1–4, December 2012
12. Attabi, Y., Dumouchel, P.: Emotion recognition from speech: woc-nn and class-interaction. In: 2012 11th International Conference on Information Science, Signal Processing and their Applications (ISSPA), pp. 126–131, July 2012
13. Razak, A.A., Komiya, R., Izani, M., Abidin, Z.: Comparison between fuzzy and nn method for speech emotion recognition. In: Third International Conference on Information Technology and Applications, 2005, ICITA 2005, vol. 1, pp. 297–302, July 2005
14. Gunler, M.A., Tora, H.: Emotion classification using hidden layer outputs. In: 2012 International Symposium on Innovations in Intelligent Systems and Applications (INISTA), pp. 1–4, July 2012
15. Bradley, M.M., Cuthbert, B.N., Lang, P.J.: International affective picture system (iaps): Technical manual and affective ratings. In: NIMH Center for the Study of Emotion and Attention, FL: The Center for Research in Psychophysiology, University of Florida (1997)
16. Bradley, M.M., Cuthbert, B.N., Lang, P.J.: International affective digitized sounds (iads): Stimuli, instruction manual and affective ratings, In: The Center for Research in Psychophysiology, University of Florida (1999)
17. Yin, L., Wei, X., Sun, Y., Wang, J., Rosato, M.J.: A 3d facial expression database for facial behavior research. In: 7th International Conference on Automatic Face and Gesture Recognition, 2006, FGR 2006, pp. 211–216, April 2006
18. Moody, G.B., Mark, R.G., Goldberger, A.L.: Physionet: a web-based resource for the study of physiologic signals. Eng. Med. Biol. Mag. IEEE 20(3), 70–75 (2001)
19. Petridis, S., Martinez, B., Pantic, M.: The MAHNOB laughter database. Image Vis. Comput. 31(2), 186–202 (2013). Affect Analysis In Continuous Input
20. Scherer, K.R.: What are emotions? and how can they be measured? In: Trends and Developments: Research on Emotions, vol. 44, pp. 695–729. Social Science Information and SAGE Publications (2005)
21. Friesen, W.V., O'Sullivan, M., Chan, A., Diacoyanni-Tarlatzis, I., Heider, K., Krause, R., LeCompte, W.A., Pitcairn, T., Ricci-Bitti, P.E., Scherer, K., Tomita, M., Tzavaras, A., Ekman, P.: Universals and cultural differences in the judgments of facial expressions of emotion. J. Pers. Soc. Psychol. 4, 712–717 (1987)
22. Russell, J.A.: A circumplex model of affect. J. Pers. Soc. Psychol. 39, 1161–1178 (1980)
23. Gerrod Parrott, W.: Emotions in Social Psychology, 1st edn. Psychology Press, Philadelphia (2001)
24. Ramirez, M.A.L., Aguinaga, A.R., Flores, B.M.R.: Classification model of arousal and valence mental states by eeg signals analysis and brodmann correlations. Int. J. Adv. Comput. Sci. Appl. (IJACSA) 6, 230–238 (2015)
25. Brodmann, K., Garey, L.J.: Brodmann's Localisation in the Cerebral Cortex, 3rd edn. Springer Science, USA (2006)

26. Fox, S.I.: Human Physiology, 7th edn. Mcgraw-Hill (Tx), Boston (2002)
27. Sherwood, L.: Human Physiology from Cells to System, 8th edn. Brooks/Cole, Cengage Learning, Belmont (2013)
28. Cecotti, H., Graser, A.: Convolutional neural networks for p300 detection with application to brain-computer interfaces. IEEE Trans. Pattern Anal. Mach. Intell. **33**(3), 433–445 (2011)
29. Pourtois, G., Schwartz, S., Seghier, M.L., Scherer, K.R., Vuilleumier, P., Sander, D., Grandjean, D.: Emotion and attention interactions in social cognition: brain regions involvedin processing anger prosody. NeuroImage Spec. Section Soc. Cogn. Neurosci. **28**, 848–858 (2005)

EmoBall: A Study on a Tangible Interface to Self-report Emotional Information Considering Digital Competences

Carolina Fuentes[(✉)], Iyubanit Rodríguez[(✉)], and Valeria Herskovic

Pontificia Universidad Católica de Chile, Santiago, Chile
{cjfuentes,iyubanit}@uc.cl, vherskov@ing.puc.cl

Abstract. Monitoring emotional information is highly complex: it is difficult to accurately register it due to subjectivity and technical complexities; and it is difficult to provide reliability and incorporate contextual information. However, it is an important problem in healthcare, since it is useful to monitor people, especially if they are at a high risk of depression or other mental illnesses. Research in affective computing seeks to generate new methodologies to help store, analyze and share this information. Several techniques have been proposed to monitor emotions. One of them is *self-report*, which is a subjective method of measuring emotions from the perspective of the individual. This work presents a new tangible interface to self-report emotions, called EmoBall, specifically designed for people with low digital competences, since it requires practically no previous knowledge of technology. We evaluated this interface and analyze the results of the evaluation, considering the digital skills of the interviewed users. We found EmoBall to be a promising first step towards a tangible interface to self-report emotions; however, we did not find evidence of digital competences affecting user perceptions of the device. This paper discusses our insights regarding the reasons for these results, as well as directions for future research.

1 Introduction

Emotional well-being is an important element in people's quality of life because emotions are part of human intelligence and they are related with different types of behaviors. Monitoring emotional information is highly complex: it is difficult to accurately register emotional information due to subjectivity and technical complexities; and it is difficult to provide reliability and incorporate contextual information. Research in affective computing seeks to generate new methodologies to help store, analyze and share this information. Several techniques have been proposed to monitor emotions. One of them is *self-report*, which is a subjective method of measuring emotions from the perspective of the individual.

The evolution of user interfaces has allowed new ways of interacting with technology. Tangible User Interfaces (TUI) allow manipulating digital information by taking advantage of human abilities to handle physical (tangible) objects [18],

© Springer International Publishing Switzerland 2015
J. Bravo et al. (Eds.): AmIHEALTH 2015, LNCS 9456, pp. 189–200, 2015.
DOI: 10.1007/978-3-319-26508-7_19

taking advantage of physical interaction to improve collaboration, communication, learning and decision making [12]. We think that TUIs could be appropriate for populations with low digital competences.

This work is a first attempt to study emotion self-reporting considering digital competences from users. For this, we created a prototype tangible interface called EmoBall that allows easy self-reporting of emotions (by pressing a ball), sharing this information with social networks and providing feedback to users through simple images that show them their registered emotions. The contributions of this work are the following ones:

1. We identify the benefits and challenges of using a TUI to self-report emotions in users with different digital competences.
2. We provide insights regarding how digital competences could affect the usability of a TUI to self-report emotions; and
3. We provide design guidelines for interfaces for self-reporting emotions.

This paper is organized as follows. First, we discuss related work, considering studies about digital skills and competences, and tangible interfaces for emotion self-reporting. Then, we describe the design and characteristics of our prototype, EmoBall. Section 4 describes our experiment, then Sect. 5 describes the results and their discussion. Finally, Sect. 6 presents our conclusions and discusses possible avenues of future work.

2   Related Work

This section presents related work: first, we review literature about digital skills and then we discuss tangible, wearable and ambient interfaces to express, view, or share human emotions.

2.1   Digital Skills

Digital skills, competences, and digital literacy are concepts that aim to identify the skills or knowledge regarding technology that users have. Technology is constantly changing, causing the skills needed to use it to become a "moving target". The concept of digital competence also involves social and emotional aspects that allow users to understand the use of digital devices [15]. Digital competences have been defined as involving "the confident and critical use of information Society technology (IST) for work, leisure, learning and communication", and requiring knowledge about computer and internet use [16].

The DIGCOMP project began in 2011 with the purpose of developing a standardized instrument to measure digital competences [16]. This instrument evaluates four relevant areas of competences: information, communication, content creation and problem solving. Four final categories of users are defined, their digital competences may either be: *no*, *low*, *basic*, or *above basic*. This proposal has been applied in a wide sample of at least 15 countries in the European community [9]. We use this instrument for our work.

2.2 Interfaces for Emotions

Tangible interfaces incorporate physical interaction into digital data manipulation [18]. This type of interface has been used to express emotions, e.g. with SubtleStone in classroom settings [1]. In this case, the device allowed students to be more aware of their own emotions during class [1]. Another use of this type of interface is for people to communicate remotely, allowing awareness of the presence and availability of others [17]. Mood Squeezer is a ball that allows users to reflect on their mood, with the goal of providing a wider range of conversations in an office environment [11].

The term Ambient Intelligence refers to a digital environment that is sensitive, adaptive and responsive to the presence of people [3]. This may encourage reflection processes that may result in better work practices and behavioral change. For example, a rabbit figure was used to provide mood visualization through its ears [14]. Results showed that different interfaces are appropriate in different situations, and that mood is affected by context. Common household objects have also been used as ambient intelligence interfaces. For example, EmotoCouch is a couch that changes color depending on user emotions, either to reinforce those emotions, comfort the user, or give feedback [13]. MoodLight [19] is another example, changing color depending on the degree of user excitement.

Wearable computing integrates computational capabilities to body-worn devices, such as clothes or accessories. A scarf was used as a wearable interface to visualize five emotions (stressed, happy, sad, excited and quiet), giving feedback through heat, vibration, and music [21].

The presented devices and systems aim to display, detect or share emotions for several purposes. However, to the best of our knowledge, there have been no studies that present tangible, wearable, ubiquitous systems that deal with emotions and study them from the perspective of users with different levels of digital competences. This is the focus of our work: to present a new interface to report and share emotions, and to understand whether a tangible interface for emotions is more appropriate for users with low levels of digital competences.

3 Design of EmoBall

The main motivation to develop Emoball was to design a simple and tangible object to report emotions. Our design was inspired in part by SubtleStone [1] as an element to register emotions in ball form. We used a LED matrix to represent positive and negative emotions with "faces" as shown in Fig. 1. To provide an interactive feedback to users EmoBall has two mechanisms: first, the ball vibrates when an emotion is registered and saved in memory to let the user know when he/she recorded data; second, self-reported emotions may be viewed in summary form or shared through Twitter when the ball is connected to a base with a touchscreen.

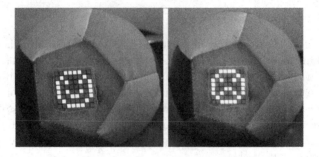

Fig. 1. EmoBall emotion faces: (a) Happy (b) Sad

3.1 System Description

The EmoBall system has two main interfaces: the ball TUI and a base with a touchscreen. Each time the user presses the ball, a LED matrix on the ball displays a face depicting a specific emotion. When the ball is pressed twice, the emotion is selected and saved, and the ball vibrates. When the ball is placed on its base, the user can see the information he/she has registered on a touchscreen. The screen has three options: a graph visualization of the latest emotions the user has reported, a text visualization in which each emotion is represented by an adjective and the total number of reported emotions of each kind, and an option to share the emotions via Twitter (a popular social microblogging site). Figure 2 illustrates the system architecture.

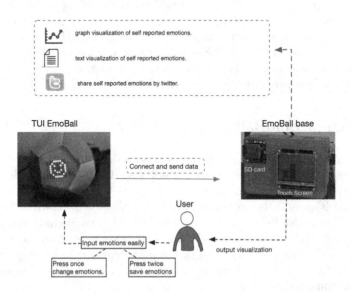

Fig. 2. General architecture of the EmoBall system.

We implemented EmoBall using a Microsoft Gadgeteer FEZSpider Kit with .NET Framework 4.0, .NET Micro Framework 4.2, GHI Electronics SDK and Visual Studio 2012. This kit was incorporated into a toy ball (Fig. 2). The following Gadgeteer modules were used for our implementation.

- **Information storage:** Information is stored in a SD card.
- **Emotion representation:** Emotions are represented with an 8×8 matrix.
- **User interaction:** EmoBall uses pressure sensors to allow users to change emotions on the ball. If the ball is pressed twice, the selected emotion is stored in memory and haptic feedback is provided through vibrations to let the user know the emotion was recorded.
- **Base:** The base was implemented with a second Gadgeteer FEZSpider Kit and a T35 touchscreen that allows visualizing the registered information.

4 Methodology

Our goal was to evaluate our interface considering the digital competences, or skills, of the potential users. To accomplish this goal, we evaluated EmoBall through focus groups, allowing users to interact with the system and collecting three types of information:

- Questionnaire results regarding digital skills (based on DIGCOMP [9]).
- Results from a usability evaluation using SUS (System Usability Scale) [5].
- Audio recordings from the focus group.

Then, we analyzed our results, to see whether our system is considered useful and usable, and how the results relate to the participants' digital skills.

4.1 Participants

Our participants were 14 women and 2 men. 6 had low digital skills, 7 had basic digital skills, and 3 had above basic digital skills. The average age of participants was 53. We conducted three focus groups: the first had 7 participants, average age: 65, the second had 6 participants, average age: 56, and the third had 3 participants, average age: 18. In our study the age of participants and the level of digital skills was correlated (higher age participants had lower digital skills).

4.2 Assessment Tools

We used the DIGCOMP instrument to measure digital competences [9], and the system usability scale (SUS) as a quick way to measure the overall usability of the system [5]. In this scale, scores below 60 indicate poor usability, while scores over 80 indicate very good usability [20]. The discussion within the focus groups was recorded and transcribed. We used thematic analysis to identify and analyze themes within the data [4].

4.3   Experiment

To evaluate the prototype and see whether results from the evaluation correlated with digital skill levels, we performed three focus groups (with 16 participants in total) during January 2015. Each focus group had the following structure:

1. One researcher gave a brief introduction about the EmoBall prototype, describing its purpose and its mode of use.
2. Participants were given time to interact with the prototype.
3. We encouraged semi-structured discussion (using questions from a guide) about the prototype.
4. Participants completed the DIGCOMP survey and the SUS questionnaire.

5   Results

This section presents our analysis of the obtained results. We discuss the usability results and the qualitative analysis of the focus group discussion.

5.1   System Usability Results

The average usability score from the SUS questionnaire was 68.5. This means that general usability of EmoBall is good. Section 5.3 discusses these results when divided into groups considering digital skills.

5.2   Analysis of Focus Groups

Two researchers transcribed the comments from the focus groups, and built a theme map (Fig. 3). We also used the transcription to build a word cloud, to see common topics emerging. We programmed a python script to remove all conjunctions, prepositions, articles, pronouns and adverbs from the transcription (in spanish), translated the remaining text, and used the WordItOut [8] service to build the word cloud (Fig. 4). We can see that the main discussed topics are emotions, people, and types of emotions (happy, sad, angry).

The thematic map allowed us to see the following topics emerge from the focus group discussions. We include some quotes (translated from spanish) from the participants.

1. **Potential users:** The focus group participants identified who they believed can benefit from using the prototype, e.g.: patients caregivers, shy people, students, people with disabilities. For example, some users believed this type of interface to be ideal for children who do not yet know how to read or express themselves clearly: *"it would be great for young children [...] to know whether the child had a normal day, a happy day or it was stressful or sad"*.
2. **Purpose:** The participants identified potential scenarios of use: at school, in the workplace, in therapy sessions, and for self-reflection: *"it helps to you to know how you're feeling, it allows you to think and analyze it and say "Oh!, I feel this way", and by end of week I can see summaries of how I felt"*.

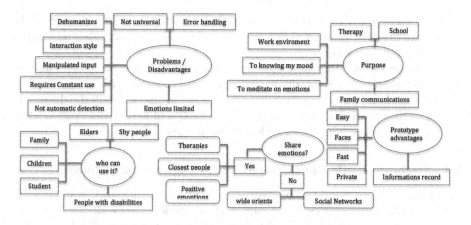

Fig. 3. Thematic map from focus group discussions

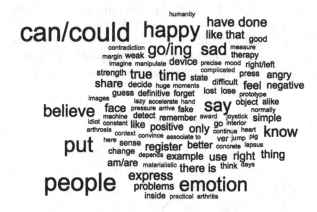

Fig. 4. Word cloud from transcription of focus group discussions

3. **Problems and Limitations:** Participants discussed interesting problems, related to ethics, privacy and ease and comfort of use. One participant was concerned with losing human abilities to express emotions. Another wanted the device to automatically detect his/her emotions, even at the risk of losing accuracy, like a "mood ring". There was also some discussion about not being able to correct errors in expressed emotions, and in having to express emotions as an additional chore to be done. The range of emotions in EmoBall is limited, which some users found to be a constraint *"You could have other faces, like intermediate options, the ball only has sad and happy moods"*. One participant commented that people with some disabilities, e.g. arthritis, would find it difficult to use the ball (as it requires physical force).

4. **Sharing and Privacy:** Sharing emotions is a privacy issue. Users do not share emotions with anyone: they share emotions with their closest family members and with therapy professionals. Some participants only want to

share their positive emotions, keeping their negative emotions private *"I do not like to share in social networks, because it is like publicly exposing myself. I feel this information is personal..."*

5. **Advantages or Benefits:** Participants mentioned that the prototype has several advantages, especially its ease of use and how quickly it can be used. It also records information privately and it is easy to see (through the displayed emoticons) which information is being saved. 60 % of participants commented on advantages or benefits that they found in EmoBall.

5.3   Usability Evaluation Concerning to Digital Competences

To understand how digital competences could affect the usability evaluation of a TUI to self-report emotions [2], our study reflects evidence of *Good* usability evaluation for participants with low digital competences ($SUS_{Low} = 64$ $Average_{age} = 63$) and basic digital competences ($SUS_{Basic=} = 64$ $Average_{age} = 53$). The group with high level of digital competences found the usability to be *very good* with scores ($SUS_{AboveBasic=} = 88$ $Average_{age} = 34$). Figure 5 show the SUS results for each focus group. We show the scores for each focus group since the format of discussion in which one participant's opinion may influence another's may explain some homogeneization within each group.

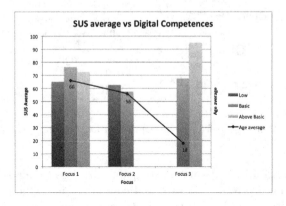

Fig. 5. SUS evaluation for each focus group

These results are counter-intuitive to our initial hypothesis, since users with higher digital competences found EmoBall to be better than users with low and basic digital competences. Although this was an unexpected result, we believe there are some possible explanations for this phenomenon: first, users with higher digital competences were younger, and more open to trying new types of devices. Future experiments should consider a homogeneous age group with different digital competences. Second, users generally found this interface to be useful, but not necessarily *for themselves*: they believed, as previously discussed, that this interface is ideal for e.g. children, people with disabilities, caregivers, or in a context of therapy or self-reflection. People with higher digital skills could perhaps more easily understand uses for the technology that did not immediately concern themselves, and thus were more positive about it. Further experiments are needed to confirm these hypotheses.

5.4 Design Insights

The analysis of the focus group discussions led us to a set of design insights to consider when designing tangible user interfaces considering digital competence of users. These are discussed below.

- *The context of use may define the interaction style.* EmoBall was implemented as a general-purpose emotion self-reporting device, based on previous works (e.g. [10]). However, we did not specify a clear context of use or target population, and this was a cross-cutting concern for all digital competence groups we interviewed. Our results agree with Edge and Blackwell's proposal [7] on methodologies for the design of tangible interfaces: an important aspect of TUI design is a clear identification of context of use, how the user will benefit, and which properties of the interface will support the activities it was designed for. We believe that a second iteration of EmoBall, designed for a specific context, may need to have additional characteristics and a different interaction style, which will help it become more successful and accepted for the specific target population.
- *Privacy concerns: Selective sharing.* A device to register and report emotions was found to be beneficial by our study participants, because they believed it is positive to reflect about their emotions, and review them afterwards. However, sharing this information has many privacy concerns. It is important to allow the user to clearly identify whether he/she wants to share this type of information, who to share it with, and which types of emotions to share (e.g. only share positive emotions).
- *Motivate users to self-report emotions and self-reflect by showing benefits of this practice.* The study participants perceived storing emotional information to be a positive aspect of EmoBall. This is similar to the results from the SubtleStone study [1], as well as other studies that have shown that TUIs for children promote participation and produce emotions in their users [22]. It is important to consider during TUI design how to encourage the user to actually use the device and clearly display the benefits of doing so. One measure of the motivation for using an interface is the Intrinsic Motivation Inventory [6], which may be used to measure an activity and how it relates to interest/enjoyment, perceived competence, effort, value/usefulness, felt pressure and tension, and perceived choice. We believe further generating spaces to self-reflect in interfaces for emotions may motivate users to actively use a device such as EmoBall.

6   Conclusions and Future Work

This work presented a proposal of a tangible interface to self-report emotions, called EmoBall. Comparing EmoBall with tangible interfaces like Mood Squeezer [11] and SubtleStone [1], there are evident similarities in the benefits and disadvantages that these devices deliver to users, e.g. they help users be more conscious about their moods, but it is difficult to incorporate a large range of emotions. EmoBall and Squeezer Mood [11] participants revealed that they did not feel comfortable with sharing their moods on social networks. On the other hand, the Squeezer Mood [11] and SubtleStone [1] studies both specify the context of use and target user, which were not available in our study. However, the study presented in this paper focuses on whether digital skills affect user experience when studying interactions with a tangible interface.

We evaluated EmoBall, finding an overall *good* level of usability evaluation (even for participants with low and basic digital competences). We also found several insights about interfaces for reporting emotions. First, users indicated they would not share this kind of information through social networks and prefer to register emotions privately. Second, our study participants suggested that the ideal scenario for this type of device may be a concrete one that can benefit from emotional information, e.g. education or mental health. Third, the device must consider all types of users in order to create a universal design.

We did not find evidence of digital competences affecting user perceptions of the device. Our experimental study had some limitations. First, we only involved 16 users, and as any study dealing with humans, the variability within these users may explain the variability of the results (or lack thereof). For example, we controlled digital competences, but we did not measure willingness to try new technologies. Second, EmoBall was a fully-implemented working device, however, it is a prototype (that e.g. requires researchers to charge it and fix any problems after use), so we could not send it to participants to use for days or weeks and analyze their experiences and activity logs afterwards. Instead, they had a short experience with the prototype before giving us their opinions. Therefore, a more extensive (and perhaps, lengthy) study, with a greater number of users, is needed to obtain more precise statistics.

As future work, it is important to study whether another type of interaction is better to report emotions, e.g. changing the squeeze interaction to touch interaction. Given the small sample size of our study, it is difficult to speak of generalizable results, so further evaluation is required. We will also apply this evaluation in specific contexts, e.g. informal caregivers, or young children.

Acknowledgements. This project was partially funded by CONICYT Chile PhD scholarship grant, CONICIT and MICIT Costa Rica PhD scholarship grant, Universidad de Costa Rica and LACCIR Project Grant R1212LAC001.

References

1. Balaam, M., Fitzpatrick, G., Good, J., Luckin, R.: Exploring affective technologies for the classroom with the subtle stone. In: Proceedings of the SIGCHI Conference on Human Factors in Computing Systems, CHI 2010, pp. 1623–1632. ACM, New York (2010). http://doi.acm.org/10.1145/1753326.1753568

2. Bangor, A., Kortum, P., Miller, J.: Determining what individual sus scores mean: adding an adjective rating scale. J. Usability Stud. **4**(3), 114–123 (2009)

3. Botta, M., Catenazzi, N., Sommaruga, L.: Human centered design framework to generate novel ambient intelligence interface solutions. In: Proceedings of the 2011 Conference on Designing Pleasurable Products and Interfaces DPPI 2011, pp. 69:1–69:2. ACM, New York (2011). http://doi.acm.org/10.1145/2347504.2347580

4. Braun, V., Clarke, V.: Using thematic analysis in psychology. Qual. Res. Psychol. **3**(2), 77–101 (2006). http://dx.doi.org/10.1191/1478088706qp063oa

5. Brooke, J.: Sus-a quick and dirty usability scale. Usability Eval. Ind. **189**(194), 4–7 (1996)

6. Deci, E., Ryan, R.: Intrinsic motivation inventory (imi) (2005). Accessed, July 23, 2006

7. Edge, D., Blackwell, A.: Peripheral tangible interaction by analytic design. In: TEI 2009 Conference on Tangible and Embedded Interaction. ACM (2009). http://research.microsoft.com/apps/pubs/default.aspx?id=192903

8. Enideo: Worditout (2015). http://worditout.com

9. Ferrari, A.: Digital competence in practice: an analysis of frameworks. Technical report, Research Centre of the European Commission, September 2012. http://ftp.jrc.es/EURdoc/JRC68116.pdf

10. Fuentes, C., Hernandez, C., Escobedo, L., Herskovic, V., Tentori, M.: Promoting self-reflection of social isolation through persuasive mobile technologies: the case of mother caregivers of children with cancer. Int. J. Hum. Comput. Interaction **30**(10), 802–814 (2014). http://dx.doi.org/10.1080/10447318.2014.927279

11. Gallacher, S., O'Connor, J., Bird, J., Rogers, Y., Capra, L., Harrison, D., Marshall, P.: Mood squeezer: lightening up the workplace through playful and lightweight interactions. In: Proceedings of the 18th ACM Conference on Computer Supported Cooperative Work & #38; Social Computing CSCW 2015, pp. 891–902. ACM, New York (2015). http://doi.acm.org/10.1145/2675133.2675170

12. Ishii, H.: The tangible user interface and its evolution. Commun. ACM **51**(6), 32–36 (2008)

13. Mennicken, S., Brush, A.J., Asta, R., James, S.: Finding roles for interactive furniture in homes with emotocouch. In: Proceedings of the 2014 ACM International Joint Conference on Pervasive and Ubiquitous Computing: Adjunct Publication, UbiComp 2014 Adjunct, pp. 923–930. ACM, New York (2014). http://doi.acm.org/10.1145/2638728.2641547

14. Mora, S., Rivera-Pelayo, V., Muller, L.: Supporting mood awareness in collaborative settings. In: 2011 7th International Conference on Collaborative Computing: Networking, Applications and Worksharing (CollaborateCom), pp. 268–277, October 2011

15. OECD: The definition and selection of key competencies. Technical report, The OECD Program Definition and Selection of Competencies, Executive Summary, June 2005. http://www.oecd.org/dataoecd/47/61/35070367.pdf

16. Parliament, E., the Council: Measuring digital skills across the eu: Eu wide indicators of digital competence. Technical report, European Commission funded DIGCOMP project, May 2014

17. Quintanilha, M.: Buddywall: a tangible user interface for wireless remote communication. In: CHI 2008 Extended Abstracts on Human Factors in Computing Systems, CHI EA 2008, pp. 3711–3716. ACM, New York (2008). http://doi.acm.org/10.1145/1358628.1358918

18. Shaer, O., Hornecker, E.: Tangible user interfaces: past, present, and future directions. Found. Trends Hum. Comput. Inter. 3(12), 4–137 (2009). http://dx.doi.org/10.1561/1100000026

19. Snyder, J., Matthews, M., Chien, J., Chang, P.F., Sun, E., Abdullah, S., Gay, G.: Moodlight: Exploring personal and social implications of ambient display of biosensor data. In: Proceedings of the 18th ACM Conference on Computer Supported Cooperative Work & #38; Social Computing, CSCW 2015, pp. 143–153. ACM, New York (2015). http://doi.acm.org.ezproxy.puc.cl/10.1145/2675133.2675191

20. Tullis, T., Albert, W.: Measuring the User Experience: Collecting, Analyzing, and Presenting Usability Metrics. Morgan Kaufmann Publishers Inc., San Francisco (2008)

21. Williams, M.A., Asta, R., O'Dowd, C., Czerwinski, M., Morris, M.: Swarm: an actuated wearable for mediating affect. In: Proceedings of the Ninth International Conference on Tangible, Embedded, and Embodied Interaction, TEI 2015, pp. 293–300. ACM, New York (2015). http://doi.acm.org/10.1145/2677199.2680565

22. Xie, L., Antle, A.N., Motamedi, N.: Are tangibles more fun?: comparing children's enjoyment and engagement using physical, graphical and tangible user interfaces. In: Proceedings of the 2nd International Conference on Tangible and Embedded Interaction, pp. 191–198. ACM (2008)

Can Videogames Improve Executive Functioning? A Research Based on Computational Neurosciences

Tania Mondéjar[1,2(✉)], Ramón Hervás[1], Jesús Fontecha[1],
Carlos Gutierrez[1], Esperanza Johnson[1], Iván González[1],
and José Bravo[1]

[1] MAmI Research Lab, University of Castilla-la Mancha,
Paseo de la Universidad 4, Ciudad Real, Spain
{ramon.hlucas,jesus.fontecha,Ivan.GDiaz,
jose.bravo}@uclm.es, {Carlos.Gutierrez5,
MEsperanza.Johnson}@alu.uclm.es
http://mami.uclm.es
[2] eSmile, Psychology for Children and Adolescents,
Calle Toledo 65, Ciudad Real, Spain
Tania.mondejar@esmile.es

Abstract. Nowadays, we are living a different use and understanding of videogames. Particularly, Serious Games aim to develop specific objectives beyond entertainment, mainly, educational and training objectives. There is a novel perspective that uses serious games as an innovative tool in the field of health (health games). This paper belongs to that perspective due to its multidisciplinary perspective focused on neurosciences and computation. The main goal is to determine the frontal-lobe brain activity (executive functioning) while using videogames. The participants of the developed experiments were children from 8 to 12 years old whose executive functioning was evaluated using psychological assessments to obtain a cognitive profile and can validate the cognitive skills developed during the use of videogames, particularly, adventure-action genre. The analysis of brain activity was performed through an electroencephalography neuroheadset which collects brain signals during the physiological assessment and while users are playing videogames. The hypotheses to validate are whether videogames can develop executive functioning and whether it is possible to identify which kind of cognitive skills are developed during each kind of typical mechanics in adventure-action videogames.

Keywords: Serious games · Videogames · Health games · Executive functioning · Computational neurosciences · Cognitive rehabilitation · Assistive technologies

1 Introduction

Executive functioning is a general term for cognitive processes that includes working memory, reasoning, task flexibility, and problem solving, and planning. These functions control and manage other cognitive processes that enable self-management, environment adaptation, selective attention, and inhibitory control. Most of these functions are

© Springer International Publishing Switzerland 2015
J. Bravo et al. (Eds.): AmIHEALTH 2015, LNCS 9456, pp. 201–212, 2015.
DOI: 10.1007/978-3-319-26508-7_20

mainly developed (not necessary in a linear manner) during the preadolescence. The executive functioning is carried out, mainly but not solely sufficient, by the brain's frontal lobe.

Authors such as Piaget and Vigosky, children's games are essential to cognitive processes and personal-emotional development. The cognitive skills above are tightly related to traditional games, and can be extrapolated to videogames [1].

This paper contributes to the efficient design of Serious Games (SG). This kind of games aims to achieve goals beyond just entertaining, typically goals related to education and training. Opportunity to use simulators, virtual worlds and interactive environments brings amazing possibilities in different areas. Particularly, there is a kind of SG focused on health, i.e., games applied to learn about healthy life [2]. Expanding this concept, this paper explores the use of SG to cognitive development and rehabilitation, an innovative approach of using health games.

This is a first approach to analyse brain activity during executive function evaluation and while users are playing videogames. The games are selected because of the cognitive abilities required in each game. It proposes an initial causal relationship between both times. In addition, like Bisoglio [3] said, it necessary to attend the individual differences making a continue research to make possible to cheek if the improvements in brain activity (executive function) are consequence to play videogames complementary to natural development.

The chosen action games in psychology are justified because it can measure common elements as format, content and mechanics. For this reason, it possible to evaluate the attention, basic perception, and improve the capacity of extracting patterns [4].

2   Related Work

SG deal with the integration of educative goals with game mechanics based on well-known tests to enhance and generalize learning to become significant [5], apart from helping to discover and use information instead of just memorizing it [6]. Regarding health area, videogames are becoming a successful tool to teach and train in areas such as chronic diseases and disability. For example, the videogame Re-Mission aids children to understand cancer disease fighting against malignant cells [7]. *Insouline* helps to learn how to control blood sugar levels through metaphors of games when a child is diagnosed with diabetes [8]. More related to psychology, it is remarkable the videogame *the treasure hunt*, to support cognitive-behavioural therapies [9], RGS, a game system for cognitive rehabilitation [10], videogames to control pain perception and management [11], and games whose goal is the self-management of emotions, e.g. anger control [12].

Being aware of the state of art in the health games context, the objective of this paper is the evaluation of cognitive skills developed while using SG based on adventure-action videogames (this concept is detailed in Sect. 3.3). Unlike most of the related work, which is just backed up psychological theories and typically evaluated through qualitative experiments, this proposal is supported on computational neurosciences and it will be validated by means of a mixed qualitative and quantitative approach. Using electroencephalogram (EEG) that enables the analysis of active brain areas during cognitive exercises, both psychological assessments and videogames, we have performed the evaluation of cognitive skills. In this way, it is possible to infer what kinds of SG mechanics are needed to enhance diagnosis and improve cognitive rehabilitation.

3 Conducted Experiment

3.1 Population

The experiment was conducted with one particular cohort: healthy preadolescents aged 8–12 years of age (n = 5, boys = 2, girls = 3). The participants and their parents were informed about the scope and goals of this research and about of collected data. They received and signed the information sheet and the consent form, keeping at all times the ethical principles.

3.2 Method

This experiment has followed an empirical method to gather evidences in terms of EEG data that was analysed qualitatively and quantitatively. The formulated research question that guides this experiment is: *How can adventure-action videogames be designed to develop cognitive skills related to executive functioning?* Two hypotheses were proposed to be tested through this experiment:

Hypothesis 1: Adventure-action videogames develop the cognitive processes related to executive functioning.
Hypothesis 2: Typical mechanics involved in adventure-action videogames stimulate same areas than psychological assessments that evaluate executive functioning, making possible the correlation between videogame mechanics and cognitive skills.

The experiment consisted of two evaluation phases: psychological assessment evaluation and videogames evaluation. Both phases followed the same protocol that can be summarized as follows: (1) participants were kindly informed about what is a EEG device and what kind of data it can collect, (2) participants were required to wear the EEG headset ensuring their comfort and confidence, (3) the psychologist explained what was happening in the researcher screen (EEG data visualization software) where participants could observe their brain activity. (4) the psychologist gave instructions about the activity to perform and appeased them remarking that nobody was evaluating their abilities (apart from remark that it is impossible to read minds using EEG devices, a typical concern of the children) (5) participants performed the proposed activities with no interruptions due to the researcher observation or EEG monitoring. Participants in these two phases wore the EEG headset for approximately 40 min.

Phase one of the experiment aims to define a cognitive model which consisted of neurological patterns of executive functioning (as previously mentioned, including working memory, reasoning, task flexibility, problem solving, and planning [13]), through the psychological assessment ENFEN (Neuropsychological assessment of executive functions in children [14]). Section 3.3 describes the ENFEN assessment in detail.

In phase two, participants took part in the recording of EEG data using videogames. This phase followed the same protocol with the exception of the directions: in this case it was not necessary to guide the activities due to the natural skill of children understanding and using videogames.

Both evaluation phases were recorded using video camera (having concern of preserving participant anonymity) and the EEG dataset were generated and labelled to the data analysis. Once collected all data, next stage was the qualitative and quantitative analysis to support (or not) the defined hypotheses and, consequently, answer the main research question of this work. The data analysis was performed following two perspectives: (a) Observational method based on the psychologist expertise regarding EEG data to identify significant segments of data and characteristic cognitive patterns, and (b) Signal processing algorithms to quantify the similarity of identified segments.

3.3 Materials

For the development of this work, we used several computational and neuroscience tools and devices. Regarding the neuropsychology fundamentals, the ENFEN assessment is a battery of tests to evaluate the overall development of maturity in boys between 6 and 12 years of age stemming from the study of executive functions. It consists of four scales: fluency, trails, washers and resistance to interference, which assess mental flexibility, working memory, planning and inhibition response, respectively.

In order to collect EEG data, we used the Emotiv EPOC + neuroheadset[1]. This device features 14 EEG channels plus 2 references offering positioning for accurate spatial resolution. These channels include 8 frontal electrodes (named AF3, F7, F3, FC5 at the left hemisphere and FC6, F4, F8, AF4 at the right hemisphere) 2 temporal electrodes (T7 & T8), 2 occipital electrodes (O1 & O2) and 2 parietal electrodes (P7 & P8). The EEG headset uses sequential sampling method at a rate of 128 samples per second. It also includes gyroscope and accelerometers but they were not used in this experiment. In order to analyse the EEG dataset, we used the Xavier TechBench Software[TM] to collect and visualize the EEG signals and MatLab R2015a[TM] to develop the signal processing algorithms and metrics. Additionally, we developed a software using C# and the Emotiv EPOC+ API to improve the gathering and conversion to our dataset format. The election of this device is because Emotiv EPOC is easy to use in children during a bit time and it has a rapid calibration that is required for fast laboratory studies. Finally, students of the Faculty of Computer Science in Ciudad Real (University of Castilla-La Mancha) developed a set of simple videogames focused on specific adventure-action mechanics. Figure 1 shows a picture of the conducted experiment including the materials involved in.

Focusing on videogames, it is necessary to delimit the kind of games to include in this research. The videogames category chosen is the named *Adventure-action videogames,* a type of videogames that combines elements of the adventure game genre with

---

[1] https://emotiv.com/epoc.php.

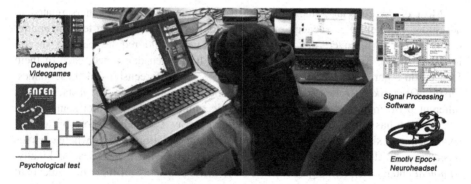

Fig. 1. Performed experiment and materials

various action game elements. It requires many of the same physical skills as action games, but also offers a storyline and other features of adventure games [15]. This genre of videogames can test out several user skills closely related to executive functioning. We can distinguish which action features are linked to processes such as concentration, attention, reflexes, short-term memory, and logical reasoning; adventure-related features are more connected to cognitive skills such as planning, long-term memory and knowledge abstraction. For this work, we have identified several typical mechanics in commercial action-adventure videogames, focusing on action-related elements. Table 1 describes the identified mechanics, including the five most representative ones. Theoretically, each of them requires different cognitive processes and skills to be successfully overcome. This statement has been tested during the experiment.

Table 1. Main adventure-action videogames mechanics

Mechanic	Description	Commercial games
Accurate actions	Player has to perform actions in a precise and careful way, typically without maximum time	Tomb Raider (climbing, jumps), Castlevania (trails, jumps), Assassin's Creed (jumps, stalking)
Timely actions (Quick Time Events)	Player has to perform single actions at the exact time according game events	God of War and Heavenly Sword (final bosses), Beyond: two souls
Mimic sequences	Player has to copy a sequence of actions that are previously defined	Zelda and Castlevania (final bosses), Fighting games (combos)
Learning patterns	Game events happen following a particular pattern that has to be understood to adapt player actions	Thief, Metal Gear, Hitman (stalking) Prince of Persia, Crash Bandicoot (traps)
Logic puzzles	Player has to plan a set of actions according to a logical problem in terms of game events	Silent Hill, Resident Evil, Tomb Raider (lever-based puzzles)

Most of commercial games mix up all those mechanics with others related to adventure features, e.g. scenery exploration, object gathering, long-term planning, dialogues, etc. Moreover, the mechanics unlocking would require playing several hours. For these reasons, several specific games have been developed, each of them focused on a particular game mechanic. Figure 2 shows screenshots of those games. Firstly, *Dreamskeeper* lies in carefully moving the mouse to avoid obstacles with different performances. *KittenQuest* is a classic running game with horizontal scroll where player has to timely miss obstacles in her/his way. *CrazyFarm* shows visual and sound sequences that have to be mimicked. *Rodrigo* is a platforms game where enemies repeat a particular pattern that have to be identified to reach next levels. Finally, *Kunoichi* entails the planning of a set of basic actions in terms of logic movements to get the exit gate.

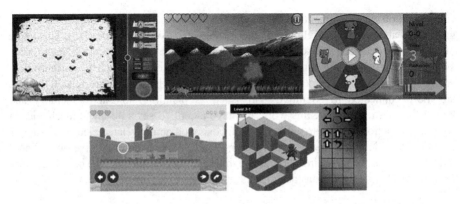

Fig. 2. Screenshot of DreamsKeeper (Accurate Actions), KittenQuest (Timely actions), CrazyFarm (Mimic sequences), Rodrigo (Learning patterns) y Kunoichi (Logic Puzzles).

3.4 Results

This section explains how observations and collected data were qualitatively and quantitatively analysed, obtaining the associated results.

3.4.1 Observational Analysis of Data

The results were evaluated by the observational method focused on electric impulses in the brain that represent an interface line emitted thought the electrodes of the EMOTIV Epoc+ headset. With this method, the electric brain activity patterns are interpreted by comparison of participants and activities. The interpretation of the results was performed by visual analysis of the graphical representation of EEG signal. Thus, the expert provides differential patterns of participants in the different areas at head surfaces as result of the evaluations in this experiment.

First of all, the results of the participants show high activity in electrodes of frontal area, (AF3, F7, F8 y AF4) the executive functioning region, as mentioned above. As we can see in Fig. 3, signals can show different levels of activation. It is observed that, compared with the rest of electrodes, there is lower activation in parietal, temporal and occipital areas. In this phase we emphasize that the level of activation in frontal lobe matches with the measure of the skills assessed in ENFEN. This was expected since that is a validated test for such purpose. In a similar way, we can see high activation in frontal area at the videogame evaluation, unlike the middle–low activation in the rest of brain electrodes. With this data we can objectively affirm that the brain significantly uses the skills located in the front area, the same as executive function, during the ENFEN activities and during the use of videogames.

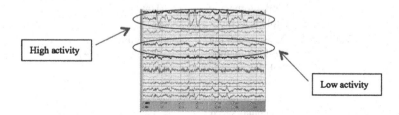

Fig. 3. Example of EEG data collected during the experiment.

To support these observations, the EEG signals visualized in the brain surface were analyzed. As Fig. 4 shows below, the remarked red zone is limited to the front surface of the head. Besides the identified similarities in the use of frontal lobe, it can be observed few differences between hemispheres that indicate more emotional presence during the use of videogames. This kind of observation is not the scope of this research and, for this reason, this aspect was not explored in detail.

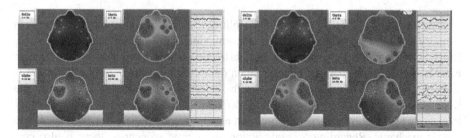

Fig. 4. Activation brainwave on trails (right) and timely action (left)

These observations occurred in the majority of the population (80 %). There is a particular case with participant 2 that resulted in uniform activation of most areas (frontal, parietal, temporal and occipital). It corresponds to a psychological profile of gifted and very distinctive creative skills (greater use of cranial surface and intensity of the electrical signal). In any case, the general observations corroborate the first hypothesis because the data demonstrated a strong relevance of executive function during the use of video games, very similar to activity during the ENFEN assessment.

Regarding the second hypothesis, Table 2 describes the specific skills in the neuropsychological assessment ENFEN and the identified matching in terms of EEG activation during the use of videogame mechanics.

Table 2. Cognitive skills related to ENFEN activities and game mechanics. Symbol (+) means the most correlated game mechanic.

ENFEN	Skills	Game mechanics
Fluency	Crystallized intelligence Working memory Explicit memory	Learning patterns (+) Timely action
Trails	Decision making Working memory Problem solving Selective attention Logical reasoning Perceptual speed Anticipation and foresight	Logic Puzzles Timely action (+)
Rings	Planning and sequencing Spatial orientation Abstraction capacity Decomposition problems	Logic Puzzles Learning patterns (+)
Interference	Selected attention Sustained attention Ability to inhibit Resistance to interference Classify	Logic Puzzles (+) Learning patterns

The findings can be summarized as follow. Fluency activity, closely related to memory and life background, has a direct correlation with learning patterns mechanic. Rings activity includes the planning and abstraction of knowledge skills that are also basic in the mechanic learning patterns again (an example is shown in Fig. 5). In Trails activity, the most characteristic skills are the selective and sustained attention in the same way that we measure timely action mechanic. Interference deals with the ability to classify information and resist to interference, as occurs in the corresponding Logic Puzzle mechanic. Regarding accurate action and mimic sequences, there is also correspondence with the four ENFEN activities. However, that correlation is softer and similar in the four activities.

3.4.2 Quantitative Analysis of Data

The EEG signals are highly non-Gaussian, non-stationary and non-linear in nature and, consequently, it is very difficult to automatically analyse even using advanced signal processing techniques. Typically, EEG signal are analysed through expert observation that can distinguish normal and abnormal states, as explained in Sect. 3.4.1. However, observational results are very general and, for this reason, we have included this second test to quantify similarity levels between EEG signals.

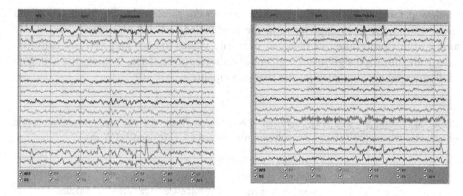

Fig. 5. Example of correlation observed by the expert: EEG Signal activation in Rings activity (right) and learning patterns (left).

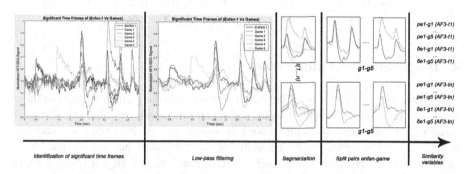

Fig. 6. Example of the anterior frontal electrode (AF3) with the participant 4 while doing activity *fluency* of the ENFEN assessment (Blue line) compared to the five studied mechanics (respectively Red, Green, Yellow, Magenta and Cyan lines). The figure shows the consecutive signal processing phases: (1) identification of significant time frames, (2) filtering through low-pass filter, (3) segmentation, (4) splitting and (5) gathering of similarity variables ($\rho e1$-gn for AF3 using Cross-Correlation Coefficient and $\delta e1$-gn for AF3 using Dynamic Time Wrapping, for each segment of EEG data)

Figure 6 shows the consecutive phases to process the significant time frames of EEG signals. This processing allows finding similar cognitive patterns. Firstly, from the expert observations, significant time frames were identified and included in datasets, both segments of ENFEN activities and videogames; typically they lasted about 5 s (640 sequential samples). The comparison was done with each ENFEN activity and each videogame, analysing each electrode separately. The signals were normalized and then, a low-pass filter ($\alpha = 0.15$) was applied. The softened signal was segmented to separate complete signal periods. Finally, these segments were analysed using two kinds of similarity methods: a statistical method through cross-correlation coefficient (CCC) and an algorithmic method named Dynamic Time Wrapping (DTW) with a window parameter of 50. All these parameters were selected by experimentation and based on our previous experience in the applications of that algorithm [16–18]. By means of this procedure, we obtained similarity values to each pair ENFEN_activity - videogame, for each significant segment of each electrode. Table 2 shows the averaged similarities taking into account the five participants.

Table 3. Averaged similarity between ENFEN_Activities (e1-e4) and adventure-action videogames mechanics (g1-g5) through non-normalized CCC (ρ) and DTW (δ).

		Videogames mechanics									
		Accurate action		Timely action		Mimic sequence		Learning patterns		Logic puzzles	
		ρ_{e-g1}	δ_{e-g1}	ρ_{e-g2}	δ_{e-g2}	ρ_{e-g3}	δ_{e-g3}	ρ_{e-g4}	δ_{e-g4}	ρ_{e-g5}	δ_{e-g5}
ENFEN	Fluency	1.77	1.01	1.58	0.98	1.98	3.42	**0.79**	**0.85**	2.31	3.08
	Trails	2.87	3.99	**0.91**	**1.59**	2.08	2.65	1.56	2.10	1.45	1.43
	Washers	2.71	2.87	1.31	2.84	2.04	2.67	**1.22**	**1.37**	1.34	2.04
	Interference	3.05	3.82	1.87	2.64	3.48	3.87	1.49	2.03	**0.76**	**1.41**

4   Discussion and Future Work

EEG signal processing is a study field in progress due to the particular nature of these signals. In this work, we firstly focused the signal processing on collecting statistical variables. Unfortunately, the findings were not conclusive. An interesting alternative is to apply advanced signal processing techniques that literature has demonstrated very valuable, e.g., different kind of entropies, Hurst exponent and Higher Order Spectra [19]. However, even proved these methods to identify anomalies associated to pathologies in EEG signals, our goal is just identifying similarities to correlate cognitive skills during activities of the ENFEN assessment and during the use of videogames. In this particular case we relied on the expert observation to collect significant time frames of data, which enable the study of similarity level in short temporal series, and we obtained relevant results through the CCC and DTW methods. However, it is not possible to distinguish which similarity value is more accurate. On one hand, CCC is better to compare signal in different scales. On the other hand, DTW allows comparing signals, which may vary over time. For this reason, we took into account both similarity coefficients.

The developed experiment and the collected datasets could be used to aid the diagnosis and treatment related to executive functioning issues. By using supervised learning techniques [20] such as Support Vector Machine (SVM) or Hidden Markov Models (HMM) it is possible to identify normal and abnormal cognitive behaviour when using videogames. This is particularly the future work to develop by means of those supervised learning techniques and increasing the population of the research, including more participants with and without diagnosed pathologies.

5 Conclusions

This work contributes to the field of computational neurosciences and serious games design. Empirically, it was possible to validate the predominant activity related to executive functioning while using adventure-action videogames that implement particular action mechanics. In fact, a transversal contribution of this paper is the described taxonomy about main mechanics in adventure-action games. This taxonomy can be useful for proper design of serious games.

Regarding to the second hypothesis linked to identify which cognitive skills are developed while using each videogame mechanic, it was observed that the relationship is not disjoint, i.e. a mechanic develops several cognitive skills and each cognitive skill is developed in several mechanics. However, it was proved the prevalence of particular cognitive skills in each game mechanic, as we showed in Table 2. Moreover, we obtained quantitative values (Table 3) that help the design of serious games with health purposes, particularly, to support the diagnosis and treatment of cognitive-related pathologies, not only in children, but also in adults.

Acknowledgments. This work was conducted in the context of UBIHEALTH project under International Research Staff Exchange Schema (MC-IRSES 316337). Thanks to the students: Laura Gutierrez, Rodrigo Marín, Carlos Vallejo, Carlos Villa and Mª Jesús Ciudad for the development of those amazing videogames. Finally and specially, many thanks to all families involved in this project.

References

1. McFarlane, A., Sparrowhawk, A., Heald, Y.: Report on the educational use of games: an exploration by TEEM of the contribution which games can make to the education process (2002)
2. Thompson, D., Baranowski, T., Buday, R., Baranowski, J., Thompson, V., Jago, R., Griffith, M.J.: Serious video games for health: how behavioral science guided the development of a serious video game. Simul. Gaming **41**, 587–606 (2010)
3. Bisoglio, J., Michaels, T.I., Mervis, J.E., Ashinoff, B.K.: Cognitive enhancement through action video game training: great expectations require greater evidence. Front. Psychol. **5**, 136 (2014)
4. Bavelier, D., Green, C.S., Schrater, P., Pouget, A.: Brain plasticity through the life span: learning to learn and action video games. Annu. Rev. Neurosci. **35**, 391–416 (2012)
5. Whyte, E.M., Smyth, J.M., Scherf, K.S.: Designing serious game interventions for individuals with autism. J. Autism Dev. Disord. (2014)
6. Garris, R., Ahlers, R., Driskell, J.E.: Games, motivation, and learning: a research and practice model. Simul. Gaming **33**, 441–467 (2002)
7. Kato, P.M., Cole, S.W., Bradlyn, A.S., Pollock, B.H.: A video game improves behavioral out-comes in adolescents and young adults with cancer: a randomized trial. Pediatrics **122**, 305–317 (2008)

8. Diehl, L.A., Souza, R.M., Alves, J.B., Gordan, P.A., Esteves, R.Z., Jorge, M.L.S.G., Coelho, I.C.M.: InsuOnline, a serious game to teach insulin therapy to primary care physicians: design of the game and a randomized controlled trial for educational validation. JMIR Res. Protoc. **2**(1), e5 (2013)

9. Brezinka, V., Hovestadt, L.: Serious games can support psychotherapy of children and adolescents. In: Holzinger, A. (ed.) USAB 2007. LNCS, vol. 4799, pp. 357–364. Springer, Heidelberg (2007)

10. Shapi'i, A., Mat Zin, N.A., Elaklouk, A.M.: A game system for cognitive rehabilitation. In: BioMed Research International (2015)

11. Sourina, O., Wang, Q., Nguyen, M.K.: EEG-based "Serious" games and monitoring tools for pain management. Stud. Health Technol. Inform. (2011)

12. Baek, Y., Ko, R., Marsh, T.: Trends and Applications of Serious Gaming and Social Media. Springer, Heidelberg (2014)

13. Anderson, P.: Assessment and development of executive function (EF) during childhood. Child Neuropsychol. **8**, 71–82 (2002)

14. Portellano, J.A., Martínez, A., Zumárraga, A.: Evaluación neuropsicológica de las Funciones Ejecutivas en niños (Neuropsychological assessment of executive functions in children): ENFEN. TEA Ediciones, Madrid (2009)

15. Rollings, A., Adams, E.: Fundamentals of Game Design. Prentice Hall, Upper Saddle River (2006)

16. Fontecha, J., Navarro, F.J., Hervás, R., Bravo, J.: Elderly frailty detection by using accelerometer-enabled smartphones and clinical information records. Pers. Ubiqui-Touscomputing **17**(6), 1073–1083 (2013)

17. Raso, I., Hervás, R., Bravo, J.: m-Physio: personalized accelerometer-based physical re-habilitation platform. In: Proceedings of the Fourth International Conference on Mobile Ubiquitous Computing, Systems, Services and Technologies, pp 416–421. Florence, Italy (2010)

18. Hervás, R., Fontecha, J., Ausín, D., Castanedo, F., Bravo, J., López-de-Ipiña, D.: Mobile monitoring and reasoning methods to prevent cardiovascular diseases. Sensors **13**(5), 6524–6541 (2013). MDPI

19. Subha, D.P., Joseph, P.K., Acharya, U.R., Lim, C.M.: EEG signal analysis: a survey. J. Med. Syst. **34**, 195–212 (2010). Springer, Heidelberg

20. Sanei, S., Chambers, J.A.: EEG Signal Processing. Wiley, Hoboken (2007)

Arousal Level Classification in the Ageing Adult by Measuring Electrodermal Skin Conductivity

Arturo Martínez-Rodrigo[1], Roberto Zangróniz[1], José Manuel Pastor[1], and Antonio Fernández-Caballero[2](✉)

[1] Instituto de Tecnologías Audiovisuales, Universidad de Castilla-La Mancha, 13071 Cuenca, Spain
[2] Instituto de Investigación en Informática de Albacete, Universidad de Castilla-La Mancha, 02071 Albacete, Spain
Antonio.Fdez@uclm.es

Abstract. Ambient intelligence is a suitable paradigm for developing daily life solutions including the health care domain. Many ageing adults who decide to live alone at home need constant monitoring to control their health status and quality of life. This paper introduces the description of a wearable device capable of acquiring the electrodermal activity (EDA) in order to obtain information on the arousal level of the elderly. The lightweight wearable device is placed in the wrist of the ageing adult to allow continuous monitoring of EDA signals. With the aim of triggering changes in the emotional state of the ageing adult, fifty pictures from the International Affective Picture System are used to assess the electronic device through a series of experiments. The initial results show that the overall system classifies people into two classes: calmed and stressed patients. The results show that through measuring the EDA events' magnitudes, the ageing adults' arousal level is classified with a global accuracy higher than 80 %.

Keywords: Wearable · Electrodermal activity · Arousal quantification

1 Introduction

In Europe, the total population older than 65 is expected to increase from 22 % by 2025 to 27.5 % by 2050, while the population aged over 80 may grow more that 4 % in the same period [1]. According to the experts, this increasing trend has a deep impact on several aspects which will affect on the quality of life and health of millions of people around the world [2]. With the aim to palliate these effects, developing countries are presenting different programmes that include changes on pensions and social security systems, among others. From a technological point of view, innovative interaction paradigms make ambient intelligence a more than suitable candidate for developing various real life solutions, including in the health care domain [3,4].

In addition, it is imperative to take advantage of emerging assistive technologies together with ubiquitous and pervasive computing in order to increase the

© Springer International Publishing Switzerland 2015
J. Bravo et al. (Eds.): AmIHEALTH 2015, LNCS 9456, pp. 213–223, 2015.
DOI: 10.1007/978-3-319-26508-7_21

health level and quality of life of ageing people who decide to stay at home [5–8]. Moreover, the innovation and development of assistive technologies might help in saving resources from the medical services. In this regard, the last reports published by the World Health Organization show that cost reduction in health care systems is one of the most promising challenges in the upcoming years [9]. In this sense, much research is focusing efforts in developing novel assistive systems based in improving health care through telemedicine equipments, fitness devices and entertainment systems [10].

However, only a few efforts have been made towards monitoring and regulating the older people's arousal state, which is indicative of stress or mental illness. Moreover, these are fundamental aspects in the self-perception of well-being [11]. The lack of human-machine interfaces in interpreting the patients' emotional states is a severe drawback in this sense [12]. Moreover, continuous monitoring of arousal levels in the ageing adult is essential for understanding and managing personal well-being regarding mental health state.

In this regard, a number of physiological features have been widely used in the literature [13]. These features measure alterations in the central nervous system [14–16]. One of these physiological markers corresponds with the electrodermal activity (EDA). EDA has been widely used to assess the arousal level of the patients, as it is able to quantify changes in the sympathetic nervous system. In order to continuously measure the EDA signal from the patients, wearable sensors are the most appropriate ones, given their performance in providing detailed user-specific information. Moreover, wearable sensors are greatly valued due to their light weight and their wireless communication capacities with either a computer or other wearable sensors [10].

The aim of the work introduced in this paper is to describe and to assess the performance of a wearable EDA-based device in classifying the arousal state in ageing adults. This is thought to be a first step in monitoring a good health status of the elder people. Firstly, the design of the electronic hardware is described. Then, the population engaged and the implemented signal processing algorithms are described. These are used to obtain the physiological markers for a robust arousal classification. Finally, the EDA features are assessed for the sake of showing the classification efficiency of the model.

2   Electrodermal Activity

Electrodermal activity (EDA) is a measure of skin conductivity. Its value is directly related with the increasing in activity of the sweat glands. Fortunately, the skin is an excellent means to conduct electricity. The sweat secretion is controlled by the sympathetic nervous system which reacts against any stress situation, pain and mental illness. Two main components are present in EDA signal morphology, which corresponds with the superposition of the spontaneous skin conductance (SSC) and the basal skin conductance (BSC). SSC is reflected in the acquired signal as a wave with a variable level of amplitude that is dependent on the intensity and duration of the stimulus [17]. Similarly, the BSC component is affected by the sympathetic nervous system and the dermal characteristics of skin in each person [18]. The electrical characteristics of these components will determine the hardware design needed for their acquisition, processing and sampling in order to develop an entire system capable of quantifying the EDA level.

Three are the standard methods for measuring electrodermal activity. The first one corresponds to the endosomatic procedure, which does not need external current to work, since potential difference is measured directly on the skin. Despite this passive method is the less intrusive and it does not need special amplifiers and coupling electrical circuits, this kind of device is rarely used. The main reason relays in that the generated signals are hardly understandable, because the obtained electrical signals can be biphasic or even triphasic. Consequently, exosomatic approaches, where small currents are injected directed on the patient's skin, are more extended. In this regard, two different schemes are used. They correspond to the direct current method (DC) and the alternate current method (AC).

Although the usage of AC methods allows measuring the capacity changes in the electrodermal responses, DC procedures are the most extended. Despite much effort has been made to standardize the use of constant voltage circuits within the DC, there does not exist an agreement for adopting a constant voltage source against a constant current voltage scheme. The use of constant voltage circuits has some advantages, which include that the skin conductance can be obtained directly from the circuit without any kind of previous transformation. However, from an electronic point of view, the use of constant current source is preferable, as the devices are more stable and exhibit less tolerance than constant voltage circuits. One of the main drawbacks of the current constant method is that the injection of excessive current throughout a small skin area could damage the sweat gland duct. To overcome this problem, the density of injected current on the skin is limited to a maximum of $10 \mu A/cm^2$. Finally, taking in consideration the aforementioned, our design will consist in an exosomatic approach based on a constant current scheme.

2.1 Wearable Acquisition Device

A lightweight wearable device is placed in the wrist of the ageing adults to allow continuous monitoring of EDA signals (as shown in Fig. 1). In this regard, the wearable system consists of an ultra-low-power, 32-bit ARM Cortex-M3 micro-controller, which acts as a system control unit (as it can be appreciated in Fig. 2). This micro-controller is selected not only because of its low power consumption, but also due to the easiness to migrate to a more powerful Cortex-M micro-controller with the same architecture. It is important to highlight that the micro-controllers' capabilities are growing exponentially nowadays, and new low power consumption devices, able to handle floating-point and digital processing calculations, are emerging every day. This is why, the right choice of the micro-controller architecture is an important factor to face.

Next, the EDA front-end is responsible for measuring the direct current (DC) exosomatic electrodermal response by using a variable-gain current-to-voltage

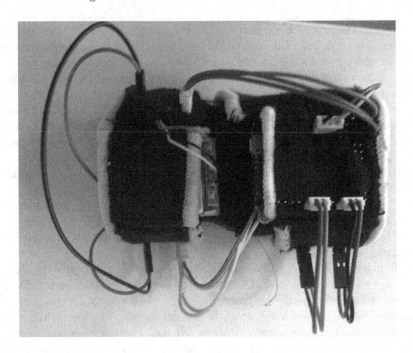

Fig. 1. A picture of the wearable device used in the present study.

operation amplifier. In addition, different filtering and amplification stages are applied to the raw data and EDA components are sampled at 20 Hz via a 12-bit analog-digital converter. A smart bluetooth protocol is used to exchange wireless data between the transceiver (installed in the wearable) and the software application. In case data transmission could not be effectuated, a data logger is

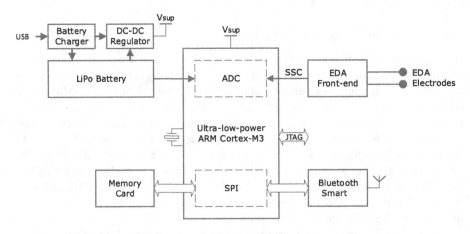

Fig. 2. General scheme of the wearable used in this study.

programmed to continuously store the physiological measurement into a removable memory card. Both bluetooth and memory card use SPI as interface with the micro-controller as can be observed in Fig. 2.

Finally, a lithium-polymer battery with a voltage of 3.7 V and a capacity of around 1500 mAh is chosen as power supply. These specifications are selected as trade-off between capacity, weight and dimensions of the battery. In this regard, the wearable is recharged by means of an integrated battery circuit, which allows recharging the battery through using an USB port. Finally, a low-dropout voltage regulator is responsible for supplying 3.0 volts from the battery to all the components of the device.

3   Methodology

3.1   Experimental Design

With the aim of triggering changes in the emotional state of the ageing adult, fifty pictures from the International Affective Picture System (IAPS) are chosen [19]. IAPS consists of a standard and categorized database of color photographs created to provide a wide range of affective stimuli. Since the mean and standard deviation of arousal level in each picture has been clearly reported [19], the criterion for choosing the photographs is the following one. Twenty-five pictures that report a mean arousal level lower than 3.26 are chosen and labeled as group A or negative stimuli. Similarly, twenty-five pictures that report a mean arousal level higher tan 5.26 are also chosen and labeled as group B or positive stimuli. It is noteworthy to remark that theses boundaries were calculated as a trade-off between the number of pictures available in the database and the number of needed pictures considering the duration of the experiment. The mean and standard deviation of the reported arousal level for each group is finally 5.87 ± 0.34 and 2.52 ± 0.22, respectively.

The display time for each picture is established on six seconds, regardless of the group the picture belongs to. Moreover, silences consisting of blank images with a fixed duration of 5 s are inserted between two consecutive images. Thus, the total duration of the experiment is 9 min from the screening of the first image. The pauses are designed to allow the patient under study to recover from the previous stimulus. In this regard, the pictures are randomly shuffled, such that the order of viewing is different for each patient, albeit keeping the silence between two consecutive pictures.

Once the pictures are selected, each patient sits in front of the experimentation monitor and the wearable is put in the right wrist. In this regard, the experimentation monitor consists of a high resolution 28 inches screen. When the technician verifies the proper functioning of the wearable and its communication with the software, the sequence of images is screened. It is important to say that the experiments are carried out in the safest possible way. Accordingly, the ageing persons are informed that they can stop visualizing the sequence in any moment by pressing a red button that stops the sequence. Moreover, the technician stays behind the elderly during the whole experiment in order to assist the patient at any time.

3.2 Study Population

Twenty-four patients (eleven men and thirteen women, aged 67.2 ± 3.5) have been enrolled in this study. All the patients are informed about the high emotional contents of the pictures and they agree to be subjected themselves to the study. At the time of reviewing the clinical history of each patient it is worthy to say that none is under heart disease treatment or antidepressant intake. The study population also declares not to suffer from any kind of pathology. Two women and one man ask for stopping the experiment. In addition, due to technical problems, data is not recorded from one man, so these patients are excluded from the results ($n = 21$, nine males, twelve females).

3.3 Finding Boundary Points on EDA

The EDA signals are acquired from the wearable at a sampling rate of 20 Hz and 12-bit resolution, as it was stated in Sect. 1. These specifications are chosen given the condition of the signals, in order not to alter their shape characteristics [20]. Given that we are interested in delineating the morphology of different events, the basal line will not be included in this study. Therefore, only the sudden skin response is considered because this signal gives the automatic response against stimuli. In this regard, EDA boundary points can be considered as those locations where the EDA response starts and it obtains its maximum amplitude, respectively.

However, EDA events can occur at the rise or decay of existing stimuli, being very difficult to determine if these responses correspond with a new stimulus or are part of previous events, thus difficult their proper delineation. Moreover, the lack of a gold standard in delineating accurately the onset and offset of EDA events, the challenge is even bigger in this task. In consequence, a developed and tested modified methodology is adopted in this study [21]. The associated algorithm has proved to be highly efficient in discriminating positive EDA stimuli [21]. In addition, given that timing of screened events are also labeled in this study, some rules associated with the duration of stimuli are designed with the purpose of decreasing the number of false positives.

Thus, considering the raw data from the wearable as $y[n]$, a new 1.5 Hz cutoff low-pass FIR filter is applied over this signal in order to decrease noise. The resulting filtered signal $\hat{y}[n]$ is calculated by means a discrete convolution as:

$$\hat{y}[n] = C_0 y[n] + C_1 y[n-1] + \ldots + C_N y[n-N] = \sum_{i=0}^{N} C_i y[n-i] \qquad (1)$$

and results of filtering can be observed in Fig. 3(a).

Next, in order to highlight the sudden changes in the signal slopes, the first derivative is calculated over $\hat{y}[n]$, such that:

$$\delta[n] = \hat{y}[n] - \hat{y}[n-1] \tag{2}$$

In this regard, the result of calculating the first derivative over the filtered signal on a random ageing person can be appreciated in Fig. 3(b). As it can be observed, an increase on the arousal level is represented as an increment of $\delta[n]$. Some kind of rule is needed in order to discriminate between positive and negative events. Considering that recorded responses can vary depending on each stimulus for each patient (in relation to his/her likes, dislikes, fears or event past experiences), a relationship between screened positive stimuli and positive responses can not be established. Consequently, an empiric methodology must be carried out to locate the positive stimuli. Thus, a threshold value equal to $0.003\,\mu S/sec$ is set as objective criterion. This threshold is calculated as a trade-off between the visually detected events and the screened positive stimuli. Thus, samples belonging to positive responses are computed as:

$$\eta[n] = \begin{cases} \delta[n] & \text{if } \delta[n] > threshold \\ 0 & \text{otherwise.} \end{cases} \tag{3}$$

Moreover, timing the screened stimuli is useful in order to decrease the number of false positives, since the duration of temporal window for each event is known. Thus, undesired double detections of the same stimulus are controlled. Bearing this in mind, a new filtering is implemented with a double purpose: on the one hand, to remove possible artifact which were not detected in the previous steps, and, on the other hand, to remove double detections of the same stimulus. Thus, events with a number of samples lower than $Fs/2$ are detected and removed from the list. Next, the last and first sample of two consecutive detected events are evaluated and the second event is unconsidered if the distance between them is lower than $Fs \times 5$, which corresponds with the total duration of a screened picture.

Finally, maximums for each event on the derivative signal $\delta[n]$ are computed. Around this peak, zero-crossings on both sides from maximum are estimated. The results are shown in Fig. 3(c). These points correspond to sudden slope changes in the original signals. Therefore, they could be used as the boundary points, so they are ported to filtered signal, $\hat{y}[n]$. In consequence, the sudden skin conductivity onset (SSC_{on}) and the sudden skin conductivity offset (SSC_{off}) are defined, as shown in Fig. 3(d).

Once the positive EDA events are detected and delineated, negative responses are also characterized by following the same methodology as described before. However, due to the fact that no changes are produced in the physiological signals when a patient shows no reaction against a stimulus, the strategy to detect these events is different. Thus, temporal windows, where negative stimuli are screened, are chosen as workspace. Then, $\delta[n]$, maximums and zero-crossings are determined over this temporal segment. In case no zero-crossings are detected at any side, boundary points are replaced by minimums in both sides.

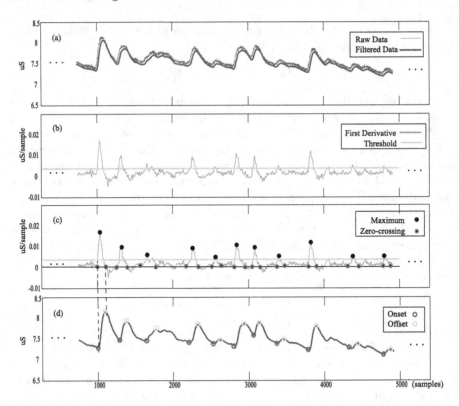

Fig. 3. Signal postprocessing. (a) Filtered signal. (b) First derivative over the filtered signal. (c) Maximums and zero-crossings on the derivative signal. (d) Sudden skin conductivity onsets and offsets.

As a result, $N = 228$ vectors of variable length, corresponding to each detected and delineated event, are computed. $N/2$ vectors correspond to positive stimuli and $N/2$ vectors to negative stimuli. Moreover, the first and the last sample for each event correspond to the onset and the offset of EDA events, respectively.

3.4   Feature Extraction

Once the EDA events are detected and delineated, different markers that might be of interest for emotion classification, are computed for each event. In this regard, Fig. 4 gives detailed information on the amplitude and time intervals that are going to be defined. Thus, for the ith detected event, skin conductivity duration (SSC_{dur}) and skin conductivity magnitude (SSC_{mag}) are defined as the distance and magnitude between its offset and onset, respectively, i.e.

$$SSC_{dur}^{(i)} = SSC_{off} - SSC_{on} \tag{4}$$

$$SSC_{mag}^{(i)} = \hat{y}(SSC_{off}) - \hat{y}(SSC_{on}). \tag{5}$$

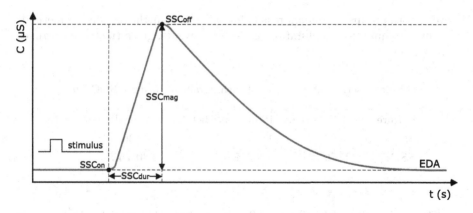

Fig. 4. EDA features extracted from a positive EDA event.

4   Results and Conclusions

Shapiro-Wilks tests have been applied. They prove that the all the studied EDA features are normal and homoscedastic. Therefore, results are expressed as mean ± standard deviation for all the events belonging to the same group. Thus, in Table 1 the statistical differences between the two groups are tested by using a one-way ANOVA test. Although the results show that both studied parameters, SSC_{dur} and SSC_{mag}, achieve a statistical significance ($\rho < 0.05$), SSC_{mag} shows a higher mean difference.

Table 1. Statistical significance between group A and group B.

Feature	Group A	Group B	ρ
SSC_{dur} (s)	1.3454 ± 1.1446	2.7615 ± 1.4295	$1.4059 * 10^{-14}$
SSC_{mag} (µS)	0.0149 ± 0.1575	0.3250 ± 0.4004	$8.8844 * 10^{-14}$

In addition, a receiver operating characteristic curve (ROC) was used in this study to assess the discriminatory power of each feature. In this regard, a ROC applies different thresholds, trying to classify correctly both groups. The true positive ratio (TP) and the false positive ratio (FP) are calculated in each iteration for each different threshold. The optimal thresholds for TP and FP are obtained when the process has completed. Table 2 shows the results for each studied parameter regarding the sensitivity, positive predictability and global accuracy. As it can be observed, SSC_{mag} reports a better discriminatory power than SSC_{dur}, achieving a global accuracy of 80.75 % in discriminating between people with low and high arousal levels, respectively. Unlike the amplitude events, the duration shows a low discriminatory power when distinguishing between both groups. The main reason for this result might rely on the methodology used to quantify the duration on negative events, given the low occurrence of EDA events.

Table 2. Discriminatory power of each parameter using a ROC curve.

Feature	Sensitivity	Positive predictability	Global accuracy
SSC_{dur} (s)	66.5 %	100 %	67.36 %
SSC_{mag} (μS)	76.19 %	91.55 %	**80.75 %**

Bearing in mind these results, we can conclude that a new hardware has been developed in order to carry out the continuous monitoring of arousal level on ageing adults. Through signal processing, two standard markers have been assessed for the sake of classifying the patients into two classes: calmed and stressed patients. The results show that through measuring the EDA events' magnitudes, the patients are classified with a global accuracy higher than 80 %.

Acknowledgements. This work was partially supported by Spanish Ministerio de Economía y Competitividad/FEDER under TIN2013-47074-C2-1-R grant.

References

1. Cortés, U., Urdiales, C., Annicchiarico, R.: Intelligent healthcare managing: an assistive technology approach. In: Sandoval, F., Prieto, A.G., Cabestany, J., Graña, M. (eds.) IWANN 2007. LNCS, vol. 4507, pp. 1045–1051. Springer, Heidelberg (2007)
2. Mowafey, S., Gardner, S.: A novel adaptive approach for home care ambient intelligent environments with an emotion-aware system. In: UKACC International Conference on Control, Cardiff, 3–5 September 2012, pp. 771–777 (2012)
3. Acampora, G., Cook, D.J., Rashidi, P., Vasilakos, A.V.: A survey on ambient intelligence in health care. Proc. IEEE 101(12), 2470–2494 (2013)
4. García-Rodríguez, C., Martínez-Tomás, R., Cuadra-Troncoso, J.M., Rincón, M., Fernández-Caballero, A.: A simulation tool for monitoring elderly who suffer from disorientation in a smart home. Expert Syst. Accepted (2015)
5. Sokolova, M.V., Fernández-Caballero, A., López, M.T., Martínez-Rodrigo, A., Zangróniz, R., Pastor, J.M.: A distributed architecture for multimodal emotion identification. In: Bajo, J., Hernández, J.Z., Mathieu, P., Campbell, A., Fernández-Caballero, A., Moreno, M.N., Julián, V., Alonso Betanzos, A., Jiménez-López, M.D., Botti, V. (eds.) Trends in Practical Applications of Agents, Multi-Agent Systems and Sustainability. AISC, vol. 372, pp. 125–132. Springer, Heidelberg (2015)
6. Sokolova, M.V., Fernández-Caballero, A., Ros, L., Latorre, J.M., Serrano, J.P.: Evaluation of color preference for emotion regulation. In: Vicente, J.M.F., Álvarez-Sánchez, J.R., de la Paz López, F., Toledo-Moreo, F.J., Adeli, H. (eds.) Artificial Computation in Biology and Medicine. LNCS, vol. 9107, pp. 479–487. Springer, Heidelberg (2015)

7. Sokolova, M.V., Fernández-Caballero, A.: A review on the role of color and light in affective computing. Appl. Sci. **5**(3), 275–293 (2015)
8. Fernández-Sotos, A., Fernández-Caballero, A., Latorre, J.M.: Elicitation of emotions through music: the influence of note value. In: Vicente, J.M.F., Álvarez-Sánchez, J.R., de la Paz López, F., Toledo-Moreo, F.J., Adeli, H. (eds.) Artificial Computation in Biology and Medicine. LNCS, vol. 9107, pp. 488–497. Springer, Heidelberg (2015)
9. World Health Organization. Ageing and Life Course (2011)
10. Hanson, M.A., Powell Jr, H.C., Barth, A.T., Ringgenberg, K., Calhoun, B.H., Aylor, J.H., Lach, J.: Body area sensors networks: challenges and opportunities. IEEE Comput. Soc. **42**(1), 58–65 (2009)
11. Fernández-Caballero, A., Latorre, J.M., Pastor, J.M., Fernández-Sotos, A.: Improvement of the elderly quality of life and care through smart emotion regulation. In: Pecchia, L., Chen, L.L., Nugent, C., Bravo, J. (eds.) IWAAL 2014. LNCS, vol. 8868, pp. 348–355. Springer, Heidelberg (2014)
12. Koelstra, S., Muhl, C., Soleymani, M., Lee, J.-S., Yazdani, A., Ebrahimi, T., Pun, T., Nijholt, A., Patras, I.: DEAP: a database for emotion analysis using physiological signals. IEEE Trans. Affect. Comput. **3**(1), 18–31 (2012)
13. Martínez-Rodrigo, A., Zangróniz, R., Pastor, J.M., Latorre, J.M., Fernández-Caballero, A.: Emotion detection in ageing adults from physiological sensors. In: Mohamed, A., Novais, P., Pereira, A., González, G.V., Fernández-Caballero, A. (eds.) Ambient Intelligence-Software and Applications, vol. 376, pp. 253–261. Springer, Switzerland (2015)
14. Healey, J.A., Picard, R.W.: Detecting stress during real-world driving tasks using physiological sensors. IEEE Trans. Intell. Transp. Syst. **6**(2), 156–166 (2005)
15. Veltman, J.A., Gaillard, A.W.K.: Physiological indicies of workload in a simulated flight task. Biol. Psychol. **42**, 323–342 (1996)
16. Nagamine, K., Nozawa, A., Ide, H.: Evaluation of emotions by nasal skin temperature on auditory stimulus and olfactory stimulus. IEE J. Trans. EIS **124**(9), 1914–1915 (2004)
17. Lidberg, L., Wallin, G.: Sympathhetic skin nerve discharges in relation to amplitude of skin resistance responses. Psychopysiology **18**(3), 268–270 (1981)
18. Venables, P.H., Christie, M.J.: Electrodermal activity. Techniques in Psychophysiology, pp. 3–67. Wiley, New York (2012)
19. Lang, P.J., Bradley, M.M., Cuthbert, B.N.: International affective picture system (IAPS): affective ratings of pictures and instruction manual. Technical report A-8, University of Florida, Gainesville (2008)
20. Martínez-Rodrigo, A., Alcaraz, R., Rieta, J.J.: Morphological variability of the P-wave for premature envision of paroxysmal atrial fibrillation events. Physiol. Meas. **35**, 1–14 (2014)
21. Healey, J.A.: Wearable and automotive system for affect recognition from physiology. Philosophical Dissertation, Massachusetts Institute of Technology (2000)

Stress Modelling Using Transfer Learning in Presence of Scarce Data

Pablo Hernandez-Leal[1](✉), Alban Maxhuni[2], L. Enrique Sucar[1],
Venet Osmani[2], Eduardo F. Morales[1], and Oscar Mayora[2]

[1] Instituto Nacional de Astrofísica, Óptica y Electrónica, Sta. María
Tonantzintla, Puebla, México
{pablohl,esucar,emorales}@ccc.inaoep.mx
[2] CREATE-NET, Via Alla Cascata 56/D Povo, Trento, Italy
{amaxhuni,vosmani,omayora}@create-net.org

Abstract. Stress at work is a significant occupational health concern
nowadays. Thus, researchers are looking to find comprehensive approaches
for improving wellness interventions relevant to stress. Recent studies have
been conducted for inferring stress in labour settings; they model stress
behaviour based on non-obtrusive data obtained from smartphones. However, if the data for a subject is scarce, a good model cannot be obtained.
We propose an approach based on transfer learning for building a model of
a subject with scarce data. It is based on the comparison of decision trees
to select the closest subject for knowledge transfer. We present an study
carried out on 30 employees within two organisations. The results show
that the in the case of identifying a "similar" subject, the classification
accuracy is improved via transfer learning.

Keywords: Stress modelling · Transfer learning · Semi-supervised
learning

1 Introduction

Over the last four decades there has been rising concern in many countries
about the growth and consequences of work-relevant stress and burnout. Recent
reports show that stress is ranked as a second most common work-related health
problem across the members of the European Union [1]; the same report shows
that individuals with high levels of stress were accompanied by physical and
psychosocial complaints and decreased work-control for the requirements placed
on them.

To date, current approaches to measuring stress rely on self-reported questionnaires [2], which can be a source of subjectivity. As such, the availability
of rich set of embedded sensors in smartphones is increasingly being used to
provide objective measures of behaviour phenomena.

The objective of this study was to model stress levels from different behavioural
variables obtained from smartphones when the labelled data for a person is scarce.

© Springer International Publishing Switzerland 2015
J. Bravo et al. (Eds.): AmIHEALTH 2015, LNCS 9456, pp. 224–236, 2015.
DOI: 10.1007/978-3-319-26508-7_22

Collected data includes information related to psychological self-assessments that are obtained from standardised validated questionnaire and the sensor data from smartphones from 30 employees in two different organisations. Our approach learns a model for each subject which is useful not only to predict but to perform comparisons among different subjects in order to obtain groups of people (clusters) that behave similarly. When a model is built for a new subject it usually contains insufficient information to have an accurate model. For this reason we use a transfer learning approach that uses data from the most similar user in order to improve the model which results in better accuracy.

We performed an experimental analysis using real data focused on predicting stress based on several smartphone sensors. The study includes 3 aspects: (i) using semi-supervised learning to complete the models for subjects with missing data, (ii) clustering the subjects based the similarity of the learned decision trees, (iii) applying transfer learning to try to improve the model of a new user with scarce data.

2   Related Work

Smartphones have already been used to detect mental health conditions, as shown in our previous work [3–6]. However, capturing what is causing an emotion change that is influenced from work-related stressors and detect the onset of stress can be quite challenging. Current methods have tried to infer stress based on physiological signals, e.g., heart-rate variability, blood pressure, body temperatures and respiration [7]. Furthermore, recent work emphasize the importance of measuring physiological signals that would help providing short-term feedback to the users in everyday activities [8]. However, these methods have as drawback that they need to be carried at all times (and in specific places in body) in order to allow accurate and continuous monitoring.

StressSense [9] proposes a method for detecting stress based on speech analysis and the variation of speech articulation. However, in real-life activities (e.g., crowded environments) this approach may lead to misinterpretation of speech and therefore of emotion.

In order to infer relation dynamics of people and behaviour changes in daily activities, smartphones have been suggested as a promising candidate to obtain user's context. Research using smartphones for long-term monitoring [10] have reported that smartphone sensing can be used to collect many types of contextual data including: physical activities, body postures and locations. In [11], the authors build a self-tracking system called MoodScope to help its users manage their mood. The system detects users mood from smartphones usage data (e-mail, call and SMS logs, application usage, web history and location changes). The authors reported their initial 66 % accuracy of 32 subjects from their daily mood and improving to 93 % after two months of training.

Another relevant work is from Bauer et al. [12] whose work aimed at recognizing stress from 7 students before and after the exam period. The assumption is that students are likely to be under stress during the exam sessions.

They acquired data from smartphones (location, social proximity through Bluetooth, phone calls and SMS logs) and they reported an average accuracy of 53 % during the exam session. In recent work, Bogomolov et al. [13] used call logs, SMS logs, proximity data, and self-reported surveys about personality traits. The authors reported detecting daily stress levels with a 72.28 % accuracy combining real life data from different sources. However, measuring stress in uncontrolled settings poses several difficulties since it requires the efforts of human annotators about their current perceived stress and other variables relevant to stress.

Building an accurate model to predict stress requires a considerable amount of labelled data. However, users tend no to answer the questionnaires all the time, and for a new user we will have few samples. Hence, to overcome these issues, in this study we use semi-supervised learning methods that use unlabelled instances and combine the information in the unlabelled data with the explicit classification information of labelled data for improving the classification performance [14]. Another related technique used to improving accuracy when available data is limited is transfer learning [15]. To the best of our knowledge, no study has applied semi-supervised nor transfer learning methods aiming at predicting work-related stress.

3   Data Acquisition

For this study, we collected data from 30 healthy employees[1] of two organisations located in the North-eastern part of Italy for a period of 8 weeks, further described in [3]. All subjects were given a smartphone[2] where the application used for this study collected data continuously as a background application. The features we extracted for each subject are categorised into two types, the first group of variables includes information of user's behaviour that was collected from the smartphone sensors during work hours, these are called *objective variables*. The second group contains *subjective* information obtained from the self-reported questionnaires, that includes mood and work-relevant stress items.

3.1   Self-reports

The self-reported questionnaire included scales that have demonstrated validity for inferring stress (the Oldenburg Burnout Inventory [16]). The survey was administrated via the smartphones and the data obtained from the participants was obtained three times a day: 9:00 am, 2:00 pm, and 5:00 pm, for a period of 8 weeks.[3]

---

[1] 16 male and 14 female; married (50 %) and not married (50 %); age ranged from 26–30(16.67 %), 31–40(60 %) and above 40(23.33 %); 33.33 % of participants had an academic degree, 36.7 % had bachelor degree and 30 % had high school education.

[2] Samsung Galaxy S3 mini 32 GB.

[3] The scales ranged from 1-to-5 and items selection has been performed considering the specificity of the Italian work-context in order to ensure their suitability.

Table 1. Overall number and percentage of Stress-responses

Variable	Level	Nr.Responses (%)	Nr.Subjects
Perceived stress	High	325 (22.18 %)	27
	Moderate	515 (35.15 %)	30
	Low	625 (42.66 %)	30
	Total responses:	1465 (100.00 %)	30

Table 2. Number of parameters and features extracted from smartphones

Category	Smartphone sensors	Attributes (Feature-Extracted)
1. Physical activity level	Accelerometer	- 3-Axis (Magnitude)
		- 3-Axis (Variance Sum [17])
2. Location	Cellular	- CellID and LACID (Number of clusters (DBSCAN) [18])
	WiFi	- Access Points (Number of clusters (DBSCAN) [18])
	Google-Maps	- Latitude and Longitude (Number of clusters (DBSCAN)[18], and distances [19])
3. Social interaction	Microphone	- Proximity interaction
		- Pitch [20], Mel-MBSES [21]
4. Social activeness	Phone calls	- Number of Incoming and Outgoing Calls
		- Duration of Incoming and Outgoing Calls
		- Most common Contact-Calls
	SMS	- Number of Incoming and Outgoing SMS
		- Duration of Incoming and Outgoing SMS
		- Most common Contact-SMS
	Calendars	- Number of Calendar-Events
	App usage	- Number of used applications (Social, System)
		- Duration of used applications (Social, System)

In Table 1, we present the overall stress responses for the whole period (8 weeks), where we include only the questionnaires obtained from (2:00 pm and 5:00 pm). The overall number of responses from both intervals was 1465. In order to simplify the measurements of the work-related stress, we have classified the stress-level into three classes: ≤ 2 as "Low-Stress", 3 as "Moderate-Stress", and ≥ 4 as "High-Stress". In Table 1 is shown that during the entire monitoring weeks, 27-subjects have perceived "High-Stress" and is about 22.18 % of the monitoring weeks.

3.2 Objective Data Acquisition and Features Extraction

In Table 2 we provide an overview of the types of smartphone data acquired for the study. In addition, we provide an overview of each category used in our study:

- **Physical Activity Level:** We measured the level of activity using accelerometer data capturing 3-axial linear acceleration continuously at a rate of 5 Hz, which was sufficient to infer physical activity levels. For extracting features, we used the method developed in the framework in [17] and we measured the magnitude and the variance sum of 26 seconds ($n = 128$-samples) from accelerometer readings. Each segment was classified into *"high"*, *"low"*, and *"none"* activity levels.
- **Location:** Location patterns and the location changes were measured using the list of WiFi access points (AP) available with their respective BSSID address, cell tower location and Google location information (latitude, longitude). We performed clustering for WiFi by means of the received signal strength (RSS) from each access point (AP). Density-based clustering (DBSCAN) [18] was used to obtain a number of different locations (clusters) in hourly basis. Similarly, DBSCAN was used to cluster Google location and cellular tower location.
- **Social Interaction:** We have used the microphone sensor embedded on smartphones in order to capture verbal interaction within the employees when they where involved in conversation in a close proximity. We have extracted two main audio features (Pitch [20] and Mel-MultiBand Spectral Entropy Signature (Mel-MBSES) [21]) to perform speech recognition. From the classifier, we obtain the values (true, false) and we measure the distribution of the interactivity in a daily basis.
- **Social Activeness:** We have included measurements from the phone usage (number and duration of phone calls, number and length of SMS messages) and the usage of two types of apps: system (Camera, Calendar, Web-browsing, Mail) and social (WhatsApp, Facebook, Skype) that were installed on the smartphones.

4   Learning and Comparison of Models

Predicting perceived stress of the user can be modelled as a classification problem. We used decision trees [22] to model subject's stress since this representation can be easily understood by a human, and this could help to have a better understanding of what causes stress. Also, using this representation we can compare the models for the different subjects, which is important for transfer learning. Our approach is to build a decision tree (can be seen as a model) to predict stress for each subject of the study. To learn decision trees we used the C4.5 algorithm using as attributes the objective variables presented in Sect. 3.2. The class to predict is the self-reported stress level (Sect. 3.1) (*Low, Mid, High*).

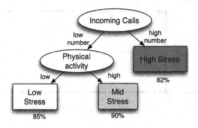

Fig. 1. Decision tree that classifies the level of Stress of one of the subjects in the study. Ovals represent decision nodes. Rectangles are leaves (terminal nodes) that give the classification value, in this case they represent low, mid or high level of stress.

In Fig. 1 we depict an example of a decision tree classifying the stress level of a subject.

Our first objective is to analyse how subjects are related to each other in terms of how similar are their models. To compare the trees, the dissimilarity measure presented in [23] is used. This measure combines the structure (the attributes of the nodes) and predictive (the predicted classes) similarities in a single value. The dissimilarity measure among two trees T_i and T_j is defined as:[4]

$$d(T_i, T_j) = \sum_{h=1}^{H} \alpha_h (1 - s_h) \frac{m_{h0}}{n} + \sum_{k=1}^{K} \alpha_k (1 - s_k) \frac{m_{0k}}{n} \qquad (1)$$

where the m_{xy} values measure the predictive similarity and the α_x and s_x values measure the structural similarity. This measure can be normalized to be in the range $[0\text{–}1]$, where 0 represents that the trees are very similar and 1 that they are totally dissimilar.

4.1 Initial Dataset

From the set of 30 subjects, we initially removed those that had a significant number of missing values (mainly in the questionnaires for self-evaluation of their stress level). Thus, having a remaining set of 18 subjects.

A decision tree was learned for each subject and using the distance in Eq. (1) we compared all pairs of models to obtain a similarity matrix. From that matrix we performed hierarchical clustering using the unweighted pair group method with arithmetic mean algorithm which yields the dendrogram depicted in Fig. 2, where a box with a colour indicates the average self-reported stress for that subject. From the figure we can observe 3 clusters with 7, 6 and 4 subjects. The largest cluster (with 7 subjects) roughly corresponds to subjects which reported low levels of stress in average (denoted by the blue boxes). The second major cluster (with 6 subjects) corresponds to subjects who reported a mid level of

---

[4] Let $1, \ldots, H$ as the leaves of T_i, and $1, \ldots, K$ as the leaves of T_j, m_{hk} is the number of instances which belong to both the hth leaf of T_i and to the kth leaf of T_j.

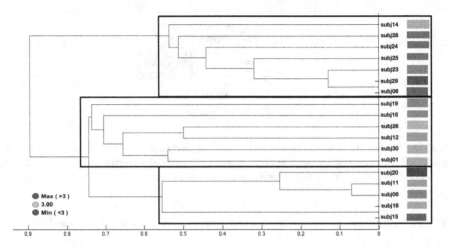

Fig. 2. Dendrogram obtained by computing similarities between models of each subject (using only 18 subjects). Three major clusters can be noted, colour boxes correspond to average stress for different subjects (Color figure online).

stress (grey boxes). The third cluster with only 4 subjects shows subjects with high and mid level of stress.

Since the initial data had a large portion of missing values (20.03 % of overall dataset), semi-supervised learning was used to fill those. In this study, we use a single classifier method called self-training [14] to classify the unlabelled data. These new data is added to the training set, the classifier is re-trained and the procedure repeated.

After applying the semi-supervised learning phase, there is enough data to compute comparisons with the 30 users of the study. A dendrogram of the similarity of all users is depicted in Fig. 3. In this case we can observe 4 main clusters. One cluster (bottom, 9 subjects) is formed by those subjects whose stress level was consistently the same for the entire study. Note, that in this case subjects were clustered by the rule of behaviour (always the same stress level) not by the prediction itself. Another cluster is formed by subjects that on average showed low and mid level of stress (6 subjects). A third cluster (with 4 subjects) contains subjects with high and mid levels of stress. The largest cluster is formed with 10 subjects which do not show a consistent level of stress.

4.2 Similarity Matrices

The process described in previous section was used to obtain a similarity matrix, depicted in Fig. 4(a), where the more similar a subject is to another the more darker that square is (subjects are ordered by clusters). Then we decided to remove 50 % of the data from all subjects (this will be useful for our transfer learning approach in the next section). The similarity matrix using this reduced

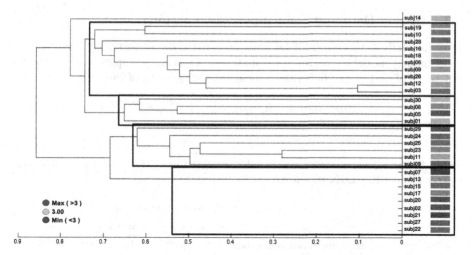

Fig. 3. Dendrogram obtained by computing similarities between models of each subject (for the 30 subjects) after using semi-supervised learning to fill missing data. Colour boxes correspond to average stress for each subject (Color figure online).

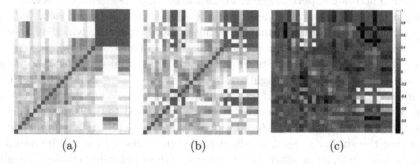

Fig. 4. Similarity matrices of 30 users using (a) all data (after semi-supervised learning) and (b) with 50 % of instances removed –darker cells indicate high similarity. (c) depicts the difference between (a) and (b); a white cell indicates a + difference, black a − negative difference, and grey no difference.

data is depicted Fig. 4(b), and in Fig. 4(c) we depict the matrix resulting from the difference of (a) and (b) where a grey value means no difference.

In summary, we have three similarity matrices with different quantity of data. For each matrix we computed the average values, the initial data with 18 subjects showed a more disperse set of distances with an average of 0.65 ± 0.18 (higher value, means subjects are more different to each other). After the semi-supervised algorithm was applied the average distance was 0.55 ± 0.16 even when number of subjects increased (30 subjects). Finally, when the data was reduced the average distance decreased to 0.49 ± 0.15, which may not happen in all cases (note that removed data was randomly selected).

4.3 Missing Data and Semi-supervised Learning

Now we analyse the effect of adding/removing data in terms of the comparisons among models, i.e. similarity matrices. Thus, we computed the absolute difference of each entry between an *original* and a *modified* matrix:

$$\Delta i, j(original, modified) = |e_{i,j}^{original} - e_{i,j}^{modified}| \tag{2}$$

Table 3. Percentage of entries whose value increased more than $\epsilon = 0.1, \ldots, 0.5$ from matrix *original* to matrix *modified*.

Data		$\Delta(Original, Modified) > \epsilon$				
Original	Modified	$\epsilon = 0.1$	$\epsilon = 0.2$	$\epsilon = 0.3$	$\epsilon = 0.4$	$\epsilon = 0.5$
Initial	Semi-supervised added data	0.39	0.22	0.14	0.07	0.05
Semi-supervised	Removed random 50 % data	0.55	0.29	0.19	0.13	0.11

Table 3 shows the percentage of entries where $\Delta_{i,j} > \epsilon$ with $\epsilon = 0.1, \ldots, 0.5$ between two matrices. After applying the semi-supervised approach, 39 % of the entries in the similarity matrix changed more than 0.1, which is a small change in similarity for a large portion of entries. In contrast only 5 % of entries changed more than 0.5. Results show that after the semi-supervised approach the similarity matrices were slightly altered with an average value of 0.12 ± 0.14, meaning there were no drastic changes in similarities. When we reduced the data by 50 % the difference between matrices increased to 0.19 ± 0.20 which is expected since the data was reduced significantly. These results are important to show that the similarity used is robust to missing values. This will be useful in the next section since we start with the reduced data but using transfer learning we can improve their accuracy.

5 Transfer Learning

Our approach assumes a set of previously learned models along with their respective data. Then, a new subject appears; however, its associated data is scarce which results in having a model with poor predictive accuracy. Information from the other subjects could be useful to improve the model. First we learn a model t_i for the new subject i and compare with the rest T using Eq. 1. The model $k = argmin_{t_j \in T} d(t_i, t_j)$ which is the most similar to t_i is selected and its data is transferred to i. A new model is learned using the original and the transferred data.

We applied the described approach on the data which has a percentage of data removed. The average distance to the nearest subject is 0.28 and there are 18 subjects that have only one nearest subject. These subjects were selected for the proposed transfer learning approach.

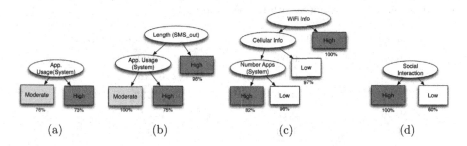

Fig. 5. Learned models of different subjects: *Subj*30 (a) and its most similar *Subj*17 (b). *Subj*29 (c) and its most similar model *Subj*05 (d).

Table 4. Classification accuracy, Δ transfer shows the difference between no transfer and transfer columns. All data shows the accuracy using all original data (upper bound). The number of initial and transferred instances is shown. The top part of the table shows the results when the distance to the closest subject is small (<0.37), while the bottom when it is large (>0.37).

Subject	No transfer	Transfer	All data	Δ Transfer	Initial I	Transf. I	$d(nearest)$
*Subj*28	57.35	63.23	77.94	5.88	35	26	0.18
*Subj*10	44.89	51.02	71.42	6.13	26	31	0.27
*Subj*12	55.93	54.23	62.71	−1.69	18	31	0.32
*Subj*18	70.27	62.16	75.67	−8.10	31	18	0.32
*Subj*24	67.14	67.14	71.42	0.00	36	31	0.36
*Subj*05	70.68	65.51	86.20	−5.17	29	37	0.36
*Subj*30	42.85	53.57	78.57	10.71	37	29	0.36
*Subj*09	57.69	73.07	76.92	15.38	18	35	0.36
Average	58.35	**61.24**	75.10	2.89	28.75	29.75	0.31
*Subj*25	85.71	83.67	89.79	−2.04	24	31	0.39
*Subj*04	81.25	71.88	84.37	−9.38	32	31	0.42
*Subj*08	57.41	50.00	55.55	−7.41	27	35	0.46
*Subj*16	61.11	62.96	74.07	1.85	30	29	0.48
*Subj*14	51.56	48.44	82.81	−3.13	32	31	0.49
*Subj*23	53.33	50.00	58.33	−3.33	32	35	0.53
*Subj*19	60.00	53.33	90.00	−6.67	33	26	0.54
*Subj*01	72.86	61.43	78.57	−11.43	41	32	0.58
*Subj*29	62.07	44.83	79.31	−17.24	29	33	0.60
*Subj*11	65.45	74.55	72.72	9.09	30	29	0.62
Average	**65.08**	60.11	76.55	−4.97	31	31.2	0.51

Table 5. Classification accuracies with different threshold for applying transfer learning and percentage of instances with transfer approach.

Transfer threshold	% Transferred instances	Average accuracy
0.00	0.00	62.09
0.30	0.11	62.76
0.37	0.44	**63.37**
0.50	0.72	62.26
1.00	1.00	60.61

We compare the results using the reduced data with and without the transfer learning approach to classify the same data. Accuracy is obtained by learning a classifier using either: the reduced data or the reduced plus transferred data, then testing that model on the data without removed instances. The results showed that using transfer did not improve the accuracy for all subjects. This happens because there is information we are ignoring of when transfer will be more useful: the distance to the nearest subject. The idea is to use transfer when the distance is small (when the model is close to another) and not when distance increases. For example, in Fig. 5(a) and (b) we depict trees that of subjects 30 and 17 which have a $d = 0.36$. In this case trees are similar in their decision nodes. In contrast we show models of subjects 29 and 5 (in Fig. 5(c) and (d)) which have $d = 0.60$, here these trees show different decision nodes.

Using transfer only when distance was less than a *transfer threshold* (in this case < 0.37) improves the accuracy from 58.35 to 61.24 (Table 4), in contrast when $d \geq 0.37$ is better not use transfer learning since the models are far from each other and this causes a negative transfer. We performed experiments varying the threshold with values $0.0, 0.3, 0.37, 0.5, 1.0$, average accuracy for all subjects is shown in Table 5. From the results we can see that the trivial approaches of not using transfer or using transfer on all subjects do not obtain the best results. However, selecting the appropriate threshold of transfer increases the accuracy.

Finally, we also performed experiments removing only 20 % of the data and repeated the transfer learning process. However, the transfer learning approach did not improve the accuracy. Preliminary analysis show that transferring all the data from the closest user is not always the best choice, a selection of the data must be applied and we leave that as future work.

6   Conclusion

Using smartphones to predict the affective state of a person, such as stress, requires a considerable amount of data to build a user-specific model. However, having enough labelled data is difficult. In this paper we have proposed an approach that combines semi-supervised and transfer learning to deal with this issue. An experimental evaluation was conducted with 30 subjects to predict stress at work. The results show that transfer from similar subjects can improve the classification accuracy, but using transfer from dissimilar persons could be detrimental. Future research ideas are to select instances of data to transfer from several similar models.

Acknowledgements. The work on this paper was partially funded by EC Marie Curie IRSES Project UBIHEALTH - 316337.

References

1. Agence européenne pour la sécurité et la santé au travail, Malgorzata Milczarek, Eusebio Rial-González, and Elke Schneider. Occupational safety and health in figures: stress at work-facts and figures. Office for Official Publications of the European Communities (2009)
2. Näätänen, P., Kiuru, V.: Bergen burnout indicator 15. Edita (2003)
3. Ceja, E., Osmani, V., Mayora, O.: Automatic stress detection in working environments from smartphones' accelerometer data: a first step. IEEE J. Biomed. Health Inform. PP(99), 1 (2015)
4. Osmani, V.: Smartphones in mental health: detecting depressive and manic episodes. IEEE Pervasive Comput. **14**(3), 10–13 (2015)
5. Ferdous, R., Osmani, V., Mayora, O.: Smartphone app usage as a predictor of perceived stress levels at workplace. IEEE **8**, 20–23 (2015)
6. Grunerbl, A., Muaremi, A., Osmani, V., Bahle, G., Ohler, S., Troster, G., Mayora, O., Haring, C., Lukowicz, P.: Smartphone-based recognition of states and state changes in bipolar disorder patients. IEEE J. Biomed. Health Inf. **19**(1), 140–148 (2015)
7. Bakker, J., Pechenizkiy, M., Sidorova, N.: What's your current stress level? detection of stress patterns from gsr sensor data. In: 2011 IEEE 11th International Conference on Data Mining Workshops, pp. 573–580. IEEE (2011)
8. Liu, K.K-L.: A personal, mobile system for understanding stress and interruptions. Master's thesis, MIT Media Arts and Science (2004)
9. Lu, H., Frauendorfer, D., Rabbi, M., Mast, M.S., Chittaranjan, G.T., Campbell, A.T., Gatica-Perez, D., Choudhury, T.: Stresssense: detecting stress in unconstrained acoustic environments using smartphones. In: Proceedings of the 2012 ACM Conference on Ubiquitous Computing, pp. 351–360 (2012)
10. Kocielnik, R., Sidorova, N., Maggi, F.M., Ouwerkerk, M., Westerink, J.H.D.M.: Smart technologies for long-term stress monitoring at work. In: 2013 IEEE 26th International Symposium on Computer-Based Medical Systems, pp. 53–58 (2013)
11. Likamwa, R., Liu, Y., Lane, N.D., Zhong, L.: Moodscope: building a mood sensor from smartphone usage patterns. In Proceeding of the 11th Annual International Conference on Mobile Systems, Applications, and Services, pp. 389–402 (2013)
12. Bauer, G., Lukowicz, P.: Can smartphones detect stress-related changes in the behaviour of individuals? In: 2012 IEEE International Conference on Pervasive Computing and Communications Workshops (PERCOM Workshops), pp. 423–426 (2012)
13. Bogomolov, A., Lepri, B., Ferron, M., Pianesi, F., Pentland, A.S.: Daily stress recognition from mobile phone data, weather conditions and individual traits. In: Proceedings of the ACM International Conference on Multimedia, pp. 477–486 (2014)

14. Zhu, X.: Semi-supervised learning. In: Sammut, C., Webb, G.I. (eds.) Encyclopedia of Machine Learning, pp. 892–897. Springer, Heidelberg (2010)
15. Pan, S.J., Yang, Q.: A survey on transfer learning. IEEE Trans. Knowl. Data Eng. **22**(10), 1345–1359 (2010)
16. Demerouti, E., Bakker, A.B.: The oldenburg burnout inventory: a good alternative to measure burnout and engagement. Handbook of stress and burnout in health care. Hauppauge, NY: Nova Science (2008)
17. FUNF - Open Sensing Framework (2014). http://funf.org/about.html
18. Birant, D., Kut, A.: St-dbscan: an algorithm for clustering spatial-temporal data. Data Knowl. Eng. **60**(1), 208–221 (2007)
19. Robusto, C.C.: The cosine-haversine formula. Am. Math. Mon. **64**(1), 38–40 (1957)
20. Hedelin, P., Huber, D.: Pitch period determination of aperiodic speech signals. In: 1990 International Conference on Acoustics, Speech, and Signal Processing, 1990, ICASSP-90, pp. 361–364. IEEE (1990)
21. Harris, F.J.: On the use of windows for harmonic analysis with the discrete fourier transform. Proc. IEEE **66**(1), 51–83 (1978)
22. Quinlan, J.R.: C4.5 Programs for Machine Learning. Morgan Kaufmann, San Mateo (1993)
23. Miglio, R., Soffritti, G.: The comparison between classification trees through proximity measures. Comput. Stat. Data Anal. **45**(3), 577–593 (2004)

Improving Social Communication Disorders Through Human-Avatar Interaction

Esperanza Johnson[1], Ramón Hervás[1(✉)], Tania Mondéjar[2],
José Bravo[1], and Sergio F. Ochoa[3]

[1] MAmI Research Lab, University of Castilla-la Mancha,
Paseo de la Universidad 4, Ciudad Real, Spain
MEsperanza.Johnson@alu.uclm.es,
{ramon.hlucas,jose.bravo}@uclm.es
http://mami.uclm.es
[2] eSmile, Psychology for Children and Adolescents,
Calle Toledo 79 1ºE, Ciudad Real, Spain
Tania.mondejar@esmile.es
[3] Computer Science Department, Universidad de Chile,
Av. Blanco Encalada 2120, 3rd Floor, Santiago, Chile
sochoa@dcc.uchile.cl

Abstract. Current assistive technologies can improve the quality of life of people who have been diagnosed with different forms of Social Communications Disorders (SCD). In this paper we describe the way in which we have approached an assistive system for improving SCD, based on human-avatar interaction. Since the final development is in progress, this paper contributes with a general taxonomy that classifies the different kinds of interaction between humans and avatars, including the relationship among them and their communication skills. These skills are typically training to treat SCD.

Keywords: Affective computing · Social communication disorder · Cognitive disabilities · Android · Human-avatar interaction

1 Introduction

The proposed project comes from a growing interest from the scientific community to help people with cognitive developmental problems (e.g., autism spectrum disorder, and attention deficit disorder). These disorders typically encompass problems with social interaction, social understanding and pragmatics (i.e., using language in proper context). Assistive systems come in the shape of those affected living more independent lives, with a lesser degree of difficulties and issues. In short, improve their quality of life in whatever way we can. In this particular case, we aim to improve it in terms of communication (social interaction) with other individuals, as well as a better understanding of themselves (introspection).

This paper proposes an application for tablets-pc that will have an interactive avatar, by which the user's action will generate a reaction from the avatar, and such a reaction will generate another reaction from the user, occurring a Human-Avatar communication. The avatar will draw the social interaction and communication with a

J. Bravo et al. (Eds.): AmIHEALTH 2015, LNCS 9456, pp. 237–243, 2015.
DOI: 10.1007/978-3-319-26508-7_23

narrative role-playing game, in which the user is immersed in the different situations. With this, the system helps the usersto know how to behave in certain situations and what emotions will occur.

2 Related Work

Concerning this research topic, we have found information mainly related to applications that act as assistive systems, as well as various focused on the design of avatars. The literature reports many assistive systems, such as smart homes that could help older adults with the ADL (Activities of Daily Living), following the performance on each activity [1, 2]; augmented reality-based systems to give guidance to people with dementia based on well-known points of interest [3]; an eye tracker system for people with severe motor disability to interact with an avatar [4]; and training systems that assist older people with mental and physical damages through the use of an avatar in their televisions [5].

In terms of avatar based interaction, there have been several interesting proposals that we have looked into, including those centered on human-avatar interaction in a simulation game, and quantifying how engaged the played is [6] and user interfaces based on 3D avatars for interactive television, and how the user interacts and reacts to it [7]. There is also a proposal of AI Framework for the supporting behavioral animation of avatars, to make them behave more realistically [8], as well as research works that discuss children's avatar preferences [9], which has been key for the idea behind the avatar creation of this paper.

3 Human-Avatar Interaction

This section will cover the aspect of human-avatar interaction. We discuss the different kinds of interaction that a person can have with an avatar, classifying them in different categories. Each kind of interaction can be useful to treat different communicative and cognitive skills. Since our primary users are children with SCD, the human-avatar communication helps to improve both verbal and non-verbal social communication skills. Particularly, these skills include responding to others, using gestures (waving or pointing), talking about emotions and feelings, taking turns when talking, staying on a topic, adjust speech to fit different contexts, etc. These skills depend on particular cognitive processes related to communication.

In this paper we have taken into account seven cognitive processes to work with those communication skills. Firstly, *joint attention (J)* is the shared focus of two individuals on a same point or look to the other in the eyes; *focused attention (F)* is the cognitive process of selectively concentrating on a discrete aspect of the communication; *emotional states (E)* are the feeling that we are seeming during the communication, *intonation (I)*, i.e., variations of spoken pitch that indicates the attitudes of the speaker; *self-control (S)*, the ability to control one behavior and desires in communication demands; *proprioception (P)*, the sense of body position (e.g., hands, arms, face) related to body-language; and, *understanding (U)*, as the general comprehension of matters in the conversation.

This taxonomy has been subdivided into implicit and explicit interactions (Table 1). This comes from careful thinking and a realization that some of the interactions that have been planned are involuntary, meaning that the gathered information and data from the user does not come explicitly in some cases, which will be exemplified shortly. From there, we have identified in the most basic human information processing: the human senses.

In terms of explicit interactions, we also refer to them as voluntary interactions, as the interactions are done by the user with full intention and knowledge to do so. Because of this way to understand explicit interactions, we have classified the following interactions as explicit: Ocular, Gestural (Facial and Body-language), Verbal, Tactile, Object and Audio Interaction.

The previous interactions show the different senses involved in such a process. In particular, ocular interaction refers to eye interaction from the user, and a clear example would be eye-tracking applications in which the user is asked to follow or fix their gaze on something on a screen. Facial Interaction would be the user moving their facial muscles to form expressions, Verbal Interaction is the action of speaking, Tactile Interaction refers to the user interaction with their hand and anything they can touch, whether it be a tactile screen, Body Interaction refers to the user moving their bodies in whichever way it would be needed, Object Interaction refers to the interaction between or with an object, and finally, Audio Interaction that is used frequently in studies that involve any reaction to audio stimulation.

The interactions we have categorized as implicit are: Ocular, Gestural (Facial and Body), Smell, and Biofeedback Interaction. The reason we have included Ocular, Facial and Body Interaction in this section, as well as the previous one, is because there are a variety of articles that study the involuntary aspects of those actions, such as the unintentional wander of the eyes to detect the degree of attention [10], as well as facial and body tics that are not a voluntary action from the user.

Then the Smell Interaction is what would be one-sided reception senses that play an important part in the interaction, but it is rarely available to output any data.

Biofeedback Interaction requires the use of peripherals and more advanced technology. It is possible to gather different vital signal to improve human-avatar inter-actions, such as blood pressure, heart rate, and brain activity. We deepen on the last one in this paper because neurological reactions to certain interactions are commonly used to observe the nature of said reaction on a deeper level. This is an obvious aspect that humans cannot control. Table 1 presents visually all the previous

Table 1. Taxonomy of the different types of interaction.

	Interaction		Involved technology	Cognitive processes
Explicit interaction (Bidirectional)	Ocular		Camera	J, F, S
	Gesture	Facial	Camera, Motion Capture Sensors	E, P, S
		Body	Camera, Movement Sensors	E, P, S

(Continued)

Table 1. (*Continued*)

	Interaction		Involved technology	Cognitive processes
	Verbal		Microphone	E, I, U
	Tactile		Tactile Sensors, Accelerometer	J, S, U
	Object		Sensors, Mobile devices	J, S, U
	Audio		Speakers, Headphones	E, S
Implicit interaction (Human to Avatar)	Ocular		Camera	F
	Gesture	Facial	Camera, Motion Capture Sensors	E, S
		Body	Camera, Movement Sensors	E, S
	Biofeedback Interaction		Headset, Vital Sign devices	E, S

information and includes the communicative and cognitive skills that can be treat with each kind of interaction.

4   Proposal for Cognitive Stimulation Through Avatars

The current project proposes an interactive avatar that will create the previously mentioned human-avatar interaction using available technology. The primary technology that will be used is a tablet-pc (Android), as our initial target audiences were children, and they are very much at ease with this technology. This is because it is a fairly extended and used device nowadays; it can be acquired without investing too much money, and has many of the elements that were mentioned in Table 1 that would be needed to create the interaction.

First design decision, based on the importance of the empathy of children that it is related to the avatar gender [9], was the creation of an androgynous avatar, so that the children themselves would decide the gender of the avatar that they are interacting with, as to draw a more positive response with such an avatar. The initial draft of the avatar is shown in Fig. 1.

Figure 1 also shows the interactions that the avatar supports, indicated by arrows that point both ways, representing bilateral communication between the human and the avatar. Particularly, voice-based communication, video and audio-based interaction refer to the Audio, Verbal, Ocular and Facial interactions that were explained in Sect. 3. Gamification and serious games refer to the narrative role playing games that the avatar will play with the human, though in this case it is unilateral as it is something that the avatar sends to the human, and any communication during the game falls within the bilateral interaction that was previously mentioned. Natural multi-interaction comes from the human, and it is specified as natural because the human reactions are not programmed, such as the avatar's interactions.

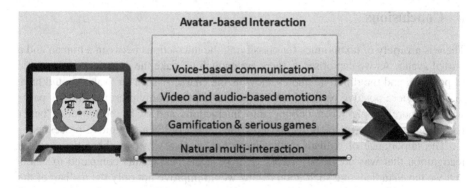

Fig. 1. Avatar-based interactions included in the system and draft of the avatar.

The interactions is implemented in a tablet-pc, and therefore the technology used will be mostly with the sensors that are available, which are a camera for Ocular and Facial Interaction, Microphone for the Verbal Interaction and Headphones/Speakers for the Audio Interaction. The Tactile Interaction is both with the accelerometer that most tablets have in place, as well as the tactile screen.

In order to maximize the *Human-Avatar Interaction*, we are including an aspect of emotion recognition, as to garner a more precise reaction from the avatar to the facial expressions of the user. This will be accomplished using Active Shape Models and Support Vector Machines that has been proven to yield good results [11], and recognizes the six basic emotions (happiness, sadness, anger, fear, disgust and surprise, as well as a neutral) that will be present during the interaction.

5 Future Development

Next step is the development of Avatar-based videogames with the mentioned interactions. The games would be narrative role playing games, by which the user would be put in a certain situation (role playing aspect of the game) and there it would advance throughout the story (narrative aspect of the game). The user would be put in day-to-day situations, so that when the time comes, they will be more used to the idea of those situations, as well as have a better set of skills to face said situation, both in general communication terms, as well as social. The interactions in these games will be mostly explicit interactions with the avatar, in terms of Ocular, Facial, Verbal, Tactile and Object, and we will also have implicit interactions with Biofeedback, using the *Emotiv Epoc* neuroheadset, which will be used in controlled environments to verify that we are gathering the results that we are expecting of this project. The user will interact with the avatar, simulating these situations, and s/he may also be asked to interact with certain objects in a room, for some of those situations.

The intention set for the future of this project is to make it as interactive as possible. It would be desirable to interact with other objects that the user would interact with (objects with NFC tags or other sensors) to maximize the options to use in the narrative role playing game mentioned in the introduction.

6 Conclusions

There is a variety of taxonomies for classifying the interactions between a human and a virtual avatar. As we can observe, there are enough to make the experience as realistic as possible, and the different studies show us the characteristics an avatar should have to draw a more positive response. We hope that the taxonomy presented in this paper will aid more people when delving into interactions and SCD, both with a better understanding of the interactions and how they affect different cognitive processes.

The importance of realism in the interaction is also why we chose the emotion recognition that was previously stated, as it gave the best results compared to others that we have studied, and such good results would improve not only the realism of the interaction between human and avatar, but also the possibilities of an improved social skill learning with a more accurate emotional reaction from the avatar for certain situations, and a better representation of said emotional state.

Acknowledgments. This work was conducted in the context of UBIHEALTH project under International Research Staff Exchange Schema (MC-IRSES 316337).

References

1. Fontecha, J., Hervás, R., Mondéjar, T., González, I., Bravo, J. Towards context-aware and user-centered analysis in assistive environments. J. Med. Syst. **39**(120) (2015)
2. Serna, A., Pigot, H., Rialle, V.: Modeling the progression of Alzheimer's disease for cognitive assistance in smart homes. User Model. User-Adap. Inter. **17**(4), 415–438 (2007)
3. Hervas, R., Fontecha, J., Bravo, J.: An assistive navigation system based on augmented reality and context awareness for people with mild cognitive impairments. IEEE J. Biomed. Health Inform. **18**(1), 368–374 (2013)
4. Adjouadi, M., Sesin, A., Ayala, M., Cabrerizo, M.: Remote eye gaze tracking system as a computer interface for persons with severe motor disability. In: Miesenberger, K., Klaus, J., Zagler, W.L., Burger, D. (eds.) ICCHP 2004. LNCS, vol. 3118, pp. 761–769. Springer, Heidelberg (2004)
5. Plischke, H., Kohls, N.: Keep it simple! Assisting older people with mental and physical training. In: Stephanidis, C. (ed.) Part I, HCII. LNCS, vol. 5614, pp. 278–287. Springer, Heidelberg, Berlin (2009)
6. Norris, A.E., Weger, H., Bullinger, C., Bowers, A.: Quantifying engagement: measuring player involvement in human–avatar interactions. Comput. Hum. Behav. **34**, 1–11 (2014)
7. Ugarte, A., García, I., Ortiz, A., Oyarzun, D.: User interfaces based on 3D avatars for interactive television. In: Cesar, P., Chorianopoulos, K., Jensen, J.F. (eds.) EuroITV 2007. LNCS, vol. 4471, pp. 107–115. Springer, Heidelberg (2007)
8. Iglesias, A., Luengo, F., Ortiz, A., Oyarzun, D.: AI framework for decision modeling in behavioral animation of virtual avatars. In: Shi, Y., van Albada, G.D., Dongarra, J., Sloot, P. M.A. (eds.) ICCS 2007. LNCS, vol. 4488, pp. 89–96. Springer, Heidelberg, Berlin (2007)
9. Inal, Y., Sancar, H., Cagiltay, K.: Children's avatar preferences and their personalities. In: Society for Information Technology and Teacher Education International Conference, pp. 4259–4266. Florida, USA (2006)

10. Galgani, F., Sun, Y., Lanzi, P.L., Leigh, J.: Automatic analysis of eye tracking data for medical diagnosis. In: IEEE Symposium on Computational Intelligence and Data Mining, CIDM 2009, pp. 195–202. IEEE, March 2009

11. Lozano-Monasor, E., López, M.T., Fernández-Caballero, A., Vigo-Bustos, F.: Facial expression recognition from webcam based on active shape models and support vector machines. In: Pecchia, L., Chen, L.L., Nugent, C., Bravo, J. (eds.) IWAAL 2014. LNCS, vol. 8868, pp. 147–154. Springer, Heidelberg (2014)

Applications and Case Studies of AmIHealth Environments

A Methodology for the Creation
of Integrated Service Networks
in Outpatient Internal Medicine

Miguel Angel Ortiz Barrios[1(✉)], Juan Escorcia Caballero[2],
and Fabián Sánchez Sánchez[2]

[1] Department of Industrial Engineering,
Universidad de la Costa CUC, Barranquilla, Colombia
mortizl@cuc.edu.co
[2] Department of Industrial Engineering,
Universidad Autónoma del Caribe, Barranquilla, Colombia
escajuan@alumni.uv.es, fsanchez@uac.edu.co

Abstract. Extended patient waiting times for medical care in outpatient internal medicine has a direct impact on patient dissatisfaction. This issue has become increasingly relevant in Colombia where patient waiting times tend to be longer. In this context, a methodology based on value stream mapping (VSM) and collaborative sceneries has been created to examine different improving alternatives focused on the design of integrated service networks in outpatient internal medicine with the participation of two hospitals with mixed-patient type environment. First, an individual diagnosis for each hospital is made through VSM to identify non-value activities in the value chain and design improvement strategies for each process. Second, a strategic platform of the network is set. Third, communication and service protocols of the network are defined. Then, a simulation model is designed and validated to conduct experiments on the structure of the network. Finally, payment and risk tables are determined and key performance indexes of the network are established. The results prove the validity of the proposed approach upon reducing 75 % of the lead time in this process creating a positive impact on population's health under satisfactory and equitable financial benefits for the participant hospitals.

Keywords: Integrated service networks · Value stream mapping · Collaborative sceneries · Outpatient internal medicine · Healthcare

1 Introduction

Currently, the challenges for improving healthcare organizations are stronger than ever. Issues like population growing, medical errors, process inefficiencies and extended lead times describe the existing state of these kinds of companies. With the increasing demand for improved healthcare, healthcare providers must consider providing more agile and quality services under constraint resources. This is related to the fact of offering more effective services under complicated circumstances. In this point, healthcare managers and decision makers are required to balance their processes with

© Springer International Publishing Switzerland 2015
J. Bravo et al. (Eds.): AmIHEALTH 2015, LNCS 9456, pp. 247–257, 2015.
DOI: 10.1007/978-3-319-26508-7_24

the needs of the patients. If this is not done, this could result in the appearance of a new disease and possible admissions to more complex and high-cost services if it was not previously necessary. Services in outpatient internal medicine are not the exception; long waiting times for a consultation are common bringing about dissatisfaction on patients and an increased probability of more serious effects in health. Specifically, in Colombia, lead time for outpatient service in Internal Medicine tend to be greater with a growing ratio of 0.58 days/appointment being highlighted as one of the specialties with need of primary intervention even though when the number of available offered appointments is insufficient [1]. Therefore, this study aims to develop a novel approach based on Value Stream Mapping (VSM) and collaborative sceneries to design integrated service networks that reunites hospitals to work in an efficient, effective and collaborative way so that patients who require outpatient internal medicine attention can be examined faster and hospitals can obtain collateral and satisfactory financial benefits under payment and risk agreements between the parties [2–4]. For this purpose, a case study of two hospitals with mixed-patient type environment has been explored as a first step to prove the validity of the proposed framework.

This paper is organized as follows: Sect. 2 briefly revises some actions that have been developed to create these kinds of structures and their implications. Section 3 presents the proposed methodology for the design of effective and integrated healthcare networks. Section 4 provides the results of using this methodology in a study case. Finally, conclusions about this research work and suggestions for further research are made in Sect. 5.

2   A Recent Literature Review

The collaborative practice makes part of improvement strategies in healthcare logistics and reflects the participation of several organizations that reunites their systems so that patient can perceive a higher quality level and agility in the service requested. Integrated healthcare systems are widely considered to provide a superior performance in terms of quality and safe, as a result of an effective communication and standardized protocols, although these results have not been extensively demonstrated [6]. In this sense, some authors have worked on the design of different collaborative models that allows creating multilateral benefits for both healthcare providers and patients. Taddei et al. [7] proposed the design of collaborative sceneries for the development of medical decisions in the diagnosis and care of congenital malformations through a teleconsultation network via internet that was used by several hospital centres in countries as Bosnia-Herzegovina, Croatia and Albany. On the other hand, Avery et al. [5] identified 5 key aspects for the effective collaboration between medical centres specialized in maternal care. They are: Impetus for the new collaboration, basic findings of collaborative care, commitment for a successful link, integration of care service and the formation of healthcare professionals in practical interprofessional environment. Grafton et al. [8] described the performance of three networks of hospitals with the public sector reforms. It was observed that the actors of the collaborative model deferred in their potential for generating efficiency and legitimist collaborative revenues, their commitment to the institutional principles and their wish of collaborating under the influence of eternal events. Campbell et al. [9] described the need of creating a collaborative care model in Canadian healthcare systems and exposed the results of an application developed in three units of Toronto East General Hospital in the improvement of patient safety, patient satisfaction and the use of resources. Upon analysing all these contributions, it is observed that a methodology for the creation of integrated service networks in outpatient internal medicine is needed since authors have not developed step-by-step approaches that guide practitioners to implement these kinds of strategies, reason by which the primary contribution of this paper will focus on the development of the required approach.

3   Methodology

3.1   Ethical Considerations

Before beginning this research, the project methodology was presented and discussed with the chief executive and the ethical committee of each hospital in study. As this study was supported in an interview with the stuff from the hospital, no formal approval by the committee was necessary. However, it was required to establish a confidentiality agreement with respect to the information handling.

The proposed methodology for the design of integrated healthcare services in outpatient internal medicine involves 7 steps (Fig. 1):

- Step 1 - *Individual diagnosis of outpatient service in Internal Medicine for each hospital*: In this stage, the current status of the process in outpatient service-Internal Medicine is described in each hospital with the purpose of establishing intervention points and design improvement strategies to prepare organizations in the efficient establishment of the integrated service network.
- Step 2 - *Establishment of the goals for the service network:* In this section, strategic objectives are defined with the purpose of accomplishing with Law # 1438 of 2011 issued by the Ministry of Social Protection where integrated Healthcare networks are legitimized besides the individual goals of the participant organizations. The law's primary aim is to strengthen the Colombian Healthcare System so that health improvement and healthy environment are achieved through quality, patient- centred and equitable services.
- Step 3 - *Definition of communication lines and service protocols:* In this phase, communication lines are defined; through them, hospitals will be interacting to each other at the moment of remitting patients. In this stage, procedures, responsible team and equipment will support the collaboration. Besides, service protocols are established according to the Law # 1438 of 2011, risk management procedures and epidemiological surveillance.
- Step 4 - *Efficient design of the service network and resource optimization:* Through the creation of a simulation model in software Arena 15.0, the integrated network of services in outpatient internal medicine is designed between the hospitals with the aim of determining future sceneries in terms of doctors required, average lead times and evaluation of caring policies.

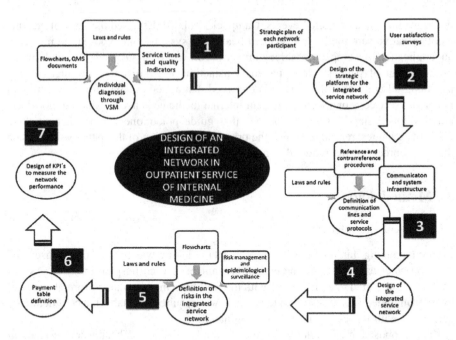

Fig. 1. Methodology for the design of an integrated service network in outpatient internal medicine (More details are explained below)

- Step 5 - *Definition of risks for the service network:* In this phase, financial, pathological and other risks are identified.
- Step 6 - *Definition of payment table in service network:* Through the use of the collateral payment model, utility distribution is defined for each hospital and possible collaboration sceneries are evaluated with the respective payment. For this purpose, a payment table is defined for possible sceneries in the integrated network in outpatient internal medicine service. This table is designed according to Musoles & Escortell [13] who proposed a collateral payment model (Eq. 1) where the utility distribution is subject to the characteristic function N = {Hospital 1, Hospital 2} that covers a collaborative game (2, v): P (N) → R. This function was adapted by the authors with the inclusion of correlation coefficient r being defined as it follows:

$$\forall S(Nv(s)) = \left[\frac{M|r|}{1+\alpha\beta}\right] (SEQ) \tag{1}$$

Where:

r: Correlation coefficient between the lead time that was increased during the collaboration and the number of remitted patients that the hospital received.

M: The amount of payment that is offered to the coalition S under specific sceneries.

α, β: Constants that represent the contribution of each type of internal medicine appointment in the total of appointments per hospital (α: first-time appointments and β: control appointments)

- Step 7 - *Design of key performance indexes for measuring service network performance:* In the final part of this methodology, KPI's are established through which the performance of the integrated service network will be measured on population in terms of revenues for the hospitals and lead time for patients. Three key performance indexes were defined to measure the behaviour of the integrated service network in outpatient internal medicine monthly: Average weighted lead time, % of effective remissions and economic participation in network.

With the application of the proposed framework, it is required to establish if collaborative sceneries between the hospitals will be beneficial for each one in terms of revenues [10–12]. By the other side, it is needed to evaluate the benefits for patients in relation to the waiting times. Finally, it is pretended to assess the equilibrium in the network in order to determine if there is some hospital with major benefits than the other.

4 Results

4.1 Case Study

A real case study for the design of an integrated network in outpatient internal medicine service is presented to prove the applicability and effectiveness of the proposed methodology. The intended network is designed with two of the most important hospitals in Barranquilla (Colombia). These hospitals have been identified as Hospital 1 and Hospital 2. Currently, Hospital 1 presents a lead time of 11.4 days/appointment with a probability of 15 % of overpassing upper control limit established by the Ministry of Health and Social Protection (15 days/appointment). In fact, Hospital 1 has performed over the limit in several months. On the other hand, Hospital 2 has a better performance than Hospital 1. This hospital has an average lead time of 4.35 days/appointment and do not have any probability of overpassing the upper limit of the process. Patients are pregnant women (20–40 years old) who are under medical treatment; in some cases, with high-risk pregnancy.

For step 1, a VSM scheme was designed for each hospital. In Hospital 1, 99.58 % of the cycle time was represented in non-value activities, while in Hospital 2 these activities represented 99.79 % of the total process time. The non-value activities were most characterized in the lead time (Amount of time that a patient has to wait in order to consult a doctor). This fact could result in an emergency admission or more complex affectations on patient's health. From the scheme, four key aspects were identified as the main causes of wastes of time: anticipated scheduling of appointments, last-minute cancelations of medical agenda, waiting times in the process of billing paper reception and medical order claim and non-delivery of clinical histories. With basis on the previous aspects, the hospitals developed some strategies to reduce the patient waiting time obtaining a 3.11 % and 16.66 % reduction for Hospital 1 and Hospital 2 respectively. However, it is recommendable to achieve a higher reduction, reason by which, collaborative sceneries have to be explored.

For step 2, Law # 1438 of 2011 issued by the Ministry of Social Protection is explored to define the strategic platform for an integrated healthcare network. This law reveals that these networks have to be designed according to the patient requirements in order to be really effective. It is also noticed that service networks must count on technical, administrative and financial capacity, health promotion services, illness prevention, diagnosis, treatment, rehabilitation that allows getting the benefit plans. Apart from the previous law, it was necessary to articulate this law with the goals of each hospital in order to establish a coherent and effective strategic platform. For this reason, the strategic plans of Hospital 1 and Hospital 2 have been explored. It is concluded that "efficiency", "opportunity" and "quality" are common concerns in all of these organizations and "satisfy patients" a common goal. Taking into account the perspectives of each actor in the service network, a scheme have been developed as a strategic framework (See Fig. 2).

It is described that the network has to be led by a board of directors composed by the same quantity of participants for each hospital. Finally, two network objectives have been defined to measure the performance of the network:

- Provide the earliest appointment to the patient reducing the risk of major affectations in his/her health.
- Increase the level of revenues for each participant upon decreasing the probability of losing patients because of delays.

For step 3, communication lines were defined. It was required to explore and follow the guidelines of reference and contrarreference procedures of each hospital and design efficient information flows to guarantee a satisfactory performance of the network.

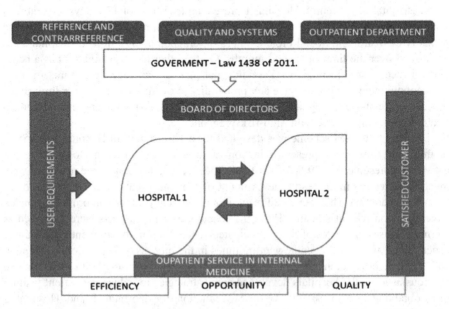

Fig. 2. Strategic platform for an integrated service network in internal medicine (Study case in Colombia)

The board of directors must define supervisors and a supervision frequency in order to detect possible errors and inefficiencies during the process. It must be noted that only patients from health companies like CAPRECOM, COMFACOR, COMPARTA and particulars can access to the benefits of network due to these companies have contracts with both hospitals, reason by which it is possible to send them in remission.

As next stage, the service network must be designed in order to determine possible impacts in each participant of the network. It is also necessary to evaluate the initial hypothesis made in methodology section in which it is wanted to determine economic implications, impacts of collaboration over the lead time of each participant in outpatient internal medicine service. To illustrate the model, a flowchart has been constructed (See Fig. 3). The network is modelled and simulated with the aid of Arena15.0 software. The results obtained with this simulation were really relevant. It is observed that Hospital 1 had a shorter lead time than Hospital 2 when initially was the opposite. This could evidence that there were collaboration between the hospitals. The weighted average lead time was 5.31 days/appointment, which is really good for patients because they will be served faster. Hospitals 1 and 2 had weighted average lead times of 4.57 days/appointment and 7.63 days/appointment respectively with zero probability of overpassing. Another analysis that was done consisted about comparing the previous status of each hospital with its current. For instance, it was demonstrated that the lead time for Hospital 1 changed with a p-value of 1.7×10^{-7}. This demonstrates that statistically, there was a reduction in internal medicine lead time for outpatient service. By the other side, the lead time for Hospital 2 changed too with a p-value of 6.4×10^{-5}. This demonstrates that statistically, there was an increase in internal medicine lead time for outpatient service. At the moment of evaluating the collaboration between the hospitals (Fig. 4), it is proved that there was collaboration with 476 patients remitted. The collaborative flow from Hospital1 (H1) to Hospital (H2) was widely bigger than H2 − H1.

Then, the collaborative model was evaluated without taking into account that doctors do not present failures in their services). This is, there are not cancelations of weekly medical agenda, lateness and last-hour absence. First, a statistic test was done to prove if there were differences between the performance of the network with and without medical failures. With a p-value of 0, there were no doubts that were differences with high reduction of the lead time. The lead time for Hospital 1 was 0.3 days/appointment and 4.58 days/appointment for Hospital 2, showing a reduction of average lead time in each hospital, even in the network with 2.54 days/appointment when it was 5.31 days/appointment. This obeyed to the fact that hospitals will have more capacity to serve their patients faster. This was confirmed at the moment of evaluating collaboration with this new condition. It is concluded that the number of collaboration was reduced to 283 patients, representing a significant reduction of collaboration activities in the network; this is explained in the fact that hospitals prefer serving their patients before sending them to another institution (If the queue size of doctor is equal to the others').

In the next phase, risks of collaboration were identified. First, there is a risk of failure in the attendance of the doctors. It is probable that when a patient gets for a consultation, the appointment could be called off. Cancelations of medical agenda could cause a loss of utility since a patient could be programmed earlier in the origin

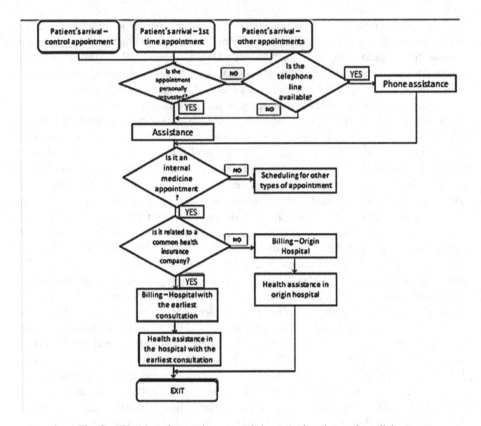

Fig. 3. Flowchart for service network in outpatient internal medicine

hospital but its lack of capacity, actives the collaboration to guarantee the better service for patients. As it was demonstrated in Step 4, this increases the lead time for the hospital. On the other hand, it could have a risk of failure in communication between the hospitals due to technical aspects. This could bring about scheduling errors such as programming an appointment with the doctor with larger queue than other (s) at a specific time.

M changes with the type of Health Company because the hospitals (H1 and H2) have agreements with different utility values. M = \$15012 for COMPARTA, M = \$30500 for CAPRECOM, M = \$31620 for COMFACOR and M = \$15637 for PARTICULAR REQUEST. α (H1) = 0.071, α (H2) = 0.9229, β (H1) = 0.068 and β (H2) = 0.932

The utility distribution is subject to the sceneries shown in Table 1.With these sceneries, payments for each hospital were calculated (See Tables 2 and 3).

Table 2 presents the payments for Hospital 1. It is noted that all the appointments will be paid with basis on the minimum rate. This reflects that correlation was insignificant since collaborative activities did not have a high influence on lead time for Hospital 1. The same case is shown with the payments for Hospital 2 (See Table 3);

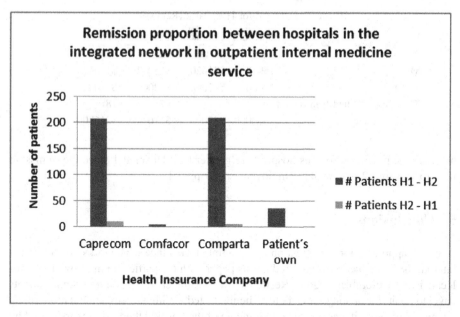

Fig. 4. Remission proportion between hospitals in the integrated network in outpatient internal medicine network

Table 1. Payment sceneries for an integrated service network studied in Colombia

		Which hospital serves the patient?	
		H1	H2
What is the origin hospital?	H1	M	H1: M − Máx {$12000;Mr/ (1 + (α + β))} H2: Máx {$12000;Mr/ (1 + (α + β))}
	H2	H2: M − Máx {$12000;Mr/ (1 + (α + β))} H1: Máx {$12000;Mr/ (1 + (α + β))}	M

Table 2. Payment for Hospital 1 (Remissions)

H1	Caprecom	Comfacor	Comparta	Patient's own
R	0.0944	0.2113	0.242	0.1172
M	$15012	$31620	$15012	$15637
V (S)	$12000	$12000	$12000	$12000
# Patients remitted from H2	23	3	7	1
Total payment	$276000	$36000	$84000	$12000

Table 3. Payment for Hospital 2 (Remissions)

H2	Caprecom	Comfacor	Comparta	Patient's own
R	0.1243	0.1111	0.2361	0.0794
M	$15012	$31620	$15012	$15637
V (S)	$12000	$12000	$12000	$12000
# Patients remitted from H1	130	4	97	18
Total payment	$1560000	$48000	$1164000	$216000

however the payments for this hospital are greater than Hospital 1 since the remission flow to Hospital 2 was widely employed by Hospital 1.

5 Conclusions

A novel approach for the creation of integrated Healthcare networks in outpatient internal medicine has been explored in this paper with the participation of two hospitals located in a Colombian region. Results show that under the existing system, patients have to wait for a long time before being tested. With the implementation of an integrated network it was observed that in one of the hospital the lead time increased by 75 % while its partner reduced it by 150 %. This results in a reduction perceived by patients, who will have low probabilities of requesting emergency services and other complex services. However, some of the hospitals will always have an increased patient waiting time. This has to be carefully compensated economically taking into account that collaboration is not the only variation source. In this case, poor correlations were not awarded through the characteristic function. For this reason, a new framework was developed adapting collateral payment model to the need and implications of the model. It is also remarkable to note that when doctor failures are avoided, the collaboration level decreases. This is explained in the fact that each hospital prefers gaining M than just a portion of it; although it was proved that it is better to remit a patient to obtain a part of M instead of 0. This framework will guide practitioners and decision makers in healthcare services to obtain better results under the current projections of population growing and trends in outpatient service in some specialties. For future work, it is recommendable to explore networks with more hospitals, more decision variables if considered and other specialties or processes that require an immediate intervention.

References

1. Ortiz Barrios, M., Felizzola Jiménez, H., Nieto Isaza, S.: Comparative analysis between ANP and ANP- DEMATEL for six sigma project selection process in a healthcare provider. In: Pecchia, L., Chen, L.L., Nugent, C., Bravo, J. (eds.) IWAAL 2014. LNCS, vol. 8868, pp. 413–416. Springer, Heidelberg (2014)

2. Zimmerman, J., Dabelko, H.I.: Collaborative models of patient care: new opportunities for hospital social workers. Soc. Work Health Care **44**(4), 33–47 (2007)
3. Katon, W.J., Lin, E.H., Von Korff, M., Ciechanowski, P., Ludman, E.J., Young, B., McCulloch, D.: Collaborative care for patients with depression and chronic illnesses. New England J. Med. **363**(27), 2611–2620 (2010)
4. Thota, A.B., Sipe, T.A., Byard, G.J., Zometa, C.S., Hahn, R.A., McKnight-Eily, L.R., Community Preventive Services: Collaborative care to improve the management of depressive disorders: a community guide for systematic review and meta-analysis. Am. J. Prev. Med. 42(5), 525–538 (2012)
5. Avery, M.D., Montgomery, O., Brandl-Salutz, E.: Essential components of successful collaborative maternity care models: the ACOG-ACNM project. Obstet. Gynecol. Clin. N. Am. **39**(3), 423–434 (2012)
6. Casey, J.J.W.: *A lean enterprise approach to process improvement in a health care organization* (Doctoral dissertation, Massachusetts Institute of Technology) (2007)
7. Taddei, A., Gori, A., Rocca, E., Carducci, T., Piccini, G., Assanta, N., Ricci, G.: Tele-consulting for collaborative diagnosis and care of heart malformations. In: Computing in Cardiology, pp. 253–256. IEEE, September 2011
8. Grafton, J., Abernethy, M.A., Lillis, A.M.: Organisational design choices in response to public sector reforms: A case study of mandated hospital networks. Manage. Account. Res. **22**(4), 242–268 (2011)
9. Campbell, B., Fryers, M., Devitt, R., Vestal, K.: Towards a collaborative model of care. In: Healthcare Management Forum, vol. 22(3), pp. 27–31. Elsevier, November 2009
10. Gorbaneff, Y., Torres, S., Contreras, N.: Anatomía de la cadena de prestación de salud en Colombia en el régimen contributivo. Gerencia y Políticas de Salud 3(6), 88–106 (2004)
11. Varkey, P., Reller, M.K., Resar, R.K.: Basics of quality improvement in health care. In: Mayo Clinic Proceedings, vol. 82(6), pp. 735–739. Elsevier, June 2007
12. Leng, M., Parlar, M.: Allocation of cost savings in a three-level supply chain with demand information sharing: A cooperative-game approach. Oper. Res. **57**(1), 200–213 (2009)
13. Musoles, M.B., Escortell, A.I.: Matemáticas de las operaciones financieras:(teoría y práctica) (1994)

NI-CHIC: A Model for Academic Engagement with Industry

Jonathan Synnott[1(✉)], Stephen McComb[2], Chris Nugent[1],
and James McLaughlin[2]

[1] School of Computing and Mathematics, University of Ulster, Belfast, UK
{j.synnott, cd.nugent}@ulster.ac.uk
[2] School of Engineering, University of Ulster, Belfast, UK
{sj.mccomb, jad.mclaughlin}@ulster.ac.uk

Abstract. The Northern Ireland Connected Health Innovation Centre has been established to promote business led collaborative Connected Health research between academia, industry and government. Established in June 2013, the Centre currently has 26 members from backgrounds including hardware development, software development, data analytics, and domiciliary care provision. The projects have also utilized partnerships with public health and charity-based organizations. To date, the Centre has completed four calls for proposals, resulting in tangible outputs in the form of novel hardware and software, field trials, data, and shared insight. This paper describes the Centre in detail, provides two case studies demonstrating completed projects, and discusses the challenges, lessons learned and impact thus far.

Keywords: Connected health · Collaboration framework · Industry engagement

1 Introduction

In February 2015, UK Life Sciences Minister George Freeman launched a strategic foresight report in Belfast, Northern Ireland. This laid out the need for a stronger alignment of health, academia and business to address emerging healthcare needs and the growth of the economy. He stated *"We know that we need a more 'joined up' approach to maximize the potential of the life and health sciences."* [1]. This approach of a joined up or triple helix is not a new concept but something reflected in policy, economic and journal papers throughout the last couple of decades. Etzkowitz [2] refers to interactive models and the need to move from beyond single interactions between industry and academia and develop and incubate ideas. The Five Year Forward View strategy document, published by the National Health Service (NHS) in October 2014, discusses a need for even wider partnership beyond the triple helix with linkage to voluntary and commercial organizations [3]. This is reflected in the emergence of Academic Health Science Networks in England which support a greater engagement across sectors to address emerging healthcare needs [4].

As part of the strategic context of Northern Ireland, the Department of Enterprise Trade and Investment (DETI) [5] brought Industry, Academia and Government

© Springer International Publishing Switzerland 2015
J. Bravo et al. (Eds.): AmIHEALTH 2015, LNCS 9456, pp. 258–263, 2015.
DOI: 10.1007/978-3-319-26508-7_25

together to investigate five sectors in Northern Ireland and explore how these sectors could be further developed. This was completed under the guidance of a group called MATRIX: Northern Ireland Science Industry Panel [6], which was launched in February 2007 [7]. Life and Health Sciences was one of these five areas where it was recognized that there was expected economic growth and existing local capability. A subcommittee for Life and Health Sciences was formed, called the Horizon Panel, who then commissioned investigations in this area and identified Connected Health as an area with focus. A £5 million fund was allocated by the Northern Ireland government to create a competence centre which explored in this area. As a result, the Northern Ireland Connected Health Innovation Centre (NI-CHIC) [8] was then formed to deliver this business led research.

Section 2 describes NI-CHIC in detail, including its formation and processes. Section 3 provides two case studies demonstrating representative projects and outcomes from the Centre. Section 4 discusses the challenges, lessons learned and impact of the Centre thus far, and Sect. 5 provides concluding remarks.

2   The Northern Ireland Connected Health Innovation Centre

NI-CHIC was established in June 2013. The Centre is funded by Invest NI and is based at Ulster University's Jordanstown campus. The core team is comprised of two existing research groups: The Smart Environments Research Group (SERG) and the Nanotechnology and Integrated Bioengineering Centre (NIBEC). These research groups share a common interest in the area of Connected Health, yet share fundamentally different focusses and areas of expertise. SERG, led by Prof. Chris Nugent, has a focus on the development and trial of novel software applications that typically incorporate leading edge off-the-shelf sensor technology for use in the areas of assisted living and integrated care. NIBEC, led by Prof. James McLaughlin, has expertise in the development of novel hardware with application in the areas of vital signs and point of care diagnostics. The collaboration of these research groups within NI-CHIC has resulted in a diverse and complimentary team of researchers capable of producing novel holistic solutions spanning many areas of Connected Health. The model can also support research beyond the core researchers where there is a business need.

Member companies are invited to become NI-CHIC members. Such a membership provides access to invitations to participate in project submissions, networking events, and information days providing awareness of upcoming external funding opportunities. Membership fees are based on company size, and commercial care organizations are exempt from any fees as they represent potential customer insight. A number of formal and informal agreements are in place with charity and public health organizations to encourage participation in the research where there is a mutual interest with specific projects.

The Centre currently has 26 members from a range of backgrounds including hardware development, software development, data analytics, diagnostics, and domiciliary care provision. The NI-CHIC executive board is business led, and consists of representatives from member organizations, SERG and NIBEC (Fig. 1).

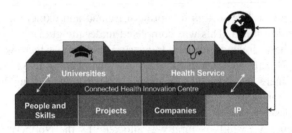

Fig. 1. An overview of the elements brought together by NI-CHIC

Projects are initiated through calls for projects. Previous calls have focused on: "Vital Signs technology", "Point of Care Diagnostics" and "Integrated Care and Assisted Living". Submitted proposals are reviewed internally to ensure they align with the Centre's core themes and criteria, with successful projects involving three or more partners and typically demonstrating sector and domain knowledge sharing and linkage to government policy. All NI-CHIC projects require a 25 % member contribution which may be in the form of staff time contribution or hardware or software contribution. Accepted proposals undergo a 5 day Alpha phase before being reviewed externally and moving to the core stage of research. Funded projects fall under two categories. Feasibility studies, which have the purpose of exploring potential market opportunities or new technology options, last under one year and receive between £25,000 and £100,000 funding. Full research and development studies typically last one to three years and receive funding of £250,000 to £1 million. The establishment of a core group of researchers has allowed for a more dynamic start, stop and continue approach where new projects can be initiated quickly and where necessary ended earlier than anticipated to release resources.

3 Case Studies

The Centre has currently completed four calls for proposals and has resulted in 8 successfully completed projects with several ongoing projects. This section provides two examples of successful NI-CHIC projects.

3.1 Case Study 1 – Unobtrusive Monitoring of Home-Based Activities Through Thermal Sensing Technology

This project comprised of three companies: IoT Tech [9], a hardware platform manufacturer; I+ [10], a software platform developer, and Extra Care [11], a domiciliary care provider. Each company shared an interest in the use of novel technology to assist with the unobtrusive monitoring of activities in the home of an older adult. When the project began, IoT Tech was involved in the early stages of the development of a novel thermal sensor platform. This platform was capable of recording and transmitting low resolution thermal data using a sensor placed in the ceiling of a room. The company wanted to assess the potential for the sensor to record activities in a household and generate alerts if a dangerous scenario was detected. I+ had an existing software platform which was designed to be used by older adults to generate activity reminders and to record metrics such as blood pressure and weight. The company wanted to assess the ability to integrate the novel thermal sensor with their existing platform. Finally, Extra Care wanted to gain knowledge in the domain of Connected Health in order to assess the feasibility of integrating sensor technology and software into their existing service offerings.

The project ran for 11 months. Regular project meetings were held, consisting of either project consortium meetings involving all members of the project consortium, or one-to-one meetings between one company and NI-CHIC. The project successfully produced a prototype system capable of collecting, storing, analyzing and visualizing data from multiple thermal sensors simultaneously. The system was capable of outputting metrics describing the number of room occupants and the amount of movement of the occupants. Additionally, early stage fall detection was demonstrated. An approach was developed to visualize these metrics over time. This approach was developed in a way that could be easily integrated with I+'s existing software platform and provided an intuitive overview of home activity that could be used by Extra Care's care staff to assess the wellbeing of clients while care staff are not present.

Other outputs from the project included academic publications [12], and the creation of a promotional video used by IoT Tech to demonstrate product potential to potential customers and collaborators, and by NI-CHIC to facilitate recruitment of new members. This work has formed the foundation of subsequent NI-CHIC projects.

3.2   Case Study 2 – Rapid Diagnostics for Consumer Use

This project comprised of three companies: CIGA Healthcare [13], CMASS [14], and Atto Partners [15]. CIGA Healthcare specializes in the manufacture of self-test products under the brand Suresign. The company supplies approximately 40 % of pregnancy tests purchased in the UK, and provides other tests including alcohol screening, blood pressure, diabetes and temperature. CMASS provides electro-mechanical contract manufacturing and software media duplication services for customers globally. Atto Partners are a team of designers and developers with expertise in web applications and cross platform design.

The project focused on the area of rapid diagnostics to be used within products sold directly to end consumers. Prof. James McLaughlin and his research team provided expertise in device creation, medical sensors and clinical chemistry while CIGA provided in depth market knowledge and insight to guide the scope, direction and selection of various components of the solution. CMASS provided insight into the manufacturing processes considerations and circuit board build that would typically not be available to a research laboratory. Atto partners offered different perspective as their experience was in digital user engagement. The project demonstrated a healthy tension of academic insight and commercial experience working together for a common goal. The outputs from the project were working demonstrators of sufficient quality to allow the companies to present the products to potential customers and investors.

4   Challenges, Lessons Learned and Impact

The projects completed by NI-CHIC thus far have provided new knowledge within technical domains and the area of Connected Health. Additionally, these projects have provided valuable insight into the challenges associated with collaborations of such diverse consortia and aligning the needs of academia, industry and government.

Traditional applied academic research and development can attempt to be entrepreneurially focused, with a degree of success in the area of technology transfer however they often reflect a technology push model. NI-CHIC projects strived for a more collaborative working relationship. Healthcare providers and commercial organizations have recognized that Academia is rewarded by publications which can emphasize academic silos based on disciplines which may not take into account a wider need to consider deployment issues. Therefore a key challenge was to develop a way of working with Academia that utilized the consortia investment but also worked within the structures in place to reward academics.

Collaboration with public organizations, such as healthcare providers, can also be challenging due to operational hurdles such as competing operational demands which may result in last minute changes and the loss of project momentum. Additionally, transformative projects can challenge the status quo and budget boundaries and procurement barriers may create difficulties in creating positive working relationships. Finally, businesses are driven by profit and loss and therefore have limited tolerance of risk without clearer understanding of the outcomes. This can manifest itself in frustration as the hurdles of business case approval, multiple decision makers and often a lack of decision making can add additional layers of delay. The companies have welcomed faster initiation of projects and a more responsive focus to their needs. Open communication and frequent engagement with all members of project consortia was key to successfully maintaining the moment of projects. Additionally, early identification of project objects and clear commitment agreements resulted in a minimization of complications and changes in scope within the later stages of projects. Consortium members typically consist of higher level employees at CEO or director level, however it was found that direct contact with appropriate mid-level employees was essential for quickly progressing technical elements.

The results from projects completed to date have been very well received. The outputs from the projects detailed in both Case Studies are leading on to further commercial discussions globally with significant interest. IoT Tech provided the following quote in relation to their experience with NI-CHIC: *"The work produced by CHIC researchers has been invaluable in moving forwarded our internal development goals. [...] CHIC is a great example of a well thought out organization lead by people who understand at a deep level the various needs of both the customer (HSC) and the producers and acts as the "oil" to lubricate the 'wheels of engagement'."*

With regards to the project outlined in Case Study 2, the Chief Executive of CIGA provided the following quote: *"The partnership with CHIC has complemented our market knowledge with technical and scientific insights which has created an attractive market proposition which we are investigating with our customers in North America and other world markets."*

5   Conclusion

NI-CHIC was established to facilitate collaborative projects which align the needs of academia and industry with government. Since the Centre was first established in June 2013, the number of members has increased to 26, and four calls for proposals have been successfully completed. Projects completed to date have included hardware manufacturers, software developers, and domiciliary care providers. These projects have resulted in tangible outputs and knowledge gained in the successful cultivation of such diverse consortia. Two case studies have been provided, providing details of two successfully completed projects. Additionally, the challenges, lessons learned and impact of the Centre have been discussed.

Acknowledgements. Invest Northern Ireland is acknowledged for supporting this project under the Competence Centre Program Grant RD0513853 - Connected Health Innovation Centre.

References

1. Invest NI. https://www.investni.com
2. Etzkowitz, H.: Incubation of incubators: innovation as a triple helix of university-industry-government networks. Sci. Public Policy. **29**, 115–128 (2002)
3. NHS England. http://www.england.nhs.uk/ourwork/futurenhs
4. NHS England. http://www.england.nhs.uk/ourwork/part-rel/ahsn/
5. Department of Enterprise, Trade and Investment. http://www.detini.gov.uk/
6. MATRIX Northern Ireland Science Industry Panel. http://matrixni.org/
7. Invest NI. http://www.investni.com/news/launch-of-matrix-life-and-health-sciences-foresight-report.html
8. Northern Ireland Connected Health Innovation Centre. http://www.ni-chic.org/
9. IoT Tech Ltd. http://www.iottech.co.uk/
10. I+ SrL. http://www.i-piu.it/website/index.php
11. Extra Care. http://extra-care.org/
12. Synnott, J., Nugent, C., Jeffers, P.: A thermal data simulation tool for the testing of novel approaches to activity recognition. In: Pecchia, L., Chen, L.L., Nugent, C., Bravo, J. (eds.) IWAAL 2014. LNCS, vol. 8868, pp. 10–13. Springer, Heidelberg (2014)
13. CIGA Healthcare. http://www.cigahealthcare.com/
14. CMASS. http://www.cmass-ni.com/
15. Atto Partners. http://www.attopartners.com/

Simulation Results of a Model to Provide Consistent Functionality and Performance in a Healthy Smart City

Gabriel Urzaiz[1]([⊠]), Eric Murillo-Rodríguez[2], Jaime Zaldívar-Rae[3], Ramón Hervas[4], Jesús Fontecha[4], and José Bravo[4]

[1] División de Ingeniería y Ciencias Exactas, Universidad Anáhuac Mayab, Mérida, Yucatán, Mexico
gabriel.urzaiz@anahuac.mx
[2] Escuela de Medicina. División de Ciencias de la Salud, Universidad Anáhuac Mayab, Mérida, Yucatán, Mexico
eric.murillo@anahuac.mx
[3] Vicerrectoría Académica, Universidad Anáhuac Mayab, Mérida, Yucatán, Mexico
jaime.zaldivar@anahuac.mx
[4] Universidad de Castilla-la Mancha, Ciudad Real, Spain
{ramon.hlucas,jesus.fontecha,jose.bravo}@uclm.es

Abstract. This paper presents simulation results of a model aimed to obtain uniform functionality and performance of the services provided within a healthy smart city. Simulation results were useful to demonstrate the model usefulness and the possibility to enhance the quality of the services. However, this enhancement was observed in a generalized manner, and it was not yet possible to concentrate efforts in those zones with the poorest quality of service. Further work is needed to achieve consistency.

Keywords: Healthy smart cities · Smart environments · Health services

1 Introduction

We define a *healthy smart city* as a place in which modern Information and Communication Technology (ICT) is used to provide health services in a way that seeks economic development, high quality of life, and a wise management of natural resources.

There is a lot of work being done to offer alternatives to improve the infrastructure of the smart cities and to help them evolve towards intelligent dynamic infrastructures that serve citizens fulfilling the criteria of energy efficiency and sustainability [1]. To mention some examples, an architecture for smart cities is presented in [2], where city management, community service providers and citizens have access to real time data by integrating various ICT into the artifact of the city. A grid platform is presented in [3] as an aggregation of micro smart grids, enabling a better management of the available resources.

© Springer International Publishing Switzerland 2015
J. Bravo et al. (Eds.): AmIHEALTH 2015, LNCS 9456, pp. 264–269, 2015.
DOI: 10.1007/978-3-319-26508-7_26

There are also advances in communications technology and energy efficiency. A good example is the 802.11p protocol, which is an amendment of the 802.11 protocol to support Intelligent Transportation Systems applications and to add wireless access in vehicular environments. Yet a further low-latency version of the 802.11p protocol is presented in [4] improving performance and throughput. Another example is the utility function model presented in [5] in order to choose the best access point in a heterogeneous network aiming to save energy for the smart mobile devices and to reduce computational time when the network is overloaded.

Heterogeneity is also a major topic being addressed. Smart cities require the possibility to communicate a variety of devices with a wide variety of communication technologies. Several solutions arise, such as UniGate [6], a modular universal wireless communication gateway to enable inter-connectivity between devices using different wireless technologies and to serve as a virtual computing resource for all connected devices.

Despite of these advances, there are still major challenges to be addressed, such as consistency of the services provided within the smart city. Increasing population density in urban environments demands adequate provision of services and infrastructure [2]. This explosion in city population implies a variation in the quality of the services along the smart city. Consistency is undoubtedly a major challenge.

2   Previous Work

In a previous work [7] we presented a high-level model to be used as a guide for the Mexican city of Mérida to become a healthy smart city. This model could also be adapted for other cities in the world. The primary objective of the proposed model was to provide a structure for a healthy smart city to enhance the quality of life of patients and caregivers, and to achieve a regional competitive advantage by allowing that any patient who is within the city limits is continuously monitored and supported by all the people and services that he or she needs at any time.

Quality of services in different parts of the city can vary significantly. Our strategy to assess the proposed model was based on the effectiveness to provide the same functionality and performance regardless of the physical location where the user is located, provided that it is within the smart city boundaries.

We decided to implement an overlay network in order to provide a robust communication platform to offer the same functionality and performance along the city. The model included three components: network layer, semantic layer, and application layer. The network layer was mainly used to provide enhanced network services by implementing two combined enhancement techniques: route optimization and information optimization. The semantic layer was responsible for providing important features such as the automatic responses or actions in case of routine decisions that do not need any human intervention, and others. The application layer provided a user interface, and it was also responsible for the control and the management of the information and the users.

3 Development of the Model Components

A piece of software was developed to implement the three model components. The software was developed in the C programming language, and it was based on the idea of having service requesters to be connected to service providers by means of the enhanced network communication platform. Depending on the desired topology, it is possible to have one or more service requesters connected to one or more service providers. At this development stage, neither specific services nor specific behaviors were yet considered.

4 Simulation

We included three types of participants: patients, caregivers and health services. Patients and caregivers were simulated as service requesters, and the health services were simulated as service providers.

We also defined three zone types that were classified as type 0, 1 or 2, depending on their characteristics. Patients, caregivers and health services may be unevenly distributed along the different zones of the city (Table 1).

Table 1. Distribution of patients, caregivers and health services in different zones.

Zone	Patients	Caregivers	Health services
0	Some	Some	Many
1	Some	Some	Some
2	Many	Few	Few

For simulation purposes, we interpreted the terms "few", "some", and "many" as 10, 20 and 50 respectively.

4.1 Metrics

We defined specific metrics to evaluate functionality (service coverage and offering density) and performance (success rate and average response time).

Service coverage was calculated as a percentage of the requirements of services that received a corresponding offering within the maximum time, with reference to the total number of requirements. Offering density was defined as the average of the offers received within the maximum time, divided by the number of requirements of services that received a corresponding offering within the maximum time.

Success rate was defined as the number of successful services divided by the total number of solicited services, and the average response time was calculated as the average response time for all successful services.

4.2   Simulation Scenario

The simulated scenario (Fig. 1) consisted of one type 0 zone, one type 1 zone, and one type 2 zone.

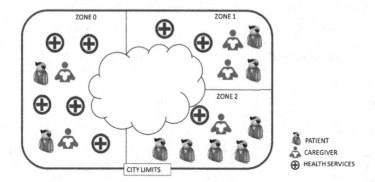

Fig. 1. Simulated scenario

Besides the differences in the distribution of patients, caregivers and health services, we also considered that each zone may have different characteristics.

From the provider (health services) side, the response time was calculated by adding the link latency to the node latency. Link latency and node latency were simulated according to Table 2.

Table 2. Link latency and node latency in different zones

Zone	Link latency (s)	Node latency (s)
0	0.2	Between 0.1 and 1.5
1	1.0	Between 0.1 and 1.5
2	3.0	Between 0.1 and 1.5

In general, it was also considered that the model reduced the link latency in 30 % but increased the node latency (overhead) in 10 %.

From the requester (patient and caregiver) side, the requested response time was simulated as a random number between 0.1 and 2.0 s, and it was considered that an offer was received only if it was received in 3.0 s or less.

4.3   Simulation Results

The simulation was to compare the results obtained by applying the model with the results obtained in the original situation. Simulation results are graphically represented in Fig. 2.

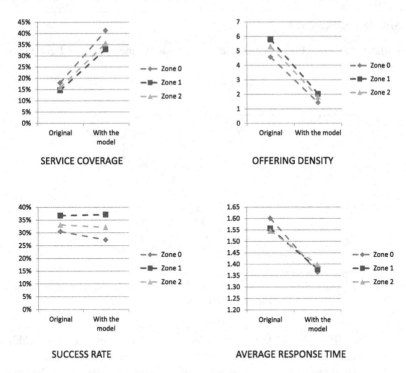

Fig. 2. Simulation results

The use of the model helped to enhance the service coverage and the average response time in all zone types, and success rate remains almost unaltered. It can be noticed that the model produced worse numbers in the case of offering density, probably because of the implicit overhead.

5 Conclusion

Simulation results were useful to demonstrate the model usefulness and the possibility to enhance the quality of services by providing a better functionality and performance, which translates into better health services and higher quality of life within the smart city.

However, this enhancement was observed in all zones in a generalized manner. It was not yet possible to provide a selective enhancement, which is needed to achieve the original aim of the model of providing a balanced and uniform functionality and performance of the services provided among the different zones within a healthy smart city. Our original hypothesis considered the possibility to concentrate the enhancement effort as needed, especially in those zones with the poorest quality of service. The model must be capable to provide enhancement selectively in order to obtain uniform functionality and performance of the services provided within a healthy smart city. Further work is needed to better understand the specific factors that have impact on functionality and performance depending on the different zone types.

References

1. Pellicer, S., Santa, G., Bleda, A.L., Maestre, R., Jara, A.J., Gomez Skarmeta, A.: A global perspective of smart cities: a survey. a. innovative mobile and internet services in ubiquitous computing (IMIS). In: 2013 Seventh International Conference on Digital Object Identifier, pp. 439–444 (2013). doi:10.1109/IMIS.2013.79
2. Jalali, R., El-khatib, K., McGregor, C., Smart city architecture for community level services through the internet of things. In: 2015 18th International Conference on Intelligence in Next Generation Networks (ICIN), pp. 108–113, 17–19 Feb 2015. doi:10.1109/ICIN.2015.7073815
3. Menniti, D., Sorrentino, N., Pinnarelli, A., Burgio, A., Brusco, G., Belli, G.: In the future smart cities: coordination of micro smart grids in a virtual energy district. In: 2014 International Symposium on Power Electronics, Electrical Drives, Automation and Motion (SPEEDAM), pp. 676–682, 18–20 June 2014. doi:10.1109/SPEEDAM.2014.6872123
4. Nasrallah, Y.Y., Al-Anbagi, I., Mouftah, H.T.: A quality of service model for IEEE 802.11p communication protocol in a smart city. In: Global Information Infrastructure and Networking Symposium (GIIS), pp. 1–3, 15–19 Sept 2014. doi:10.1109/GIIS.2014.6934257
5. Mazza, D., Tarchi, D., Corazza, G.E.: A user-satisfaction based offloading technique for smart city applications. In: Global Communications Conference (GLOBECOM), 2014 IEEE, pp. 2783–2788, 8–12 Dec 2014. doi:10.1109/GLOCOM.2014.7037229
6. Felemban, E., Murad, M., Manzoor, M.A., Sheikh, A.A.: UniGate: modular universal wireless gateway. In: 2014 World Congress on Computer Applications and Information Systems (WCCAIS), pp. 1–3, 17–19 Jan 2014. doi:10.1109/WCCAIS.2014.6916657
7. Urzaiz, G., Hervas, R., Fontecha, J., Bravo, J.: A high-level model for a healthy smart city. In: Pecchia, L., Chen, L.L., Nugent, C., Bravo, J. (eds.) IWAAL 2014. LNCS, vol. 8868, pp. 386–389. Springer, Heidelberg (2014). doi:10.1007/978-3-319-13105-4_55

Web Application for Doctor-Patient Communication in the Treatment of Mental Disorders

E. Pérez-Brito[1], A. Quesada-Arencibia[1(✉)], C.R. García[1], and A. Pérez-Brito[2]

[1] Institute for Cybernetic Science and Technology,
University of Las Palmas de Gran Canaria, Las Palmas, Spain
perezbritoe@gmail.es, {aquesada, rgarcia}@dis.ulpgc.es
[2] Fundación Canaria Contra La Leucemia Alejandro Da Silva,
Santa Cruz de Tenerife, Spain
anapbrito@cop.es

Abstract. For this project we have used new technologies to create a new channel of communication between doctors and patients in the treatment of mental disorders. We have created a web application using an adaptable design accessible from any mobile device, which allows doctors to adapt their patients' therapy to real-time knowledge of their current condition. In turn, patients can express their mood state with respect to the component elements of their therapy.

Keywords: Web application · Doctor-patient communication · Emotional diary · Psychological test · Therapeutic adherence

1 Introduction

Mental illnesses rank amongst those that cause the greatest impact to the patient and their family. One of the main shortcomings in the treatment of mental disorders is the lack of real-time information on the status of the patient. Through this project we aim to provide a new channel of communication between doctors and patients, using the Internet and new technologies, to facilitate the adaptation of patient therapy to their needs by receiving real-time updates on their condition.

These real-time updates on the mood state of the patient in relation to the component elements of their therapy will enable the doctor to perform an immediate adjustment to the therapy to improve patient outcomes.

This project was developed in the context of the public health system of the Autonomous Community of the Canary Islands. No similar tool is currently used by this health service. Only the drago system[1] is used to obtain information on scheduled visits and to view clinical and medication history.

---

[1] Canary Islands Primary Care administrative and clinical management system. For management of diaries, appointments, service portfolio, performance of care, waiting lists, reuptakes, interdisciplinary consultation and requests for additional tests in the field of Specialised Care.

© Springer International Publishing Switzerland 2015
J. Bravo et al. (Eds.): AmIHEALTH 2015, LNCS 9456, pp. 270–278, 2015.
DOI: 10.1007/978-3-319-26508-7_27

In the private sector there are various psychological care websites (none of them psychiatric) offering online emotional care (entire treatment) or a first consultation method.

Email is also used frequently as a tool for monitoring and/or virtual consultations between two appointments that are very far apart.

Currently, various techniques based on new technologies are being employed in the field of healthcare. These include, specifically, the field of cognitive software, specialised in stimulating and enhancing mental skills associated with the processes of learning, visual memory or linguistic stimuli. This type of software permits the tests to be configured to parameters defined by the patient's needs, taking into account aspects such as modality (visual or audible instructions), level of difficulty or response time. Some examples of cognitive software are:

- Telepsychology
- Virtual reality
- Augmented reality
- Video Games
- Telecare
- Robots.

2 eHealth

eHealth represents a change in our approach to healthcare. Technology at the service of everyone so we can live a healthier life. We can monitor our vital signs and keep track of our treatments for better therapy compliance and even use remote medical consultation. This change is enabling data collection which, when analysed, will offer a more accurate and reliable diagnostic and therapeutic approach.

Mobile applications and new online communication tools are undergoing exponential growth as we seek immediate answers to all our health queries.

The technologies that have been adopted to improve doctor-patient communication have brought some benefits, although they have also introduced new medical-legal and patient privacy risks.

One of the main advantages of eHealth is access to reliable quality information that helps resolve general queries about the health of the patient when they arise. The patient becomes the protagonist of the process, able to store all information on their condition in their own medical history that they can share with the therapists.

Another advantage is the ability to stay in contact with therapists with waiting times that are shorter than under the current system. It reduces delays and unnecessary travel for all kinds of administrative tasks and consultations that can now be done online.

Finally, it facilitates learning so that the patient becomes increasingly autonomous in caring for their own health and for that of their dependants. Some of the advantages of eHealth are:

- Speed.
- Low Cost.

- Asynchrony.
- Accessibility.
- Permanence.
- Without barriers.
- Reduces unnecessary visits.

3 Doctor-Patient Communication Model

Doctor-patient communication conforms to several models that define how to handle conversations involving situations related to the patient's health and how to make them see the reality that surrounds them.

To carry out these communications various models have been defined that determine how the doctor achieves this reality approach when establishing contact with the patient.

Following these models, we can define this relationship as a meeting between two people, one of them the patient who needs help to recover their health, the other the doctor who is trained to provide this help. This relationship depends on the cultural, scientific and technical circumstances of each time and place.

Of all the models of doctor-patient communication, we have selected the Robert Veatch model [1] for the purposes of this project. This model considers that the contract to be established is a consensus or agreement based on the theme that motivates the meeting: the health of the patient.

The diagnosis is made by the doctor, but the responsibility for the therapy is shared. There is respect for the autonomy of the patient who is informed in order to be able to make an informed choice.

This model is the one that seems best suited to the nature of this project; when attending therapy, doctor and patient can agree on the steps to be taken, but the doctor cannot force the patient to follow them as directed. Another significant aspect of this model of communication is the importance that is given to the feedback that the patient gives to the doctor with respect to the therapy, an essential aspect in reinforcing the rationale of the project: real-time therapy adjustments according to the patient's needs.

Communication models follow several phases as the therapy progresses, according to renowned doctor Laín Entralgo [2]. These phases are summarised below.

Cognitive Moment. Stage at which the link between doctor and patient is established. The interest that binds both sides of this relationship is represented by the desire to recover health, but the person suffering from the condition is the patient, not the doctor.

In this interaction the doctor employs scientific knowledge to name, describe and set out what ails the patient; at the same time, the patient contributes with his or her ideas and emotions. The result is a medical diagnosis.

Operative Moment. Refers to the therapeutic activity of the doctor, from empathic listening at the start until the final send-off.

Therapeutic action begins when the patient decides to seek medical advice, before the actual appointment, and does not end until final discharge. The moment of diagnosis is also therapeutic.

Affective Moment. The author argues that there are two forms of affectional bonding between the doctor and the patient:

- **Medical camaraderie:** both the doctor and the patient seek to remedy the condition and achieve good health, but with little personal commitment. The patient, if cured, is grateful and becomes emotionally attached to the doctor, albeit not very deeply, because of the service provided.
- **Medical friendship:** characterised by trust whereby the patient can confide their innermost thoughts and emotions in the doctor.

4 Design and Development

In the analysis phase we identified three different types of actor who interact with the web application. The most general user type is the "unregistered user", all those who are not "registered users". Within the registered users we have the roles "Doctor" and "Patient".

- **Unregistered user:** Users who access the application without identifying themselves. May register if they want to see a doctor, or log in to identify themselves and access the corresponding features, be they doctor or patient.
- **Doctor:** Uses the features provided by the Doctor module. Has a profile with personal, professional and login information. Is responsible for creating Patient user profiles. Organises patient information, managing their history, treatment and clinical information.
- **Patient:** Uses the features provided by the Patient module. Can edit login information and some basic fields in their medical history through their profile. Responds to events generated by their treating doctor and can generate others in turn through their emotional diary.

The design of the web application separates the system functions into three modules, each module covering the actions that can be performed by each user. The modules that have been developed are as follows:

- **Application:** Contains the public part of the web application, displays information on the project features and on some mental illnesses and their effects on the family. Has access to login area and, for doctor users, user account creation.
- **Doctor:** Contains the private part intended for doctor users. Permits administration of all information pertaining to patient records, clinical history and emotional diary. Also contains psychological test editor (Fig. 1).

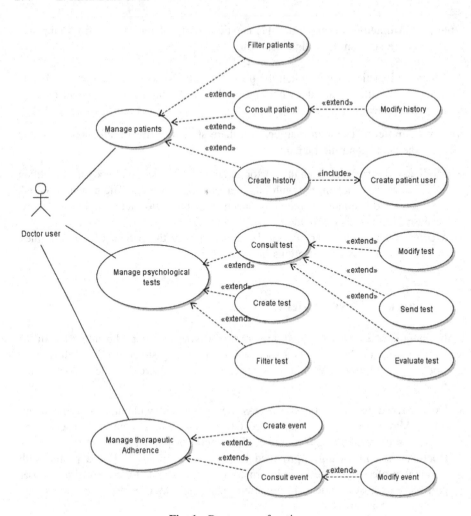

Fig. 1. Doctor user functions

- **Patient:** Contains the private part intended for patient users. In this module the patient can manage elements of their emotional diary and send feedback on elements of their therapeutic adherence.

4.1 Emotional Diary

The emotional diary is a very useful tool to complement the therapy of a patient suffering from a mental disorder. This tool is usually incorporated as an extra element as part of a broader package of measures to assist in certain problems that are emotional or have their origins in emotion.

The purpose of this record is not to provide a solution to every feeling, but to identify it and give it its exact name (Fig. 2):

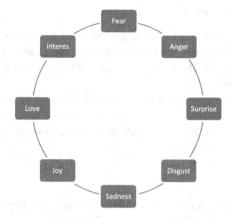

Fig. 2. Primary emotions

The emotional diary aims to elicit pure emotional expression, as this allows patients to better understand themselves in order to build self-assurance, reduce their fears and anxiety in new situations, learn to resolve problems, understand how to identify and self-regulate emotions.

Writing down these experiences will increase the patient's perception of different situations and the correct way to deal with them, because it will enable them to recognise what they are feeling in certain situations and to create behavioural patterns that they will then analyse so that they can decide how to act or react. It also provides the doctor, over time, relevant information about the patient's evolving management of their emotions.

4.1.1 Emotional Diary on the Web Application

To reflect the emotional diary on the web application, the patient is provided with a range of features to express their mood state using three methods:

- **Write a diary entry:** As if it were a physical diary, the patient has a section in which they can type up an entry in their emotional diary. As with a normal diary the patient can add the date, title and development to the diary entry.
- **Create new mood state:** Another addition to the emotional diary is an indication of mood state. When the patient suffers any mood change and wants to communicate it to the doctor they can do so in this section. Options are available here to indicate when the mood arose, give it a name, define what primary emotion most adequately describes their emotions, describe its intensity and explain the whole episode by reporting it.
- **Create new mood state associated with an image:** The patient is provided with this alternative way of describing a mood state. In this case a mood is also described with the aforementioned features, but the explanation is reinforced by uploading an image.

4.2   Therapeutic Adherence

In addition to following medical advice, a number of changes in patient habits, life-style, thoughts and abilities are required to increase the efficacy of the treatment and obtain a better quality of life as the outcome. This combined approach is called "therapeutic adherence".

The web application project seeks to group all elements of the patient's therapy in one place. All elements of the patient's therapy can be managed under the label of therapeutic adherence (consultations, medication, tests, workshops and bibliotherapy).

4.3   Feedback

In all the aforementioned sections, once the doctor has read the patient's message they can send a reply if they consider it appropriate. The patient, in turn, can send a message to their doctor about any element of their therapy whenever necessary. Both actors will be notified by the system of any entry or reply.

4.4   Psychological Test Editor

One of the most salient features of this project is the psychological test editor that allows the doctor to create and modify tests adapted to the needs of each patient.

With this editor the doctor can create tests with various types of questions:

- Simple
- Yes/No
- True/False
- Relationship/Cause
- Likert Scale

The editor has other features such as creating private entries for the doctor or a system to evaluate the test results, either as a whole or the individual answer to each question.

5   Results and Conclusions

The web application we have developed (Fig. 3) provides a number of essential tools for functional improvement of communication between doctors and patients. Some of the most salient features are

- Psychological test editor
- Doctor-patient communication system
- Emotional diary
- Combining medical and clinical history

The tool represents an advance in patient proximity and provides more continuous monitoring outside doctor visits. It offers the possibility of adjusting or changing

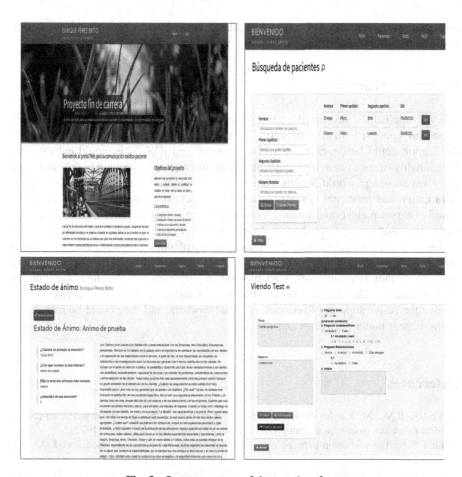

Fig. 3. Screen captures of the user interface

medical and psychological treatment in a simple, fast way that reinforces patient autonomy.

Despite this being a tool that will enhance therapy there are certain types of patient with whom it should not be used. Patients who may potentially suffer from using this tool are those who suffer from certain obsessive compulsive disorders, who are exhibiting signs of severe depression or patients with symptoms of paranoia.

All psychological therapies including cognitive behavioural counselling, systemic therapy, humanistic therapy…all apart from psychodynamic therapy. Furthermore, it could also be used in psychiatry by doctors and liaison nurses who are mental health specialists in home care programmes and day care units.

The web application could be used by patients with severe psychopathologies who remain under the care of their families; in these cases, the latter would have access to this channel of communication with health professionals in order to provide information on changes and/or new requirements that arise between scheduled visits. This would improve one of the major shortcomings of the Canary Islands Health System, in particular, but one that also affects healthcare nationally: overlong waiting times between doctor-patient visits as a result of an overloaded health system.

6 Future Work

The web application developed for this project has many features that can be expanded upon and improved. Instead of opting to use an adaptable design, a native mobile application could be developed for both Android and iOS. This would enhance the functionality of the system. For example, the representation of a mood in the emotional diary via an image would benefit from mobile device geolocation. Currently, patient information and treatment is stored in a database developed in SQL. A way could be found to export patient information by creating a format that presents the information in such a way that it may easily be transferred to another professional. Similarly, it would be useful to add a feature that allows the sharing of information on therapies; or to create a method by which a psychologist can make an online inquiry to another colleague if they have any doubts about a patient's therapy. Finally, new stakeholders can be added to the system. As noted above, in some therapies it is convenient to receive the active support of relatives or social workers, and they could be introduced to the system under new roles and functions.

References

1. Veatch, R.M.: Models for ethical medicine in a revolutionary age. What physician-patient roles foster the most ethical realtionship? Hastings Cent. Rep. **2**(3), 5–7 (1972)
2. Laín, E.P.: The friendship between physician and patient in hippocratic medicine. J. Art. **47**, 1–18 (1962)
3. Miranda, C.M., Jadresic, M.E., Chomali, G.M., Miranda, C.E., Cáceres, I.C.: The use of e-mail in the communication between physicians and their patients (2013)
4. Garvi Soler, P., Villanueva Rodríguez, C., Andrés Martínez, E.: Launching a consultation by email, to provide solutions, not to create problems (2014)
5. Bobes, J., González, M.P., Sáiz, P.A., Bascarán, M.T., Bousoño, M.: Universidad de Oviedo - Área de Psiquiatría. Instrumentos básicos para la práctica de la psiquiatría clínica (2002)

Metrics for Health Environments

Processing EEG Signals Towards the Construction of a User Experience Assessment Method

Ivan Carrillo[✉], Victoria Meza-Kubo, Alberto L. Morán, Gilberto Galindo,
and Eloisa García-Canseco

Universidad Autnóma de Baja California, Ensenada, Baja California, Mexico
{ivan.carrillo,mmeza,alberto.moran,gilberto.galindo.aldana,
eloisa.garcia}@uabc.edu.mx

Abstract. This paper proposes a neural network to identify pleasant and unpleasant emotions from recorded electroencephalography (EEG) signals, towards the construction of a method to assess user experience (UX). EEG signals were obtained with an Emotiv EEG device. The input data was recorded during the presentation of visual stimulus that induce emotions known a priori. The EEG signals recorded were preprocessed to enhance the differences and then used to train and validate a Patternet neural network. The results indicate that the neural network provides an accurate rate of 99.61 % for 258 preprocessed signals.

Keywords: EEG · Emotions · Elderly · IAPS · Neural networks

1 Introduction

The increasing incidence of diseases such as the Alzheimer's disease have moved researchers to look for alternative non-drug treatments, including technologies supporting cognition, that seek to maintain the cognitive status of the elderly through cognitive stimulation [1,2]. To this end, diverse intelligent environment applications that seek to promote cognitive stimulation (CS) have been proposed [2]. However, due to the characteristics of this group of users, caused by their decline in their physical and cognitive skills, it is necessary to assess what is the elderly perception regarding the use, acceptance and adoption of these applications.

In the literature, several usability and user experience (UX) evaluations have been reported in order to assess the perception of the users regarding the use of technology [3], however, conducting this kind of assessments may be a difficult task due to the inherent limitations of the evaluation methods themselves. For example, it is well known that in techniques based on self-report, participants tend to respond what the researcher wants to hear, or tend not to be sincere and improve their perception of the results because they felt assessed, or because they have forgotten the details of their experience [4]. Because of this, the results of these evaluations may not be very reliable.

© Springer International Publishing Switzerland 2015
J. Bravo et al. (Eds.): AmIHEALTH 2015, LNCS 9456, pp. 281–292, 2015.
DOI: 10.1007/978-3-319-26508-7_28

As an alternative to traditional UX assessment techniques, we propose to record brain electrical activity of the participants by means of a low-cost electroencephalogram (EEG) device, to infer pleasant and unpleasant emotions in an automated manner using a Patternnet neural network. The goal is to introduce a method with which we could identify emotions using EEG signals and based on these data determine the UX. In this paper we present the neural network designed and the processing techniques used for emotions recognition towards the construction of a method to assess UX.

2   Related Work

There are several ways of recording psychophysiology data from humans, for example Galvanic Skin Response (GSR), Electromyography (EMG), Electrocardiogram (ECG) and Electroencephalography (EEG) [5]. Inferring emotional states from EEG has received considerable attention as EEG has rapid response time, could directly reflect emotional states and is less expensive than other related methods, so it is widely used to monitor brain activity in BCI research [6,7].

In recent years, there have been a growing number of efforts to recognize a person's emotion in real time using EEG. For example, EmoRate developed as a commercial product (Emotiv Corp.) detects the flow of the emotional state while the user is watching a film [8]. Brown et al. proposed an EEG-based affective computer system that measures the state of valence and transmits it via a wireless link [9]. Petrantonakis [10] analyzed EEG signals and used neural networks to classify them in six emotions based on emotional valence and arousal, with a 61 % success rate.

Chai [11] evaluates three mobile phone applications using three self-report questionnaires to obtain subjective data as well as recording brain activity using EEG of participants. These data were used to determine the positive and negative states in the UX of the applications used. Hakvoort [12] evaluated the UX of a brain-computer interface (BCI) game based on the expectation of users, they used an evoked visual response as stimuli, and an EEG to register physiological data.

In a similar fashion, in this work we propose to identified pleasant and unpleasant emotions by means of a neural network fed with EEG data.

3   Emotions

Emotions can be positive or negative. At all times, no matter the context of the situation people experience a range of emotions whether positive (e.g. joy, gratefulness, sympathy, happiness, love, etc.) or negative (e.g. displeasure, irritability, disgust, anger, sadness, etc.) [13,14]. Positive emotions are associated with the activation of regions of the left hemisphere while negative emotions relate to the activation of regions of the right hemisphere [15–18].

In the frequency domain, the spectral power in various frequency bands has been implicated in the emotional state. The asymmetry analysis of the alpha power is recognized as a useful procedure for the study of emotional reactivity [19]; further, it is common to find asymmetries in the frontal region of the brain, which may be perceived on a subject since childhood [20]. In a study conducted in [21] a spectral analysis of the electrical activity obtained through an EEG demonstrated that the alpha power varies depending on the emotion present (positive or negative).

In order to determine experimental stimuli to induce emotions different modalities including the visual, auditory, tactile, or odor stimulation have been used. A recurrent technique to induce emotions is to use the standard stimulus sets such as the International Affective Picture System (IAPS) or the International Affective Digitized Sound System (IADS). The IAPS and IADS provide a set of normative pictures (IAPS) or sounds (IADS), for emotional stimuli to induce emotional changes and attention levels [22,23].

In this work the IAPS pictures have been used to induce emotions in the subjects; EEG signals are acquired using the Emotiv EEG device; and a Patternnet neural network was designed in order to identify pleasant an unpleasant emotions.

4   Methodology

In order to define a method that interprets a set of UX emotions using an EEG, we conducted a preliminary study that presents selected pictures to stimulate known a priori emotions and recorded the EEG response. Then, the EEG was filtered and processed to design a trained neural network used to identify the UX from two basic emotional states: pleasant or unpleasant. For the study we used the International Affective Picture System (IAPS). A subset of the pictures proposed in Bradley [23], which evoke specific emotions were used. The following categories of emotion in pictures were used (see Fig. 1): (A) fear (10), (B) pleasant (10), (C) unpleasant (10), and (D) neutral (29).

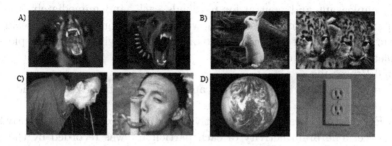

Fig. 1. Example of selected pictures from the IAPS. (A) Fear pictures. (B) Pleasant pictures. (C) Unpleasant pictures. (D) Neutral pictures.

Participants. Participants were eight older adults, 2 male and 6 female, aged 60 to 83 (AVG 72.3 years, SD 8.46 years). Participants received coffee services and a gift (equivalent to approximately $5 dlls) for their participation in the study. Inclusion criteria were: aged over 60 years, not having suffered a head trauma, absence of moderate or severe cognitive problems and absence of visual problems (i.e. being able to see well without glasses at a distance of 30–50 cm). To determine that participants did not have cognitive problems, we applied the Mini Mental State Examination (MMSE).

Materials.

- The Emotiv EEG headset was used to acquire EEG data; Emotiv EEG obtains and records brain activity through 14 electrodes (AF3, F7, F3, FC5, T7, P7, O1, O2, P8, T8, FC6, F4, F8, AF4). The electrodes were placed according to the International 10–20 System, which sets the position of the electrodes on the cranial surface corresponding to cortical areas.
- Software; the Camtasia Studio Software was used to record the facial expressions of each participant; the Emotiv EEG Control Panel application was used to calibrate the device; the TestBench software was used to record data from brain activity with the 14 electrodes; the EEGExProc was used to display images; and the EEGLAB to process the EEG data [25].

Procedure.

- Introduction. First the participants where introduced individually to the experiment, and the characteristics of the Emotiv EEG headset were explained. They were also asked to sign a consent form, and the MMSE was applied.
- Emotiv EEG calibration. For best performance of the device, this was calibrated for each participant by recognizing facial gestures and by manipulating a virtual 3D cube through brain interaction using the Emotiv EEG control panel application.
- Brain signals acquisition. In this stage, each participant, wearing the Emotiv EEG device, was presented with a set of pictures according to the proposal in Bertron [24]. Pictures were presented in the following arrangement: pleasant, fear, unpleasant and neutral for 6 seconds each, and immediately, the participant was asked to indicate what was his/her impression upon seeing the picture answering 1 to 4 according to one of the following categories: pleasant, unpleasant, neutral and fear.
- Signal Processing
  The process followed for reduction and analysis of the EEG is divided into four phases
  1. EEG Capture. Brain electrical activity was captured using the Emotiv EEG device. The brain activity of each participant was recorded by the Test-Bench software and a label was inserted into the recorded signal indicating the category of emotion presented for the future signal segmentation. The EEG signal frequency acquired bands were: alpha, beta, and theta.

2. Signal Preprocessing. Prior to extracting the characteristics of the signal, an artifact removal procedure was applied.
   The preprocessing techniques applied to the signal were:
   - Average elimination and the best linear fit of the signal mean.

$$B = A - Ai \tag{1}$$

Where A = the original data, Ai= the data mean

$$C = detrend(B) \tag{2}$$

   - A Hamming window was applied to the signal.
   - A Finite Impulse Response (FIR) bandpass filter was applied (1 Hz–30 Hz).

3. Signal Feature Extraction. In this phase the Fast Fourier Transform (FFT) was applied to the brain signals in order to obtain the signal characteristics.
   - FFT

$$C(x) = \sum_{j=1}^{N} c(j) W_N^{(j-1)(x-1)} \tag{3}$$

Where i = imaginary data, N = Data size.
The features extracted from the signal were:
   - Frequency
   - Magnitude

$$P = abs(\sqrt{real(C_{ij})^2 + imag(C_{ij})^2}) \tag{4}$$

   - Power

$$H = (P_{ij})^2 \tag{5}$$

   - Divided by brain wave (alpha, beta, theta).

$$M\alpha = \begin{pmatrix} \alpha_{11} & \cdots & \alpha_{1n} \\ \vdots & \ddots & \vdots \\ \alpha_{m1} & \cdots & \alpha_{mn} \end{pmatrix} \tag{6}$$

$$M\beta = \begin{pmatrix} \beta_{11} & \cdots & \beta_{1n} \\ \vdots & \ddots & \vdots \\ \beta_{m1} & \cdots & \beta_{mn} \end{pmatrix} \tag{7}$$

$$M\theta = \begin{pmatrix} \theta_{11} & \cdots & \theta_{1n} \\ \vdots & \ddots & \vdots \\ \theta_{m1} & \cdots & \theta_{mn} \end{pmatrix} \tag{8}$$

- Signal Average.

$$\bar{M}\alpha = \sum_{i=1}^{n} \sum_{j=1}^{k} Ma_{ij} \qquad (9)$$

$$\bar{M}\beta = \sum_{i=1}^{n} \sum_{j=1}^{k} Mb_{ij} \qquad (10)$$

$$\bar{M}\theta = \sum_{i=1}^{n} \sum_{j=1}^{k} Mt_{ij} \qquad (11)$$

- Signal maximum value for each band.

$$Max\alpha = max(\bar{M}\alpha) \qquad (12)$$

$$Max\beta = max(\bar{M}\beta) \qquad (13)$$

$$Max\theta = max(\bar{M}\theta) \qquad (14)$$

- Signal minimum value for each band.

$$Min\alpha = min(\bar{M}\alpha) \qquad (15)$$

$$Min\beta = min(\bar{M}\beta) \qquad (16)$$

$$Min\theta = min(\bar{M}\theta) \qquad (17)$$

- Standard deviation for each band.

$$ds\alpha = \frac{\sqrt{\sum_{i=1}^{n} \sum_{j=1}^{k} (Ma_{ij} - \bar{M}\alpha)^2}}{n(k)} \qquad (18)$$

$$ds\beta = \frac{\sqrt{\sum_{i=1}^{n} \sum_{j=1}^{k} (Mb_{ij} - \bar{M}\beta)^2}}{n(k)} \qquad (19)$$

$$ds\theta = \frac{\sqrt{\sum_{i=1}^{n} \sum_{j=1}^{k} (Mt_{ij} - \bar{M}\theta)^2}}{n(k)} \qquad (20)$$

4. Classification. Finally, the characteristics obtained were used to train a neural network (Fig. 2) which will be used to identify the emotions. A Patternnet neural network was used. Patternnet recognition networks are feed forward networks that can be trained to classify inputs according to target classes. The neural network was trained using the brain signals from pleasant and unpleasant emotions (explained in the next section).

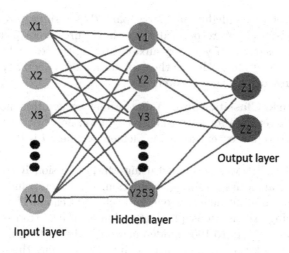

Fig. 2. The structure of the neural network.

5   Results

Participants Verbal Responses. According to the verbal classification reported by each participant (see Table 1), we obtained that the answers to the selected pictures to provoke pleasant emotions matched 91 % of the times. Additionally, responses to unpleasant pictures agreed 84 % of the times. In both cases, the pictures converge to the categories of the established test. By contrast, responses to the pictures selected to evoke fear agreed 49 % of the times, while for those selected as neutral their responses corresponded 57 % of the times, this means, that the responses in these categories were not reported as expected. For additional results see Carrillo et al. [26]. Given these results, only the pleasant and unpleasant signals brain recorded were used to train and test the neural network.

Table 1. Match averages reported by participants.

Participants									
IAPS pictures	P1	P2	P3	P4	P5	P6	P7	P8	Match
Unpleasant (10)	10	8	7	10	8	8	8	P1	84 %
Pleasant (10)	9	10	10	8	10	7	10	P1	91 %
Neutral (29)	17	11	17	26	10	14	20	P1	57 %
Fear (10)	8	8	4	7	7	0	0	P1	49 %

P: Participant; Match %: Indicates the percent were the verbals answers match with the pictures category

It is important to highlight that participant P7's results were removed. P7 was a special case, as she responded that all pictures were pleasant. It was observed that participant P7 was very anxious during the test, which along with a possible missunderstanding during the explanation of the activity could caused her to always provide the same answer.

Neural Network Classification. A Patternnet recognition neural network was used. The target data for patternnet recognition networks should consist of vectors of all zero values except for a 1 in element i, where i is the class they are to represent.

The neural network was developed using Matlab version R2013b. The data for the network categories (training, validation, test) were randomly selected. The network had 10 input neurons (one for each EEG channel) and two output neurons identifying two emotions: pleasant and unpleasant. After several settings for the neural network (10 to 1000 hidden neurons), the best result was with 253 neurons. The network was trained with 258 inputs obtaining the setting showed in Table 2.

Table 2. Neural network elements.

Neural network elements	Setting
Hidden layer neurons	253
Percent training data	80 %
Percent validation data	10 %
Percent ratio data	10 %
Training function	trainscg
Performance function	crossentropy

In order to validate the results obtained with the neural network, a lineal regression was performed with data from each section (training, validation, and test) (see Fig. 3).

Figure 4 shows the confusion matrix for the three kinds of data combined (training, testing, and validation). The network outputs are very accurate, as can be seen by the high number of correct responses (derived from neural network outputs vs pictures prior category) in the green squares (upper left and in the middle) and the low number of incorrect responses in the red squares (upper middle and first in second row). The lower right blue squares (bottom rigth) illustrate the overall accuracies (99.61 %).

Discussion. From the results obtained from verbal responses it was interesting to observe that for the elderly, the standardized pictures not always evoked the particular emotions expect. For instance, the worst case was for the fear category, only 49 % of the responses indicated that the pictures evoked this emotion, 39 % of responses indicated unpleasant and 10 % of responses were classified as neutral.

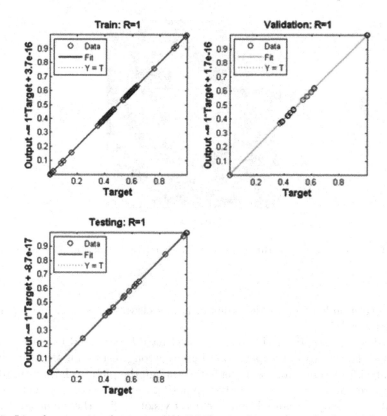

Fig. 3. Lineal regression for trained, validation and test data. It shown that R=1, thats mean that there is a correlation between trained, validation and test data with the output data.

From this group of pictures, picture 59, which shows a skeleton, was the only one that did not evoked fear; 40 % of participants responded with neutral and 30 % responded with unpleasant. For pictures in the neutral category, only 57 % of these were classified as neutral, 40 % of them were reported as pleasant and 3 % were reported as unpleasant.

Regarding the pictures in the unpleasant category, it can be observed that over 84 % evoked unpleasant emotions to participants, while 11 % were reported as neutral, 3 % as fear and 2 % as pleasant. Participant P3 indicated that picture 31, which showed a hand surgery, was perceived as pleasant to him as he was a medical doctor, so that it could be concluded that the activities being undertaken by participant P3 as a professional affected his answer.

Finally, the best results were for the pictures in the pleasant category, as expected, 91 % of the responses were reported as pleasant, 7 % as neutral and 2 % as fear (see Table 1). The results show that participant P4 expressed that picture 45 evoked fear to her; in this case the picture corresponded to 3 girls smiling, so it could be a coding error by the participant; while for picture 51,

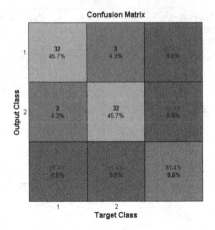

Fig. 4. Confusion matrix for three kinds of data combined (training, testing, and validation).

which corresponded to an older woman, it was classified as neutral by participants P1 and P6.

Considering that the IAPS pictures used have been tested to cause known emotions, then a possible explanation for the wrong results for the fear (49 %) and neutral (56 %) pictures could be that although the pictures have been tested with children and adults, the elderly population leaves the common perception; this difference may be caused by the elderly vision of life, the whole context of the participants' live, and, of course, the natural decline that participants may have. Given these results to identify fear and neutral pictures by participants, the corresponding brain signals were not used as input to the neural network.

Concerning the neural network, after the preprocessing of the brain signals, 258 pre-known signals were used, 129 corresponding to pleasant emotion, and 129 of unpleasant emotion.

It is important to mention than the input vector included an average from the 10 EEG channels and not for each neuron separately. An analysis for this configuration must be performed later in order to compare the differences of the results obtained.

6   Conclusions

This paper presents preliminary results of our proposal to determine a set of emotions through brain signal (EEG) records. The results of participant's verbal responses validated the emotional presence of pleasant and unpleasant emotions, especially when the selected pictures to evoke these emotions were presented.

These records where used as input in a Patternnet neural network with 253 neurons hidden layer and an accurate rate of 99.61 % for 258 characteristics of the preprocessed signals.

Our future work includes performing the analysis using the 10 nodes from the electrodes separately. In addition, we must use the validated neural network to identify pleasant or unpleasant emotions using the brain signals from users of CS applications in order to assess the UX.

Acknowledgements. We acknowledge the support of UABC, in the form of the Programa de Servicio Social 212, Proyecto Interno 231, and CONACYT by scholarship number 538130 for the first author. We also acknowledge the elderly participants from Ensenada, B.C., México for their support and participation in the study.

References

1. Buiza, C., Soldatos, J., Petsatodis, T., Geven, A., Etxaniz, A., Tscheligi, M.: HERMES: pervasive computing and cognitive training for ageing well. In: Omatu, S., Rocha, M.P., Bravo, J., Fernández, F., Corchado, E., Bustillo, A., Corchado, J.M. (eds.) IWANN 2009, Part II. LNCS, vol. 5518, pp. 756–763. Springer, Heidelberg (2009)
2. Meza-Kubo, V., Morán, A.L.: UCSA: a design framework for usable cognitive systems for the worried-well. Pers. Ubiquit. Comput. **17**(6), 1–11 (2012)
3. Meza-Kubo, V.: Guías para el diseño de aplicaciones de estimulación cognitiva utilizables por el adulto mayor. Ph.D. thesis, Universidad Autónoma de Baja California (2012)
4. Arhippainen, L., Tähti, M.: Empirical evaluation of user experience in two adaptive mobile application prototypes. In: Proceedings of the 2nd International Conference on Mobile and Ubiquitous Multimedia (2003)
5. Sohaib, A.T., Qureshi, S., Hagelbäck, J., Hilborn, O., Jerčić, P.: Evaluating classifiers for emotion recognition using EEG. In: Schmorrow, D.D., Fidopiastis, C.M. (eds.) AC 2013. LNCS, vol. 8027, pp. 492–501. Springer, Heidelberg (2013)
6. Kim, M.-K., Kim, M., Eunmi, O., Kim, S.-P.: A review on the computational methods for emotional state estimation from the human EEG. Comput. Math. Methods Med. **2013**, 13 (2013)
7. Nasehi, S., Pourghassem, H., Isfahan, I.: An optimal EEG-based emotion recognition algorithm using gabor. WSEAS Trans. Sig. Proc. **3**(8), 87–99 (2012)
8. Sourina, O., Liu, Y.: A fractal-based algorithm of emotion recognition from EEG using arousal-valence model. In: Biosignals, pp. 209–214 (2011)
9. Brown, L., Grundlehner, B., Penders, J.: Towards wireless emotional valence detection from EEG. In: 2011 Annual International Conference of the IEEE Engineering in Medicine and Biology Society, EMBC, pp. 2188–2191. IEEE (2011)
10. Petrantonakis, P.C., Hadjileontiadis, L.J.: Emotion recognition from EEG using higher order crossings. IEEE Trans. Inf. Technol. Biomed. **14**(2), 186–197 (2010)
11. Chai, J., Ge, Y., Liu, Y., Li, W., Zhou, L., Yao, L., Sun, X.: Application of frontal EEG asymmetry to user experience research. In: Harris, D. (ed.) EPCE 2014. LNCS, vol. 8532, pp. 234–243. Springer, Heidelberg (2014)
12. Hakvoort, G., Poel, M., Gurkok, H.: Evaluating user experience with respect to user expectations in brain-computer interface games, pp. 1–4 (2011)
13. Fredrickson, B.L., Losada, M.F.: Positive affect and the complex dynamics of human flourishing. Am. Psychol. **60**(7), 678–686 (2005)

14. Rodriguez, J.-A.P., Linares, V.R., Gonzalez, A.E.M., Guadalupe, L.A.O.: Emociones negativas y su impacto en la salud mental y física. Suma Psicológica **16**, 85–112 (2009)
15. Mosquera, G., Daniel, S.: Adquisición de señales electroencefalográficas para el movimiento de un prototipo de silla de ruedas en un sistema BCI. Ph.D. thesis (2012)
16. Harmon-Jones, E., Gable, P.A., Peterson, C.K.: The role of asymmetric frontal cortical activity in emotion-related phenomena: a review and update. Biol. Psychol. **84**(3), 451–462 (2010)
17. Simón, V.: Mindfulness y neurobiología. Revista de Psicoterapia **66**, 5–30 (2007)
18. Winkler, I., Mark, J., Jager, M., Mihajlovic, V., Tsoneva, T., Winkler, I., Mark, J.: Frontal EEG asymmetry based classification of emotional valence using common spatial patterns. Worls Acad. Sci. Eng. Tech. **45**, 373–378 (2010)
19. Cicchino, A.N.B.: Técnicas de procesamiento de EEG para detección de eventos. Postgradofcm. Edu.Ar (2014)
20. Navarro, F.S., Pedro, J., Lapuente, R.: Amígdala, corteza prefrontal y especialización hemisférica en la experiencia y expresión emocional. Universidad de Murcia Servicio de Publicaciones, Murcia (2004)
21. Kostyunina, M.B., Kulikov, M.A.: Frequency characteristics of EEG spectra in the emotions. Neurosci. Behav. Physiol. **26**(4), 340–343 (1996)
22. Mikels, J.A., Fredrickson, B.L., Larkin, G.R., Lindberg, C.M., Maglio, S.J., Reuter-Lorenz, P.A.: Emotional category data on images from the international affective picture system. Behav. Res. Methods **37**(4), 626–630 (2005)
23. Bradley, M.M., Lang, P.J.: The international affective picture system (IAPS) in the study of emotion and attention, pp. 29–46 (2007)
24. Bertron, A., Petry, M., Bruner, R., Mcmanis, M., Zabaldo, D., Martinet, S., Cuthbert, S., Ray, D., Koller, K., Kolchakian, M., Hayden, S.: International affective picture system (IAPS): technical manual and affective ratings (1997)
25. Delorme, A., Makeig, S.: EEGLAB: an open source toolbox for analysis of single-trial EEG dynamics including independent component analysis. Elsevier **134**, 9–21 (2004)
26. Carrillo, I., Meza-Kubo, V., Morán, A.L., Galindo, G., García-Canseco, E.: Emotions identification to measure user experience using brain biometric signals. In: Zhou, J., Salvendy, G. (eds.) ITAP 2015. LNCS, vol. 9193, pp. 15–25. Springer, Heidelberg (2015)

Reduction of Average Lead Time in Outpatient Service of Obstetrics Through Six Sigma Methodology

Miguel Ortiz Barrios[1](✉) and Heriberto Felizzola Jiménez[2]

[1] Department of Industrial Engineering, Universidad de la Costa CUC,
Barranquilla, Colombia
mortiz1@cuc.edu.co
[2] Department of Industrial Engineering, Universidad de la Salle,
Bogotá, Colombia
healfelizzola@unisalle.edu.co

Abstract. In hospital services, operations efficiency and healthcare quality are two critical factors since both define the financial sustainability of the hospitals as well as patient health, safety and satisfaction. For this reason, it is necessary to explore different strategies for the improvement of quality and efficiency indicators in the provision of healthcare services. Specifically, this paper focuses on the application of Six Sigma methodology as an important option to solve this problematic. This methodology begins with the identification of improving opportunities that are aligned with the organization goals. Then, a portfolio of potential improvement projects is created. Later, these projects are prioritized with basis on multicriteria decision making techniques, with the purpose of choosing the project with the highest impact on the organization quality and efficiency. Finally, the selected project is developed through DMAIC cycle. An application case related to the process of obstetric outpatient in a maternal-child hospital located in the city of Barranquilla (Colombia) is presented to prove the validity of the proposed approach. The results show that the average lead time in the obstetric outpatient service in which pregnant women are monitored, was reduced from about 7 days/appointment to approximately 4 days/appointment.

Keywords: Average lead time · Six sigma · Obstetric outpatient · Healthcare quality

1 Introduction

Currently, healthcare organizations face two main challenges. The first challenge is referred to the reduction of the high costs related to the inclusion of advanced technology and new medical treatments for diagnosis and intervention processes. Second, the growing demand of services with high quality standards and patient safety that implies having an adequate staff, medical equipment and processes [1, 2].

To provide a safe, quality and low-cost healthcare service, hospitals and clinics must have efficient processes, trained and committed staff, advanced technology and a strategic platform that integrates these aspects effectively.

© Springer International Publishing Switzerland 2015
J. Bravo et al. (Eds.): AmIHEALTH 2015, LNCS 9456, pp. 293–302, 2015.
DOI: 10.1007/978-3-319-26508-7_29

In last decade, Six Sigma has become in a successful strategy for those organizations that want to achieve operational excellence, get high standards of quality and reduce non-quality costs in order to be more efficient and become in world-class companies. The healthcare sector is not the exception, and despite Six Sigma was initially focused on production contexts, many healthcare organizations have implemented it as a strategy to reduce operation costs and process inefficiencies, increase service levels, make administrative processes more efficient, diminish medical errors and make good use of installed capacity [3].

This work explains the methodology and presents the results of a Six Sigma project implemented in a maternal-child hospital whose primary aim was to reduce the lead time in the outpatient service of its obstetric department. The results show the effectiveness of Six Sigma methodology to achieve meaningful improvements in services provision.

This paper is organized as follows: Sect. 2 briefly presents a background related to Six Sigma applications on healthcare services. Section 3 presents the proposed methodology for the effective implementation of Six Sigma in care processes of clinics and hospitals. Section 4 provides the activities and results of execution phase of this methodology in a study case. Finally, conclusions about this research work and suggestions for further research are made in Sect. 5.

2 Literature Review

There are multiple applications of Six Sigma methodology on the quality and productivity improvement in hospital sector. The first implementation case of Six Sigma in healthcare sector has been registered in The Commonwealth Health Corporation in 1998. Some achieved results are the increase of 33 % in throughput, a cost reduction of 21.5 % in radiology; also savings of US$2.5 million were achieved [4].

In the United States, "Mount Carmel" healthcare system, a set of 3 hospitals located in Columbus (Ohio) that has 7300 employees and a staff of 1200 doctors in different specialities, had a financial state that was experiencing a crisis that threatened the stability of the company. Given this, the directors of this organization decided to implement Six Sigma methodology since guaranteed a significant and continuous benefit projection in time. This decision meant a return of $3.1 million of dollars with increasing expectations; moreover, dissatisfaction level and stuff frustration were also reduced through meaningful operational improvements [5].

Another large-scale application case of Six Sigma was presented in The Red Cross Hospital in Netherlands. Between 2002 and 2004, 116 people were trained in Green Belt level and about 70 projects were developed. The results showed a total saving of €1.2 million at the end of 2004. Some of the projects were: Improving patient scheduling operating theatre Reducing accounts receivable; Optimizing technical maintenance; Reducing formation of physiotherapists Revision of terms of payment; Reducing admission time hip replacement Reducing admission time after delivery; Improving logistics linen distribution; Availability ambulatory files; and Reducing waiting times first contacts cardiology [2–6].

3   Methodology

For a successful implementation of Six Sigma methodology, it is necessary to take into account a series of factors such as: project articulation with organization goals, manager commitment, Six Sigma training, the conformation of a team for project development, the selection of key projects, among others [7–10]. Therefore, prior to developing any Six Sigma project, it is fundamental to consider the factors mentioned above with the aim of increasing the success probability at the moment of implementation. The present proposed approach is constituted by 4 phases (See Fig. 1) as it is shown below:

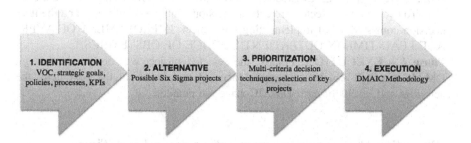

Fig. 1. Methodology for the effective implementation of Six Sigma projects

- **Phase 1- IDENTIFICATION:** To identify key improvement areas, it is necessary to analyze three aspects in any organization: Voice of customer (VOC), strategy goals and organization policies and the processes together with the key performance indexes (KPIs). The voice of customer analysis is done by the identification of critical to satisfaction (CTS). For this, a survey was designed and carried out with the aid of Health Service Companies (customers) which point out the most relevant quality characteristics in the provision of hospital services. After obtaining customer perceptions, organizational policies, goals and their importance and key performance indexes are defined. KPIs should be definite in terms of a current and future state with the purpose of evaluating the effectiveness of the Six Sigma projects that will be finally selected for their implementation.
- **Phase 2 – ALTERNATIVES:** The creation of Six Sigma project alternatives is done by linking each organizational goal with the different improvement points detected in VOC analysis, generating a Six Sigma project portfolio that is coherent and measurable with respect to the organization goal and current market. In this case study, these project alternatives were identified: Improvement of average lead time in Outpatient service of Obstetrics, Improvement of average lead time in Outpatient service of Internal Medicine, Improvement of User Information System, Improvement of Information System opportunity, Improvement of average lead time in Emergency Department and Optimization of Inventory System.
- **Phase 3 – PRIORITIZATION:** The Six Sigma project selection process consisting about evaluating a project portfolio, and then choosing the implementation

of one of them so that organization goals are achieved [11]. It is one of the most critical stages of a Six Sigma process since it defines a great part of project success [12]. Therefore, it is important to guarantee that projects are selected in line with the healthcare organization goals and objectives [13]. In this study case, a hybrid multicriteria decision technique called ANP-DEMATEL was used. This technique has been successfully employed in project selection and is based on pairwise comparisons of the importance and influences [14].

In the evaluation process, four criteria were defined: OPPORTUNITIES, BENE-FITS, RISKS and COSTS. Each criterion was divided in sub-criteria until completing a total of 15 sub-criteria. Additionally, three strategic objectives were defined: BUSINESS EXCELLENCE, INCOME GROWING and PRODUCTIV-ITY. To evaluate the selected projects, a decision team was conformed and the final decision consisted about implementing the project: IMPROVEMENT OF AVER-AGE LEAD TIME IN OUTPATIENT SERVICE OF OBSTETRICS.

- **Phase 4 – EXECUTION:** Finally, the selected project was developed through DMAIC CYCLE which is the main focus of this paper. In the next item, the activities and results of each DMAIC stage are detailed.

4 Execution Phase: Improvement of Average Lead Time in Outpatient Service of Obstetrics

4.1 Define Phase

In this case study, the define phase evaluates the performance of average lead time in outpatient service of Obstetrics from a maternal-child hospital located in Barranquilla (Colombia). In this phase, several employees from Quality Department, Financial Department, Outpatient Department and User Support Department were teamed up in order to have a clear project definition. To define the current state of average lead time in outpatient service of Ginecobstetrics, a line diagram has been used (See Fig. 2). This figure shows that in some months (September, March and April), the lead time was greater than the upper specification limit (8 days/appointment) given by the Ministry of Health and Social Protection of Colombia. The greatest lead time was 9.33 days/appointment and took place in April.

The above mentioned situation results in a more extended waiting time for pregnant women before being served. This increases the risk of complications during pregnancy since doctors will only be able to detect anomalies (in case of the patient have them) of these patients lately. This means that a new life can be put in danger. With this information, a project charter was designed. In it, six months were established as the duration of the Six Sigma project. On the other hand, to clarify the process of Obstetrics outpatient service, a SIPOC (Supplier – Inputs – Process – Outputs - Customers) has been designed (See Fig. 3).

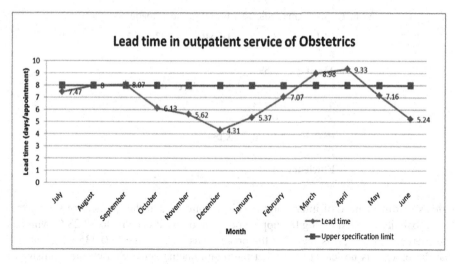

Fig. 2. Lead time in outpatient service of Obstetrics from maternal-child hospital in study

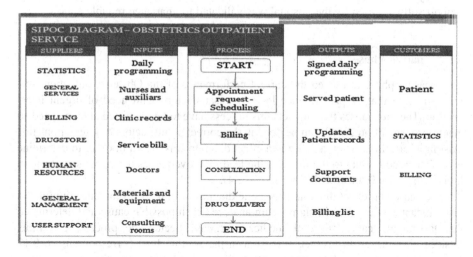

Fig. 3. SIPOC diagram for Obstetrics outpatient service

4.2 Measure Phase

In measure phase, the robustness of the process is evaluated with respect to the upper specification limit through a process capability analysis and the calculation of current sigma level, defects per million of opportunities (DPMO), process efficiency and process error (See Table 1):

Table 1 illustrates that the current process has a very low sigma level (0.71). The sigma level range is 0–6 where 0 is the worst state and 6 the best. This means that out of 1000000 appointments, 322800 will have a lead time greater than 8 days/appointment. On the other hand, this process registers an efficiency of 67.72 % which is low and

Table 1. Six sigma indicators for Obstetric outpatient service

USL	8	DPMO	322800
LSL	0		
Mean	6.89		
UCL	11.612	Sigma level	0.71
σ	1.574		
Zu	0.71		
P(Zu)	32.28 %	Cps	0.235
P(error)	32.28 %		
Efficiency	67.72 %		

reflects a primary need of intervention. This is confirmed at the moment of seeing that the probability of overpassing the upper specification limit is equal to 32.28 % which is considerable. Finally, it is seen that the process has a Cps equal to 0.235 which means that the process is not capable to meet the requirements demanded by the Ministry of Health and Social Protection. It is necessary to remark that the measure system composed by the operators of APPOINTMENT SCHEDULING DEPARTMENT and the support software used by the hospital was validated to guarantee reliable data.

4.3   Analyze Phase

The measure phase displayed the current performance of the Obstetric outpatient service, showing that its performance level is unsatisfactory with need of urgent intervention. The root causes that impacts this process have to be identified and analyzed so that improvement processes can be done in the correct points, actors or interactions that exist in it. For this reason, a cause and effect diagram was drawn in order to determine what factors contribute to the fact that the lead time overpasses the upper specification limit with 32.28 % of probability (See Fig. 4).

The cause and effect diagram (Fishbone diagram) in Fig. 4 reveals meaningful and insignificant causes. The six-sigma team analyzed each possible cause and determined that last-minute cancellation of medical agendas affected the process lead time. Besides, this causes an average extension in the waiting time corresponding to 8.12 days/appointments which impacts negatively on lead time. By the other side, a sub-specialty called *perinatology* is affecting with a correlation coefficient of 0.5459 which becomes in the main improvement point for intervention. This sub-specialty is served by just one doctor with a serving frecuency of two mornings (8 am – 12 m) in a week while the rest of the time is in charge of diverse functions that can be assumed (some of them) by a gynecologist. This sub-specialty is in charge of serving women with high-risk pregnancies and in some cases the appointment lead time is equal to 21 days. On the other hand, anticipated programming of appointment requests with a programming date equal to 3 weeks or more (control appointments) also impacted negatively on lead time. Another cause that has to be taken into account is how clinical records are being delivered to all of the doctors of this specialty. It is good to remark that a lack of clinical record could cause an appointment cancelation; reason by which,

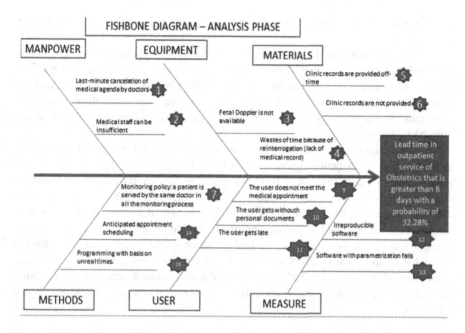

Fig. 4. Fishbone diagram for lead time in outpatient service of Obstetrics with value greater than 8 days/appointment

this event was measured by the Six Sigma team, obtaining a delivery efficiency equal to 80.58 % which is not sufficient in healthcare services; even though it is known that information flows determine the correct decision making during intervention and diagnosis processes.

4.4 Improve Phase

This phase focuses on reducing average lead time in outpatient service of Obstetrics from a maternal-child hospital. The condition of improvement is achievable though the implementation of some new policies and support software. With respect to the sub-specialty of *perinatology*, the project black belt together with the chief executive of the hospital decided to increase the installed capability of this sub-specialty so that, a high impact on the lead time of obstetrics outpatient service can be observed. For this, it was fundamental to analyze the functions of this doctor in order to verify if some of them can be reassigned to gynecologists. The analysis made recommended to reassign functions that were developed in mornings. In this way, this doctor was enabled to serve patients every day mornings. It is good to highlight that this kind of sub-specialty is not common in our country, reason by which it is difficult to hire another specialist. This fact is very delicate because directly affects women with high risk of losing their babies.

On the other hand, software for registering electronic clinic records was implemented since these records were delivered physically. This avoids wasting time looking for records in a clinic record room, interrogating patients during consultation and calling off appointments.

By the other side, the hospital decided to fine doctors who get late and cancel appointments at the last minute. If there is an absence, the Outpatient Department must verify if the excuse given by doctors is valid. This was subject to contract that the hospital has with an association of gynecologists. Finally, the scheduling of appointments with too much anticipation with respect to the requested programming date was restricted to 1 week of anticipation.

After the intervention, the indicators were recalculated. Table 2 illustrates that the current process has a better sigma level (3.16). This represents an increase of 2.45 sigma. This also means that out of 1000000 appointments, 46500 will have a lead time greater than 8 days/appointment; which indicates a reduction of 85.59 %. On the other hand, this process registers an efficiency of 95.35 % which represents an increase of 27.63 %. This is confirmed at the moment of seeing that the probability of overpassing the upper specification limit is equal to 4.65 % which is low. Finally, it is seen that the process has a Cps equal to a.054 which means that the process is capable to meet the requirements demanded by the Ministry of Health and Social Protection. On the other side, the operational cost by consultation was reduced in 12 % thanks to the intervention.

Table 2. Six sigma indicators for Obstetric outpatient service

USL	8	DPMO	46500
LSL	0		
Mean	4.08		
UCL	7.8	Sigma level	3.16
Σ	1.24		
Zu	3.16		
P(Zu)	4.65 %	Cps	1.054
P(error)	4.65 %		
Efficiency	95.35 %		

4.5   Control Phase

In this phase, it is necessary to maintain the achieved benefits. For this, it is essential to create strategies that permit a correct quality control and monitoring with the purpose of taking preventive actions before the probability of overpassing the upper specification limit (USL) gets increased. To achieve this, a control chart was designed to monitor the behavior of the lead time for Obstetrics outpatient service with a weekly frequency with the purpose of guaranteeing faster reactions in case of a reduction of sigma level. On the other hand, flowcharts from Quality Management System were updated with new policies and implementation of the software for clinical records. The six-sigma team should continue working on increasing the sigma level with the purpose of guaranteeing a sustainable quality perception by patients.

5 Conclusions

This paper focused on deploying Six Sigma through a four-phased methodology from the identification of improving opportunities to the implementation of DMAIC cycle. An application case related to the process of outpatient service of Obstetrics in a maternal-child hospital has been explored. The results prove the effectiveness of the proposed approach. The hospital achieved an increase of more than 2 sigma levels in just 6 months and a cost reduction of 12 %. With these results pregnant women will have shorter waiting times for a consultation, which reduces the risks of losing their babies. On the other side, this reduces the probability of requesting more complex services like hospitalization and emergency because it is possible to detect anomalies earlier reason by which, the recommendations and treatments indicated by the doctors will be more effective on patient's health. By the other side, it is also demonstrated that a correct selection of improvement projects has an important influence on its success due to it is related to organization goals and customer requirements. The hospital in study received a high impact on its market image, financial status and operational conditions since its primary aim is linked to maternal and child diagnosis and intervention.

This framework will guide practitioners and decision makers in healthcare services to obtain better results at the moment of intervening processes related to outpatient service in Obstetrics. For future work, it is recommendable to explore the implementation of the current methodology in other healthcare services and consider more decision variables.

References

1. DelliFraine, J.L., Langabeer, J. R., Nembhard, I.M.: Assessing the evidence of Six Sigma and Lean in the health care industry. Qual. Manage. Health Care **19**(3), 211–25 (2010). http://doi.org/10.1097/QMH.0b013e3181eb140e
2. Koning, H., Verver, J.P.S., Heuvel, J., Bisgaard, S., Does, R.J.M.M.: Lean Six Sigma in healthcare. J. Healthc. Qual. **28**(2), 4–11 (2006). http://doi.org/10.1111/j.1945-1474.2006.tb00596.x
3. Tolga Taner, M., Sezen, B., Antony, J.: An overview of Six Sigma applications in healthcare industry. Int. J. Health Care Qual. Assur. **20**(4), 329–340 (2007). http://doi.org/10.1108/09526860710754398
4. Lopez, L.: Six Sigma in healthcare: a case study with commonwealth health corporation. In: World Class Applications of Six Sigma: Real World Examples of Success (1997). http://doi.org/10.1016/B978-0-7506-6459-2.50011-1
5. Sehwail, L., DeYong, C.: Six Sigma in health care. Leadersh. Health Serv. **16**(4), 1–5 (2003). http://doi.org/10.1108/13660750310500030
6. Van Den Heuvel, J., Does, R.J.M.M., Verver, J.P.S.: Six Sigma in healthcare: lessons learned from a hospital. Int. J. Six Sigma Competitive Advantage (2005). http://doi.org/10.1504/IJSSCA.2005.008504

7. Coronado, R.B., Antony, J.: Critical success factors for the successful implementation of six sigma projects in organisations. TQM Mag. **14**(2), 92–99 (2002). http://doi.org/10.1108/09544780210416702

8. Felizzola Jiménez, H., Luna Amaya, C.: Lean Six Sigma en pequeñas y medianas empresas: un enfoque metodológico. Ingeniare. Revista Chilena de Ingeniería **22**(2), 263–277 (2014). http://doi.org/10.4067/S0718-33052014000200012

9. Ortiz Barrios, M.A., Felizzola Jiménez, H., Nieto Isaza, S.: Comparative analysis between ANP and ANP- DEMATEL for Six Sigma project selection process in a healthcare provider. In: Pecchia, L., Chen, L.L., Nugent, C., Bravo, J. (eds.) IWAAL 2014. LNCS, vol. 8868, pp. 413–416. Springer, Heidelberg (2014)

10. Sharma, S.: An analysis of critical success factors for Six Sigma implementation. Asian J. Qual. **13**(3), 294–308 (2012). http://doi.org/10.1108/15982681211287810

11. Su, C., Chou, C.: A systematic methodology for the creation of Six Sigma projects: acase study of semiconductor foundry. Expert Syst. Appl. **34**(4), 2693–2703 (2008). http://doi.org/10.1016/j.eswa.2007.05.014

12. Snee, R.D., Rodebaugh, W.F.: Frontiers of quality: the project selection process. Qual. Prog. **35**(9), 78–80 (2002)

13. Gijo, E.V., Rao, T.S. Six Sigma implementation – hurdles and more hurdles. Total Qual. Manage. Bus. Excellence (2005). http://doi.org/10.1080/14783360500077542

14. Büyüközkan, G., Öztürkcan, D.: An integrated analytic approach for Six Sigma project selection. Expert Syst. Appl. **37**(8), 5835–5847 (2010). http://doi.org/10.1016/j.eswa.2010.02.022

Author Index

Printed in the United States
By Bookmasters